Aortic Aneurysms

For other titles published in this series, go to
www.springer.com/series/7677

Aortic Aneurysms

Pathogenesis and Treatment

Edited by

Gilbert R. Upchurch Jr.
University of Michigan, Ann Arbor, MI, USA

Enrique Criado
University of Michigan, Ann Arbor, MI, USA

Foreword by Raman Berguer

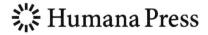 Humana Press

Editors

Gilbert R. Upchurch Jr., MD
University of Michigan
   Health System
Department of Surgery
Sec. Vascular Surgery
1500 E. Medical Center Dr.
Ann Arbor MI 48109-0329
TC2210N
USA

Enrique Criado, MD
University of Michigan
   Health System
Department of Surgery
Sec. Vascular Surgery
1500 E. Medical Center Dr.
Ann Arbor MI 48109-0329
TC2210N
USA

ISBN: 978-1-60327-203-2   e-ISBN: 978-1-60327-204-9
DOI: 10.1007/978-1-60327-204-9

Library of Congress Control Number: 2008941006

Foreword

This volume of the "Contemporary Cardiology" series updates the management of aneurysms of the descending thoracic and abdominal aorta, incorporating recent advances in the endovascular therapies that are becoming the first choice of treatment for aortic aneurysms. Aortic aneurysm has acquired new relevance in the practice of medicine. The shift from direct to endovascular repair continues to grow as the disease is diagnosed more frequently: the first wave of baby boomers passes now through the 65-year old mark and the ultrasound screening of aortas in the population at risk has become an accepted medical practice.

The dramatic differences in treatment outcomes between intact and ruptured aortic aneurysms have stimulated the search for early diagnosis and treatment. The genetics of aneurysms have established the indications for familial screening. Internists and cardiologists are usually the first physicians to identify an aneurysm and should be aware of the new options for treatment available today. The fast-evolving knowledge on aortic aneurysms is thoroughly summarized in this book edited by Drs. Upchurch and Criado, two vascular surgeons who have made important contributions to this field.

Ramon Berguer

Preface

Aortic aneurysms are increasingly common and often lethal in the aging population, making them among the leading causes of death in the United States. The incidence and prevalence of aortic disease is also increasing as life expectancy is extended. Aortic disease is often incidentally discovered when performing tests, such as ultrasonography or CT scans, for other disease processes. For this reason, it is important that physicians who deal with the aging population, such as cardiologists, are familiar with the diagnosis and management principles of aortic aneurysms. The lack of effective medical therapy makes timely surgical intervention the only viable treatment option for aortic aneurysms once they attain a certain diameter. Unfortunately, aortic aneurysms are clinically silent until patients present with catastrophic aortic rupture. Therefore, the detection of aortic aneurysms prior to rupture is critical as there is a large disparity in mortality between elective and emergent repair.

Until recently, treatment of aortic disease was primarily surgical, involving large incisions with the potential for large blood loss and life-threatening perioperative complications.

Although effective and durable, the surgical treatment of aortic aneurysms carries a relatively high mortality in this high-risk population, and is associated with prolonged convalescence and a delayed return to the preexisting level of quality of life. For these reasons, minimally invasive treatment of aortic aneurysms has become the most common therapeutic option for aortic aneurysms. During recent years, we have witnessed a progressive increase in the number of endovascular aortic repairs performed and significant technological improvements in stent graft design. The use of endovascular technology in the treatment of abdominal and thoracic-aortic pathology, in expert hands, can lower short-term mortality and morbidity. However, this comes at an increased cost because of both the cost of the stent grafts and the need for long-term serial imaging following endovascular repair of aneurysms.

This book, *Aortic Aneurysms*: *Pathogenesis and Treatment*, is part of the "Contemporary Cardiology" series. As cardiologists will be the caregivers for many patients with aortic aneurysms, the purpose of the book is to provide a concise and authorative view of the current state of the management of these patients. The book focuses on aneurysms of the descending thoracic and abdominal aorta, and peripheral artery aneurysms, and does not include the ascending aorta or the aortic arch. While the initial chapters deal with such topics as genetics, inflammation, and the management of small aortic aneurysms, the bulk of the book is meant to serve as a primer on clinical care, specifically on surgery for aortic aneurysms.

The treatment of aneurysms is a fast-evolving field. We are most grateful to all the authors for their expert and updated contributions. We hope the readers of this book and their patients will benefit from this work. We dedicate the book to the memory of Dr George Johnson Jr., a mentor to both of us.

November 2008   Gilbert R. Upchurch Jr.
University of Michigan   Enrique Criado
Cardiovascular Center
Ann Arbor, MI

Contents

Contributors

Gautam Agarwal, MD
Department of Cardiothoracic and Vascular Surgery, Medical College
of Georgia, Augusta, GA

B. Timothy Baxter, MD
Department of Surgery, University of Nebraska Medical Center
and Methodist Hospital, Omaha, NE

W.T.G.J. Bos, MD
Department of Surgery, University Medical Center Groningen, Groningen,
The Netherlands

Martin J. Carignan, M.D
Section of Vascular Surgery and Endovascular Therapy, University
of Alabama at Birmingham, Birmingham, AL

Timothy A.M. Chuter, D.M.
Department of Surgery, Division of Vascular Surgery, University of
California-San Francisco, San Francisco, CA

Enrique Criado, MD
Department of Surgery, Division of Vascular Surgery, University
of Michigan Health System, Ann Arbor, MI

Alan Dardik, MD, PhD
Department of Surgery, Division of Vascular Surgery, Yale University School
of Medicine, New Haven, CT

K. Barry Deatrick, MD
Department of Surgery, Section of Vascular Surgery, University of Michigan
Health System, Ann Arbor, MI

G. Michael Deeb MD
Department of Surgery, Division of Cardiac Surgery, University of Michigan
Cardiovascular Center, Ann Arbor, MI

Manuel Doblas, MD
Division of Vascular Surgery, Centro Hospitalario Virgen de la Salud,
Toledo, Spain

J.J.A.M. van den Dungen, MD
Department of Surgery, University Medical Center Groningen, Groningen,
The Netherlands

Jonathan L. Eliason, MD
Department of Surgery, Section of Vascular Surgery, University of Michigan
Health Systems, Ann Arbor, MI

Michael J. Englesbe, MD
Department of Surgery, Division of Transplantation, University of Michigan
Health System, Ann Arbor, MI

Guillermo A. Escobar, MD
Department of Surgery, University of Colorado Health Science Center and
Denver Health Medical Center, Denver, CO

Mark A. Farber, MD
Department of Surgery, Division of Vascular Surgery, University of North
Carolina School of Medicine, Chapel Hill, NC

Tamara N Fitzgerald, MD
Department of Surgery, Yale University School of Medicine, New Haven, CT

Angel Flores, MD
Division of Vascular Surgery, Centro Hospitalario Virgen de la Salud,
Toledo, Spain

Juan Fontcuberta, MD
Division of Vascular Surgery, Centro Hospitalario Virgen de la Salud,
Toledo, Spain

Peter Ford, M.B.B.S
Department of Surgery, Division of Vascular Surgery, University of North
Carolina at Chapel Hill School of Medicine, Chapel Hill, NC

Thomas R Gest, MD
Department of Anatomical Sciences and Medical Education, University
of Michigan Health System, Ann Arbor, MI

Jose Gil, MD
Division of Vascular Surgery, Centro Hospitalario Virgen de la Salud,
Toledo, Spain

Peter K. Henke, MD
Department of Surgery, Section of Vascular Surgery, Cardiovascular Center,
University of Michigan Health System, Ann Arbor, MI

Loay S. Kabbani M.D
Department of Surgery, Section of Vascular Surgery, University of Michigan
Medical Center, Ann Arbor, MI

Paul Knechtges, MD
Department of Radiology, University of Michigan Health System,
Ann Arbor, MI

Brian S. Knipp, MD
Department of Surgery, Section of Vascular Surgery, University of Michigan
Health System, Ann Arbor, MI

Venkataramu N. Krishnamurthy, MD
Department of Radiology, Section of Interventional Radiology, University
of Michigan, Ann Arbor, MI.

Helena Kuivaniemi, MD, PhD
Center for Molecular Medicine and Genetics, Department of Surgery, Wayne
State University School of Medicine, Detroit, MI, USA

Ignacio Leal, MD
Division of Vascular Surgery, Centro Hospitalario Virgen de la Salud,
Toledo, Spain

Guy M. Lenk, PhD
Center for Molecular Medicine and Genetics, Wayne State University School
of Medicine, Detroit, MI

John H. Lillvis, BA
Center for Molecular Medicine and Genetics, Wayne State University School
of Medicine, Detroit, MI

Peter S. Liu, MD
Department of Radiology, Division of Magnetic Resonance Imaging,
University of Michigan Medical Center, Ann Arbor, MI

William A. Marston, MD
Department of Surgery, Division of Vascular Surgery, University of North
Carolina at Chapel Hill School of Medicine, Chapel Hill, NC

Robert Mendes, M.D
Department of Surgery, Division of Vascular Surgery, University of North
Carolina at Chapel Hill School of Medicine, Chapel Hill, NC

J. Gregory Modrall, M.D.
Department of Surgery, Division of Vascular and Endovascular Surgery,
University of Texas Southwestern Medical Center,
Dallas, TX

Bart E Muhs, MD, PhD
Co-Director, Endovascular Program, Yale University School of Medicine,
New Haven, CT

Patrick J. O'Hara, M.D.
Department of Vascular Surgery, Cleveland Clinic Lerner College of
Medicine of Case Western Reserve University, Cleveland Clinic Foundation,
Cleveland, OH

Antonio Orgaz, MD
Division of Vascular Surgery, Centro Hospitalario Virgen de la Salud,
Toledo, Spain

Juan C. Parodi, MD
Department of Vascular Surgery, University of Miami Leonard M. Miller
School of Medicine, Miami, FL

Marc A. Passman, M.D
Section of Vascular Surgery and Endovascular Therapy, University
of Alabama at Birmingham, Birmingham, AL

Himanshu J. Patel MD
Department of Surgery, Section of Cardiac Surgery, University of Michigan
Cardiovascular Center, Ann Arbor, MI

Sheela T. Patel, MD
Department of Surgery, University of Miami Leonard M. Miller School
of Medicine, Miami, FL

William H. Pearce, M.D
Department of Surgery, Division of Vascular Surgery, Feinberg School
of Medicine, Northwestern University, Chicago, IL

T.R. Prins, MD
Departments of Surgery and Radiology, University Medical Center
Groningen, Groningen, The Netherlands

Kerianne H. Quanstrum, M.D
Department of Surgery, University of Michigan Health System
Cardiovascular Center, Ann Arbor, MI

Todd E. Rasmussen, MD
San Antonio Military Vascular Surgery Service, United States Air Force
Medical Center, San Antonio, TX

John E. Rectenwald, MD
Department of Surgery and Radiology, Sections of Vascular Surgery
and Interventional Radiology, University of Michigan, Ann Arbor, MI.

Paul J. Riesenman, MD, MS
Department of Surgery, Division of Vascular Surgery, University of North
Carolina School of Medicine, Chapel Hill, NC

Vera P. Shively, M.S
Department of Surgery, Division of Vascular Surgery, Feinberg School
of Medicine, Northwestern University, Chicago, IL

Gregorio Sicard, MD
Department of Surgery, Section of Vascular Surgery, Washington University
School of Medicine, St. Louis, MO

Matthew J. Sideman, M.D.
Department of Surgery, Section of Vascular and Endovascular Surgery,
Oklahoma University College of Medicine, Tulsa, OK

A.O. Sondakh, MD
Department of Surgery, University Medical Center Groningen, Groningen,
The Netherlands

James C. Stanley, MD
Department of Surgery, Section of Vascular Surgery, University of Michigan
Cardiovascular Center, Ann Arbor, MI

Houman Tamaddon, M.D.
Department of Surgery, Division of Vascular Surgery, University of North
Carolina at Chapel Hill School of Medicine, Chapel Hill, North Carolina

Kevin E. Taubman, M.D.
Department of Surgery, Section of Vascular and Endovascular Surgery,
Oklahoma University College of Medicine, Tulsa. OK

I.F.J. Tielliu, MD
Department of Surgery, University Medical Center Groningen, Groningen,
The Netherlands

Gilbert R. Upchurch, Jr. M.D.
Department of Surgery, Section of Vascular Surgery, University of Michigan
Medical Center, Ann Arbor, MI

E.L.G. Verhoeven, MD
Department of Surgery, University Medical Center Groningen, Groningen,
The Netherlands

Thomas Wakefield, MD
Department of Surgery,, Section of Vascular Surgery, University of Michigan
Health System, Ann Arbor, MI

Michael Wilderman
David M. Williams, MD
Department of Radiology, Division of Vascular and Interventional Radiology,
University of Michigan Medical Center, Ann Arbor, MI

C.J. Zeebregts, MD
Department of Surgery, University Medical Center Groningen, Groningen,
The Netherlands

Chapter 1

Genetics of Abdominal Aortic Aneurysms

John H. Lillvis, Guy M. Lenk, and Helena Kuivaniemi

Abstract Abdominal aortic aneurysm (AAA) is a multifactorial disease with a significant genetic component. Epidemiological studies have identified family history of AAA as a risk factor for both aneurysm development and rupture, making it an important consideration for targeted ultrasound screening of elderly patients and their family members. Ongoing research into the genetics of AAA is focused on identifying risk factor genes for both familial and sporadic aneurysms through the use of linkage analyses and genetic association studies, although no causative mutations have yet been identified. Additionally, microarray expression profiling and animal models of aneurysms are being used to identify genes and pathways for the design of novel therapeutics. These approaches promise to deliver a better understanding of aneurysms at the molecular level leading to improved screening and treatment.

Keywords DNA linkage, Genetic association, Chromosome 19, Chromosome 4, Animal models, Family studies, Ultrasonography screening, Microarray

Introduction

Abdominal aortic aneurysms (AAAs) contribute significantly to the disease burden of the elderly population, with as much as 10% of the population over the age of 65 harboring an aneurysm.[1] Between 1999 and 2004, AAA was the 17th leading cause of death in the United States, with approximately 15,000 deaths per year.[2] Advances in screening and endovascular surgical techniques have contributed to modest decreases in AAA mortality, but further developments are still necessary. The current treatment of choice, elective surgical repair, is highly effective when performed, with a mortality of less than 5% as compared with up to a 90% mortality associated with rupture.[3,4] However, since most AAAs do not produce symptoms until rupture, early detection is necessary for effective therapy. Additionally, due to age or comorbidities, some patients may not be appropriate candidates for surgery. Improvements in detection and therapy are therefore necessary to identify and treat aneurysms prior to their growth and rupture. One promising area of research that may lead to such developments is the study of AAA genetics.

G. Upchurch and E. Criado (eds.) *Aortic Aneurysms, Contemporary Cardiology*
DOI: 10.1007/978-1-60327-204-9_1, © Humana Press, a part of
Springer Science+Business Media, LLC 2009

There is strong evidence to suggest a genetic component to AAA. AAAs frequently show familial clustering, even when they are not associated with heritable disorders, such as the Marfan syndrome or the type IV variant of the Ehlers-Danlos syndrome. In an examination of over 125,000 Veterans Administration patients, Lederle et al.[5] found family history of AAA to be one of the best predictors of aneurysms, with an odds ratio of 1.93 (95% confidence intervals: 1.71–2.18) for small aneurysms and 1.94 (95% confidence intervals: 1.63–2.32) for large aneurysms, with only smoking being a stronger risk factor. Interviews with AAA patients and ultrasonography examinations of their first-degree relatives have shown that approximately 15% have at least one first-degree relative with the disease[6–9] (Tables 1 and 2). Examination of 952 brothers and 771 sisters of AAA patients by ultrasonography showed that 19.5% of brothers and 5.7% of sisters had AAA[22–25,27–30,32–34,36–38] (Table 2). In addition, AAA exhibits many characteristics consistent with being a genetic disease. Segregation analysis, a statistical approach to examine heredity, has been used to study cases of AAA in two populations.[16,17] One study suggested a dominant and the other a recessive mode of inheritance for AAA, possibly representing genetic heterogeneity, but each study concluded that a single gene defect is likely to cause the disease within a family. In addition to the formal statistical analyses supporting the genetic nature of AAA, several collections of AAA families have been reported, the largest one describing 233 families with multiple affecteds.[39]

AAA also demonstrates characteristics of being a multifactorial genetic disease with respect to gender. One feature of multifactorial diseases is gender discrepancy in prevalence, a phenomenon that is well documented in diseases such as pyloric stenosis, many congenital heart defects, neural tube defects, and cleft lip.[40] For AAA, the prevalence is about six times higher in males than females, perhaps due to hormonal protection in females. However, when females do present with an aneurysm, it would presumably be due to having a greater genetic or environmental liability and would therefore represent the more severe end of the spectrum of disease.[41] This

Table 1 Familial prevalence of AAA based on interviews.

Study	Patients surveyed (N)	Patients with positive history (N)	Familial prevalence (%)
Norrgård et al., 1984[10]	87	16	18.4
Johansen and Koepsell, 1986[11]	250	48	19.2
Powell and Greenhalgh, 1987[12]	56	20	35.7
Johnston and Scobie, 1988[13]	666	41	6.1
Cole et al., 1989[14]	305	34	11.1
Darling et al., 1989[15]	542	82	15.1
Majumder et al., 1991[16]	91	13	14.3
Verloes et al., 1995[17]	313	39	12.5
Lederle et al., 1997[18]	985	91	9.2
Lawrence et al., 1998[19]	86	19	22.1
Salkowski et al., 1999[20]	72	19	26.4
Rossaak et al., 2001[21]	248	48	19.4
Total	3701	470	
Combined prevalence			12.7

Modified with permission from Kuivaniemi and Tromp[9]

Table 2 Prevalence of AAA among first-degree family members based on ultrasonography screening.

Study	Country	Brothers[a] (%)	Sisters[a] (%)	Other[a] (%)
Bengtsson et al., 1989[22]	Sweden	10/35 (28.6)	3/52 (5.8)	
Collin and Walton, 1989[23]	UK	4/16 (25.0)	0/15 (0)	
Webster et al., 1991[24]	USA	5/24 (20.8)	2/30 (6.7)	7/103 (6.8)
Adamson et al., 1992[25]	UK	5/25 (20.0)	3/28 (10.7)	
Bengtsson et al., 1992[26]	Sweden			9/62
van der Lugt et al., 1992[27]	The Netherlands	16/56 (28.6)	3/52 (5.8)	
Adams et al., 1993[28]	UK	4/23 (17.4)	1/28 (3.6)	6/23 (26.1)
Moher et al., 1994[29]	Canada	9/48 (18.8)		
Fitzgerald et al., 1995[30]	Ireland	13/60 (21.7)	2/65 (3.1)	
Larcos et al., 1995[31]	Australia			0/52 (0)
Baird et al., 1995[32]	Canada	7/26 (26.9)	3/28 10.7)	
Jaakkola et al., 1996[33]	Finland	4/45 (8.9)	1/78 (1.3)	
van der Graaf et al., 1998[34]	Netherlands	26/210 (12.4)		
Salo et al., 1999[35]	Finland			11/238 (4.6)
Rossaak et al., 2001[21]	New Zealand			4/49 (8.2)
Frydman et al., 2003[36]	Australia	64/150 (42.7)	20/126 (15.9)	
Ogata et al., 2005[37]	Canada	11/98 (11.2)	4/147 (2.7)	0/31 (0)
Badger et al., 2007[38]	Northern Ireland	8/136 (5.8)	2/122 (1.6)	0/42 (0)
Total		186/952 (19.5)	44/771 (5.7)	37/638 (5.7)

[a] Number of individuals identified with AAA/number of individuals examined by ultrasonography. Other refers to relatives other than sisters and brothers of the AAA patient, or the categories of relatives were not specified. Modified with permission from Kuivaniemi and Tromp[9]

is supported by the fact that females have an increased operative mortality for both intact and ruptured AAAs compared to males.[42,43] Additionally, if the liability is genetic, one would expect to see a higher prevalence among females inheriting the mutations. In one study of 542 AAA patients, the 82 (15.1%) patients who had a positive family history were compared to the 460 sporadic cases.[15] When examined for gender distribution, the sporadic cases showed an expected 86%:14% male-to-female ratio, whereas 35% of the familial cases were female, despite no differences in smoking, hypertension, or coronary artery disease. An investigation of rupture rates of the patients with a positive family history, as well as their first-degree relatives, found that 22/73 (30.1%) aneurysms in females ruptured as compared to 23/136 (16.9%) in males. Finally, it was also found that the males with a family history were significantly younger than the males with sporadic aneurysms, another characteristic consistent with genetic diseases. Similar results were reported in a different study of 300 AAA patients that showed a higher rate of rupture among familial cases of AAA.[44]

Based on the research described above, it is clear that AAA is a complex multifactorial disease with genetic and environmental risk factors (Fig. 1). Because of technological and statistical advances in the past several years, studying the genetics of multifactorial diseases like AAA has become quite feasible. Figure 2 shows the so-called "four pillars" for the study of AAA genetics. These four approaches can each provide valuable information as well as complement each other to help unlock the genetics of AAA.

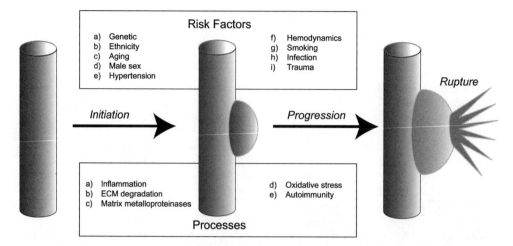

Fig. 1 Abdominal aortic aneurysm (*AAA*) pathogenesis with associated risk factors. Risk factors (*above the arrows*) contributing to and biological processes (*below the arrows*) observed in AAA formation, growth, and rupture are summarized. How AAAs form, grow, and rupture is not fully understood, but it is clear that AAA is a complex disease with both genetic and environmental risk factors. Many of the same risk factors and processes are involved in initiation and progression as well as rupture. *ECM*, extracellular matrix.

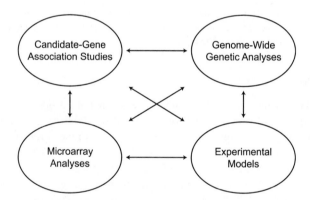

Fig. 2 Four pillars of abdominal aortic aneurysm (*AAA*) research. Unraveling the pathophysiology of AAA and identifying the specific risk factors for AAA will require interdisciplinary approaches. Each approach is described in the text and specific examples on how they are applied to AAA research are also presented.

Clinical Management and the Genetics of AAA

Despite the strong evidence for a genetic component to AAA, clinical recognition of this aspect is still largely lacking. Nakka et al. identified poor documentation concerning the counseling of patients on the occasional familial nature of AAA.[45] Additionally, "Practical Genetic Counseling", a commonly used genetic counseling reference, only describes familial aneurysms due to type III collagen defects.[46]

The primary clinical implication of understanding AAAs as a genetic disease is targeted screening with imaging techniques. In addition to being a risk factor for developing an aneurysm, family history has been shown in both epidemiological and aortic modeling studies to be a risk factor for aneurysm rupture.[47,48] Currently, the screening guidelines for AAA are conflicted as to whether family history should be included in the criteria for targeted screening. The US Preventive Task Force recommends screening only men between the ages of 65 and 75 who have smoked, citing concerns over psychological harm and early treatment. However, the guidelines acknowledge that screening can be considered in patients with a strong family history of the disease.[49,50] In contrast, the Society for Vascular Surgery and the Society for Vascular Medicine and Biology recommend screening all patients over the age of 50 with a family history of aneurysms.[51] In a study of familial aneurysms, Le Hello et al. similarly recommend screening of all patients with two or more affected relatives.[52] Since a positive family history can vary from multiple siblings or parents of both genders to a single brother who smoked, targeted screening based upon family history should rely on a careful patient interview and clinical judgment. Additionally, referral to a genetic counselor or medical genetics specialist may be useful if the patient exhibits a particularly strong family history of aneurysms.

In the future, the clinical management of AAA may be fundamentally altered by an improved understanding of the genetics of the disease. Identification of risk alleles will help identify individuals more likely to develop the disease. Additionally, targeted therapeutics may be developed as new genes and pathways important to the development of AAA are found.

Identification of AAA-Susceptibility Loci by Genome-Wide DNA Linkage Analyses

Linkage is a genetic concept referring to the coinheritance of a polymorphic DNA marker, a variation in the DNA sequence, with a DNA mutation conferring susceptibility for a phenotype or disease.[53] Linkage indicates that the marker is in proximity to the causative mutation since the distance between two points on a chromosome is proportional to the frequency of crossing over. The use of linkage analysis to identify the genetic causes of lethal, late-age-at-onset diseases, such as AAA, has been difficult at best and has required several technological advancements to make the undertaking of such studies a reality. First, the use of noninvasive diagnostic imaging, such as ultrasonography screening studies carried out on the relatives of AAA patients, has allowed the identification of far more family members with AAA prior to rupture (Table 2). As a result, there are far more living, affected members available for genetic studies. Second, the development of highly informative markers that can be easily analyzed using PCR has greatly enhanced the power of any linkage study. Third, the large number of linkage studies being performed on complex human diseases has refined and advanced the methods and models for linkage analyses. Fourth, there have been theoretical and applied advances in the linkage methodology itself.[53]

Recently, two published reports identified genetic loci linked to AAA using a method of DNA linkage analysis known as the sib-pair approach.[54,55] By relying upon a feature of sibling relationships, namely the sharing of 0, 1, or 2 identical alleles at any genetic locus, the distribution of alleles expected by chance can be easily predicted. Although sibling pairs are perhaps the most commonly used, this approach can be extended to other relationships such as cousin–cousin or child–grandparent. The sib-pair approach is useful for studying late-age-at-onset, lethal diseases like AAA for two important reasons (Fig. 3). First, sib-pair linkage analyses require only two individuals from one generation of each family to be alive and willing to contribute to the study, whereas conventional family-based studies require affected individuals to be available for study from at least three generations. Many individuals diagnosed with AAA have parents who have died, but children too young to develop an aneurysm, therefore making it difficult to find two, let alone three, generations living with aneurysms (Fig. 3). Second, conventional linkage analyses rely on the ability to accurately distinguish between affected and unaffected individuals. Since AAA is a late-age-at-onset disease, its incidence increases with age, a phenomenon known as age-dependent penetrance. However, by using a type of sib-pair analysis known as affected sib-pair (ASP), problems of penetrance are avoided because all subjects being studied have been diagnosed with the disease.

In the first published linkage analysis of AAA, Shibamura et al.[54] used an affected relative pair (ARP) approach to carry out a genome-wide screen and identified linked regions on chromosomes 4 and 19. This analysis was carried out in two phases using 235 ARPs (213 ASPs) from 119 families with at least 2 individuals per family (mean = 3.2, range 2–7). In the first phase, genomic DNA from 75 ARPs (62 ASPs) in 36 families was used in a whole-genome scan of 405 microsatellite markers. From the initial scan, 12 regions were identified as significant. In the second phase, additional microsatellite markers in those 12 regions were genotyped using the original set of ARPs and 160 additional ARPs (151 ASPs). The combined data were then analyzed using sex, number of affected individuals, and their interaction as covariates to allow for genetic heterogeneity. This analysis showed two regions with significant linkage, one on chromosome 19q13 with a logarithm of odds (LOD) score of 4.64 and another on chromosome 4q31 with a LOD score of 3.73 (Fig. 4). A second study by van Vlijmen-Van Keulen et al.[55] also demonstrated linkage

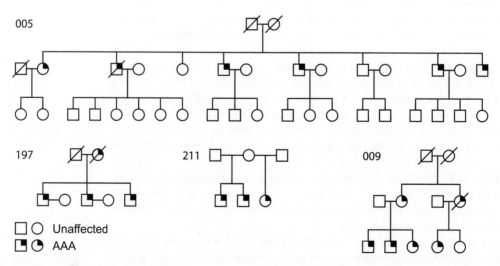

Fig. 3 Representative abdominal aortic aneurysm (*AAA*) families from our collection of 233 families. Slash across symbol means death. Squares and circles with the upper right quadrant darkened indicate male and female members, respectively, diagnosed with AAA.

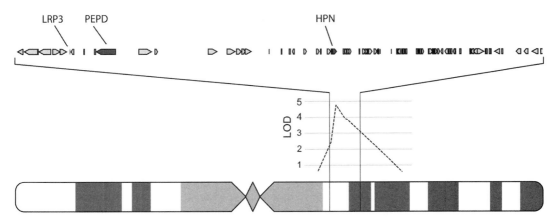

Fig. 4 Genetic-susceptibility locus on chromosome 19 for abdominal aortic aneurysm (*AAA*). This genetic region was identified in a genome-wide DNA linkage study using affected relative pair approach. The bottom of the figure shows chromosome 19 with the linked region bracketed. The middle plot shows the logarithm of odds (*LOD*) score within the region. At the top of the figure, the locations of genes in the region have been indicated by arrows. The locations of three candidate genes, low density lipoprotein receptor-related protein 3 (*LRP3*), peptidase 3 (*PEPD*), and hepsin (*HPN*), have been highlighted.

to chromosome 19q13 (nonparametric, multipoint linkage score = 3.95) by a different statistical method when analyzing 22 ASPs from three large Dutch families. However, when 79 additional ASPs from 55 families were included in the analysis, this method failed to demonstrate linkage, likely due to genetic heterogeneity.

The chromosome 19 and 4 loci have been designated as the AAA1 and AAA2 loci in the Online Mendelian Inheritance in Man (OMIM) database, respectively.[56] Note that DNA linkage studies on thoracic aortic aneurysms and dissections (TAAD) have identified completely different genetic regions suggesting that the two aortic aneurysm subtypes are genetically different.[57] These findings are not too surprising considering the differences in the clinical characteristics of patients who have TAAD versus those who have AAA; TAAD patients are much younger and there is a much smaller gender difference (1.7:1 male-to-female ratio). There are also differences in the pathobiology of these aneurysms, TAADs being characterized by medial necrosis also known as "Erdheim's cystic medial necrosis," mucoid infiltration, and cyst formation with elastin degradation and vascular smooth muscle apoptosis.[58]

Genetic Association Studies: From Candidate Gene Studies to Genome-Wide Analyses

Genetic association studies, using methods similar to other forms of case-control studies, compare two groups of individuals, those with a disease and those without, with respect to frequency of a sequence variant from the gene of interest.[53,59] The comparisons are usually carried out using both genotype and allele frequencies for the particular variant. If the frequency is statistically higher or lower in the cases, it is suggestive of a causative or protective effect, respectively. Testing for one genetic variant per gene is not usually sufficient unless a biologically important role for the tested variant has been established in functional studies. Also, in many genetic association studies the exact sequence variant responsible for the disease susceptibility has not been sought for extensively. Rather, the genotyped markers are being used as surrogate markers for variants with true functional effects. Identifying the causative variants requires an extensive analysis of the surrounding genomic sequences, which is often beyond the scope of the study.

Like other case-control studies, association studies have limitations. Selection of controls for genetic association studies must be done carefully. If independent samples of affected and unaffected individuals are used, factors such as population stratification can lead to mathematical associations that have no relationship to the underlying genetics of the disease being studied. One possible approach is the use of spouses as controls since spouses tend to be from the same ethnic and socioeconomic groups, and will have shared many environmental factors. On the other hand, using "overmatched controls" or "supercontrols" will lead to difficulty in estimating the population attributable risk for the identified genetic variants. For this reason, some investigators are advocating the use of population-based controls representative of the "general" population in the geographic area where the study is performed. In such studies, means for testing for potential stratification must be devised, and the so-called "genomic control" method has been used widely. In this approach, stratification can be tested by using genetic markers genotyped from other chromosomal regions.[60] Alternatively, genetic markers known to show population differences can be used to show that the case and control populations do not differ at those markers even when an association is detected in a specific candidate gene being tested.[61]

Another common limitation of genetic association studies is the sample size. These studies require large sample sizes, and results obtained with fewer than 250 cases and 250 controls must be viewed with skepticism. Even larger sample sizes are needed if variants with low allele frequencies are being tested, larger number of variants are being tested, or the study intends to investigate gene–environment interactions. Yet another potential complication is multiple testing since many research groups are interested in testing their study population for multiple genes and genetic variants. It is possible to design these studies so that a preliminary screening of all variants is first carried out, followed by testing only those variants which were found to be statistically significant in the initial screening in a second independent set of samples. This approach reduces the number of tests being done in the follow-up study. It must be emphasized that replication of the findings in an independent sample set is extremely important to eliminate false positives, although it is plausible that population-specific disease-susceptibility alleles exist and that replication in a different ethnic population will not support the initial findings. Detailed recommendations on how to design, conduct, interpret, and report on genetic association studies have been published recently.[62]

Tables 3 and 4 summarize the genetic association studies for AAA reported to date. These studies have examined many genes encoding for proteins known to be important in AAA or vascular biology, such as matrix metallopeptidases (MMPs), tissue inhibitors of metallopeptidases (TIMPs), angiotensin-converting enzyme (ACE), and nitric oxide synthase 3 (NOS3). Table 4 summarizes studies on a particularly intense area of study, human leukocyte antigen (HLA)

Table 3 Candidate genes for AAA tested in genetic association studies.

Study	Gene(s) studied[a]	Ethnicity	Number in the study — Cases (subgroups)	Number in the study — Controls (subgroups)	Reported findings — Polymorphism (minor allele)	Significance[b]
Powell et al., 1990[63]	HP	UK	44	83	Variant a-chains a^1/a^2	$p < 0.05$
St. Jean et al., 1995[64]	MMP9	USA	127	94	nt −131 to −90 CA repeat	$p = 0.36$
Hamano et al., 1999[65]	ACE	Japan	125	153	Intron 16 287-bp I/D (D)	$p = 0.774$
Wang et al., 1999[66]	TIMP1, TIMP2	Mixed Caucasian	84 (64 male) (20 female)	51 (29 male) (22 female)	TIMP1, nt 434 C > T	$p = 0.5005$ (males) $p = 0.0019$ (females)
					TIMP2, nt 573 G > A	$p = 0.0156$
Yoon et al., 1999[67]	MMP3, MMP9, SERPINE1	Finnish	47	174	MMP3 nt −1621 5A/6A (5A)	$p = 0.1641$
					MMP9, nt −131 to −90, CA-repeat	$p = 0.8171$
					SERPINE1, nt −675 4G/5G (4G)	$p = 0.9421$
Brunelli et al., 2000[68]	MTHFR	Italy	58	60	nt + 677 C > T	NS
Kotani et al., 2000[69]	NOS3	Japan	34 (surgical)	410	Intron 4 27-bp repeat	$p < 0.01$ (surgical vs control)
			24 (nonsurgical)			NS (nonsurgical vs control)
						$p < 0.05$ (surgical vs nonsurgical)
						NS (all AAA vs control)
Rossaak et al., 2000[70]	SERPINE1	New Zealand/ European	39 (FAAA) 151 (SAAA)	163	nt −675 4G/5G	$p = 0.024$ (FAAA vs SAAA)
						$p = 0.032$ (FAAA vs control)
Pola et al., 2001[71]	ACE	Italy	56 (NT) 68 (HT)	112	Intron 16 287 bp I/D	OR = 5.31 (HT AAA vs NT control)
						OR = 3.63 (NT AAA vs HT AAA)
						OR = 1.46 (HT AAA vs NT control)
Schillinger et al., 2002[72]	HMOX1	Austria	70	61 (controls)	nt −258 to −195 GT repeat	$p = 0.04$ (AAA vs control)

(continued)

Table 3 (continued)

Study	Gene(s) studied[a]	Ethnicity	Number in the study		Reported findings	
			Cases (subgroups)	Controls (subgroups)	Polymorphism (minor allele)	Significance[b]
				70 (PVD)		$p = 0.006$; OR = 0.38 (AAA vs CAD)
				70 (CAD)		$p = 0.01$; OR = 0.35 (AAA vs PVD)
Unno et al., 2002[73]	PLA2G7	Japan	131	106	nt + 994 G > T	$p = 0.015$
Jones et al., 2003[74]	MMP9	New Zealand	414	203 (controls)	nt −1562 C > T	$p = 0.013$ (AAA vs PVD)
				172 (PVD)		$p = 0.334$, OR = 1.53 (AAA vs control)
Bown et al., 2003[75]	IL1B, IL6, IL10, TNF	UK	91	100	TNF nt −308 G > A	$p = 1.00$
					IL1B nt 3953 C > T	$p = 0.13$
					IL6 nt −174 G > C	$p = 0.92$
					IL10 nt −1082 G > A	$p = 0.03$
					IL10 nt −592 C > A	$p = 0.24$
Ghilardi et al., 2004[76]	CCR5	Italy	70	172 (controls)	nt 794–825 deletion	$p = 0.064$ (AAA vs Control)
				76 (PVD)		$p = 0.012$ (AAA vs PVD and carotid stenosis)
				62 (carotid stenosis)		
Massart et al., 2004[77]	ELN, ESR1, ESR2, PGR, TGFB1	Italy	99	225 (male)	ESR2 nt 1730 A > G	$p < 0.05$, OR = 1.82
					Five other polymorphisms	NS
Fatini et al., 2005[78]	ACE, AGTR1	Italy	250	250	Intron 16 287 bp I/D	$p < 0.0001$
					nt + 1166 A > C	$p = 0.4$
Fatini et al., 2005[79]	NOS3	Italy	250	250	nt + 894 G > T	$p < 0.0001$
					Intron 4 27 bp repeat	$p < 0.5$
					nt −786 T > C	$p = 0.6$

Study	Genes	Population			Polymorphism	Results
Ogata et al., 2005[80]	MMP1, MMP2, MMP3, MMP9, MMP10, MMP12, MMP13, TIMP1, TIMP2, TIMP3, TGFB1, ELN, COL3A1	Belgian, Canadian	387	425	TIMP1 nt 434 C > T	p = 0.0047 (males w/o family history)
					TIMP1 rs2070584 T > G	p = 0.015 (males w/o family history)
Schulz et al., 2005[81]	ABCC6	Austria	133	910 total (controls) 54 (PXE)	TIMP1 TT haplotype 31 mutations	p = 0.036 NS
Golledge et al., 2007[82]	SPP1	Australia	689	3538	rs1126772, rs9138, rs4754, rs1126616, rs11730582	All NS
Armani et al., 2007[83]	MMP9	Italy	146	156	nt −1562 C > T nt −131 to −90 CA repeat	NS
Bown et al., 2007[84]	IL10	UK	389	404	nt −1082 G > A	p = 0.014 (A allele) p = 0.004 (AA genotype) NS when adjusted for covariates
Smallwood et al., 2007[85]	IL6	Australia	677	656	nt −174 G > C	OR = 5.78 (−572 CC genotype in recessive model)
					nt −572 G > C	OR = 1.55 (h.211 haplotype)
Helgadottir et al., 2008[86]	ANRIL	Several	2017	16,639	nt −597 G > A rs10757278-G	p = 0.000003 (excluding known CAD)
Jones et al., 2007[87]	AGT, ACE, AGTR1, BDKRB2	New Zealand, Australia, UK	1226	1723	rs10811661-T AGT rs699	NS p = 0.2

(continued)

Ta ble 3 (continued)

Study	Gene(s) studied[a]	Ethnicity	Number in the study		Reported findings	
			Cases (subgroups)	Controls (subgroups)	Polymorphism (minor allele)	Significance[b]
					ACE rs4646994	p = 0.03 (heterozygote), p = 0.05 (homozygote)
					AGTR1 rs5186	p = 0.000012 (heterozygote) p < 0.002 (homozygote)
						NS
Götting et al., 2008[88]	XLYT1	Austria	129	129	BDKRB2 rs6223 nt 343 G > T nt 1989 T > C	p = 0.011 p = 0.274

HP= haptoglobin; TIMP1/TIMP2/TIMP3= tissue inhibitor of matrix metallopeptidases gene family; ACE= angiotensin-converting enzyme; MMP1/MMP2/MMP3/MMP9/MMP10/MMP12/MMP13= matrix metallopeptidase gene family; SERPINE1= serpin peptidase inhibitor, clade E, member 1 (plasminogen activator inhibitor type 1); NOS3= nitric oxide synthase 3 (endothelial cell); MTHFR= 5,10-methylenetetrahydrofolate reductase; PLAG27= phospolipase A2, group VII (platelet activating factor acetylhydrase, plasma); HMOX1= heme oxygenase (decycling) 1; IL1B/IL6/IL10= interleukin gene family; TNF= tumor necrosis factor-alpha; CCR5= chemokine receptor 5; ELN= elastin; ESR1/ESR2= estrogen receptors 1 and 2; PGR= progesterone receptor; TGFB1= transforming growth factor-beta 1; AGTR1= angiotensin II receptor, type 1; COL3A1= collagen, type III, alpha 1; ABCC6= ATP-binding cassette, subfamily C (CFTR/MRP), member 6; SPP1= secreted phosphoprotein 1 (osteopontin); PVD = peripheral vascular disease; NS = not significant; HT = hypertensive; NT = normotensive; FAAA = familial AAA; SAAA = sporadic AAA; PXE = pseudoxanthoma elasticum

[a]Gene symbols used are HGNC-approved symbols obtained from http://www.genenames.org/
[b]p-values as reported in original studies. The statistical tests and actual comparisons vary. Some studies corrected for multiple testing, others did not

Table 4 Genetic association studies for AAA using variants in the HLA genes.

Study	HLA loci (number of alleles)	Population studied	Cases	Controls	Findings		
					Allele/Haplotype	Statistic
Norrgård et al., 1984[89]	HLA-A (7) HLA-B (11)	Sweden	48	368	NS	NS
Rasmussen et al., 1997[90]	HLA-DR B1 (13) HLA-DQ B1 (5)	USA/White	37	90	HLA-DR B1*15 HLA-DR B1*0404 HLA-DQ B1 alleles	$p = 0.035$ $p = 0.032$ NS
Hirose et al., 1998[91]	HLA-DR (12)	Japan	46	50	HLA-DR2 (15) Other HLA-DR alleles	$p < 0.005$ NS
Hirose and Tilson, 1999[92]	HLA-DQ (4)	Japan	36	39	HLA-DQ3	$p = 0.014$
Rasmussen et al., 2001[93]	HLA-DR B1 (12)	USA/White	112 (degenerative) 40 (inflammatory)	118	HLA-DR B1*02 (inflammatory) HLA-DR B1*02 (degenerative) HLA-DR B1*04 (inflammatory) HLA-DR B1*04 (degenerative)	OR = 3.6 OR = 2.2 OR = 2.5 OR = 2.0
Rasmussen et al., 2002[94]	HLA-DR B1	USA/White	142	118	HLA-DR B1*02 HLA-DR B1*04	OR = 2.5 OR = 2.1
Ogata et al., 2006[95]	HLA-DQA1	Belgian/Canadian	180 (Belgian)	269 (Belgian)	HLA-DQA1*0102 (Belgians)	$p = 0.019$ (Empirical)
	HLA-DQB1		207 (Canadian)	157 (Canadian)	HLA-DQA1-DRB1 (Begians)	$p = 0.0003$ (Asymptotic)
	HLA-DRB1, 3–5				All others	$p = 0.049$ NS
Badger et al., 2007[96]	HLA-A HLA-B HLA-DR	Northern Ireland	241	1000	All comparisons	NS

HLA human leukocyte antigen, *NS* not significant

types. Note that many early association studies were small and did not have adequate power to definitively exclude or prove an association. More recent studies have overcome this problem by using larger groups of cases and controls. Another important point is that for some polymorphisms, different studies have published conflicting results. For example, in three studies on a polymorphism in *ACE*, two studies reported an association [71,78] whereas one did not.[65] Similarly, a polymorphism in the gene *SERPINE1* (also known as plasminogen activator inhibitor 1) was found to have an association with AAA in the New Zealand population[70] but not in the Finnish population.[67] Possible explanations for these discrepancies are variation in genetic risk factors between populations, and false positives or false negatives from small sample sizes (type I and II errors).

Despite the problems with association studies on AAA mentioned above, there is convincing evidence for polymorphisms in several genes contributing to the development of AAA. Although there is conflicting evidence for a polymorphism in *ACE*, the largest and most recent study with 250 Italian cases and controls demonstrated a significant association.[78] A study by the same group also showed a significant association for one polymorphism in the *NOS3* gene.[79] *TIMP1* is another gene that shows possible association, although one study reported association only in females,[66] whereas a second larger study found association only in males without a positive family history.[80] Finally, in one of the two largest studies of HLA alleles, Ogata et al. found association with HLA DQA*0102 in the Belgian population.[95] Early studies on HLA DRB1 reported significant association, but both Ogata et al. and a recent study by Badger et al.[96] with 241 cases and 1000 controls did not confirm these results.

The next phase of genetic association studies will involve the entire genome. These genome-wide association studies, commonly referred to as the acronym GWAS, will require even larger samples sizes, but will give a better understanding of the genetic architecture of AAA.[62] They are also more feasible than family-based studies for complex and deadly diseases such as AAA since samples from extended families are not required.

Microarray-Based Global Gene Expression Profiling: An Unbiased Approach to Identify Signaling Pathways Altered in AAA

Expression profiling is the characterization of a tissue by which genes are expressed in it and how highly they are expressed. Although several methods have been developed to study gene expression profiles, the current standard is whole-genome microarray platforms available from several manufacturers. Microarray experiments compare gene expression patterns between tissues or cells, such as between an aneurysmal aorta and a nonaneurysmal one. The changes in gene expression can then be used to identify biological processes relevant to the disease being studied. This can be done by categorizing differentially expressed genes by function, such as gene ontology (GO) category[97] or Kyoto Encyclopedia of Genes and Genomes (KEGG) pathway,[98] and determining the categories or pathways that are statistically enriched.

Although microarrays have the potential to be a powerful tool for analysis, they are also subject to some limitations. First, as with other types of gene analysis, sample replicates are necessary to account for sample variability. This can be problematic if the cost of the microarrays is prohibitive or if obtaining multiple tissue samples is difficult. Another limitation is incomplete annotation for gene function; GO categories and KEGG pathways are only useful for genes with known function. Additionally, microarrays only test for levels of mRNA and may not represent what is occurring on the protein level. Therefore, it is important that microarray findings be followed-up using different methods such as immunohistochemistry. Finally, there are several statistical considerations for the analysis of microarray data such as how to define differential expression or account for the large number of false positives generated when looking at thousands of genes. For a detailed discussion of microarray data analysis, the reader is referred to Allison et al.[99]

There have been five array-based studies published on AAA.[100–104] The four earliest studies were performed using older, so-called macroarrays that hybridized radiolabeled sample cDNA to gene-specific cDNA clones spotted on a nylon membrane, between 275 and 1185 probes. The major drawback to these arrays was that they simply did not probe enough genes to study which biological processes and pathways were altered. Additionally, the measurement of expression relied upon densitometry, which is less sensitive than current fluorescence-based methods. However, these studies were able to confirm some previously known expression changes (e.g., MMP9, IL8) and provided limited expression information for future comparisons. Furthermore, three of the studies compared AAA to other disease processes. Armstrong et al.[101] compared AAA with aortic occlusive disease and showed some differences between the diseases, but the number of genes ($n = 265$) studied was too small to make any generalizations. In a similar study, Yamagishi et al.[103] compared expression of 375 cytokine genes between AAA and carotid artery stenosis. Absi et al.[102] determined the genes that are differentially expressed between thoracic aorta and thoracic aortic aneurysms (TAA) and then compared these with the genes whose expressions change in AAA. This analysis was able to show that AAA is characterized by changes in genes related to inflammation, whereas TAA is characterized by changes in cell survival, proliferation, and programmed cell death.

In contrast to the three earlier papers, Lenk et al.[104] reported the only whole-genome comparison of AAA and control aorta using two different microarray platforms. From a reference list of 18,057 genes common to the two microarrays, 3274 genes were found to be differentially expressed between AAA ($N = 7$) and control tissue ($N = 7$), even after correction for multiple testing (Fig. 5). These differentially expressed genes confirm previous work implicating genes such as MMPs, *IL1B*, and cathepsins in the pathogenesis of AAA, as well as point to new genes for study such as *RUNX3* and *SOST*. Analysis of the differentially expressed genes using KEGG pathways showed several pathways related to immune function to be enriched in AAA, including "natural killer cell-mediated cytotoxicity," "leukocyte transendothelial migration," and "T cell-receptor signaling pathway." This confirms previous histological work showing immune activation to be important in the development of aneurysm and suggests that this area merits further study.

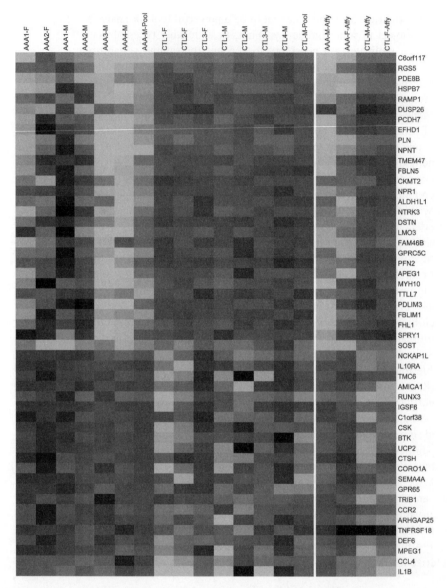

Fig. 5 Whole-genome expression profile for AAA tissue. The 50 most significantly different genes between AAA and control tissue are shown as determined by the Illumina microarray platform in ascending order (the most differential genes are located on the top and bottom, with decreasing difference toward the center). To show consistency of the results between two platforms (Affymetrix and Illumina), data from both Illumina (15 left columns) and Affymetrix (4 right columns) platforms are presented. Sample IDs are on top of each column (AAA1-F = female aneurysm patient, CTL1-F = female control, etc.). The "Pool" samples were age, sex, and ethnicity-matched pools of RNA. All four samples run on Affymetrix arrays were pooled samples. Data were log2-transformed and gene-centered for each individual platform. Gene IDs shown on the right represent official IDs found at http://www.genenames.org/. For details, see study by Lenk et al.[104] (*See Color Plates*)

Microarray analysis of AAA is an area of research that is still very much in its infancy, with many possible studies that could provide useful information about the disease. The early array studies suggest that comparison of AAA to other disease processes bears repeating on a whole-genome scale.

Additionally, comparison of abdominal aorta to other arteries may be useful in understanding what makes that region susceptible to aneurysms. Such studies and others can hopefully be expected in the near future, given improved and more affordable array technology.

Animal Models Provide Important Information About Pathogenesis of AAA

Studying the development of aneurysms in genetic knockout animals can help determine the genes that contribute to AAA development. To date, no naturally occurring mutant mouse with a phenotype resembling human AAA has been identified. Similarly, genetically engineered mutant mice do not spontaneously develop AAA, but aneurysms must be induced with additional insults such as elastase-perfusion, angiotensin II infusion, or calcium chloride ($CaCl_2$) treatment.[105,106] Currently, there is no consensus on which model is best as each has its advantages and disadvantages. For instance, elastase-perfusion causes aneurysms to develop very quickly, which may not be representative of the slow dilatation of human AAAs, but does allow faster completion of studies. In contrast, aneurysms from angiotensin II infusion develop more slowly, but they are not specific to the infrarenal aorta and often show signs of dissection. Additionally, this model uses an apolipoprotein E (*Apoe*) knockout background and relies on nonphysiological concentrations of angiotensin II. As a compromise, some investigators advocate the $CaCl_2$ model since the aneurysms develop at a medium rate and can be induced in wild-type mice. Two additional mouse models of AAA have been reported; one using a high fat diet in *Apoe* knockout mice and the other using Balb/C donor allografts in a recipient of a different strain.[105,107] However, several studies with the diet model have not produced aortic changes consistent with aneurysms, but instead showed either arteriomegaly or microaneurysm phenotypes.[108–110] The allograft model does produce true dilatations, but it has not been widely used making it difficult to judge its merits compared to other models. The major problem with all of these models is that we do not yet understand the underlying causes of aneurysm formation to design an ideal animal model.

Table 5 summarizes the gene knockouts tested in aneurysm models. Three of the five aneurysm models, elastase, $CaCl_2$, and angiotensin II models, have been used extensively in these studies. There is some agreement between the models as knockouts for *Mmp9* and *Ccr2* show similar effects in multiple models.[112,115,118,130] In contrast, two examples do exist of gene knockouts having an effect in one model, but not in another.[112,120,123,127] However, as no divergent effects have been found, it is unclear whether these results were due to differences between models or experimental design. It is also noteworthy that the genetic background has been found to influence results in that mice with a 129/SvJ or 129/SvEv background are resistant to aneurysm formation, whereas FVB and B/6 mice are susceptible.[106]

Many of the gene knockout studies have helped to characterize biological systems previously studied in aneurysm formation, such as extracellular matrix remodeling and immunity. For instance, several studies have tested knockouts of MMPs and TIMPs. Pyo et al.[112] showed that knockout of *Mmp9* decreased susceptibility to elastase-induced aneurysm formation, an effect that could be reversed with bone marrow reconstitution from wild-type mice. Longo et al.[115]

Table 5 Use of gene knockouts in AAA mouse models.

Study	Model	Strain[a]	Knocked-out gene[b]	Change in AAA susceptibility[d]
Daugherty et al., 2000[111]	AngII	C57BL/6J	*Apoe*	Increased
Pyo et al., 2000[112]	Elastase	129S/SvJ	*Mmp12*	None
		129/SvEv	*Mmp9*	Decreased
Chen et al., 2001[113]	Diet	NR	*Nos3*[c]	None
Lee et al., 2001[114]	Elastase	C57BL/6J	*Nos2*	Increased
Longo et al., 2002[115]	CaCl₂	129/SvEv	*Mmp9*	Decreased
		C57BL/6	*Mmp2*	Decreased
Bruemmer et al., 2003[116]	AngII	C57BL/6J	*Spp1*[c]	Decreased
Deng et al., 2003[117]	AngII	C57BL/6	*Apoe/Plau*	Decreased
			Plau	Decreased
			Apoe	Increased
Ishibashi et al., 2004[118]	AngII	C57BL/6Jx129/SvJae	*Ccr2*[c]	Decreased
Shimizu et al., 2004[107]	Allograft	129/SvEv	*Ifngr1/Il4*	Decreased
			Ifngr1	Increased
			Ifng	Decreased
			Cd4	Decreased
Xiong et al., 2004[119]	CaCl₂	C57BL/6	*Alox5*[c]	Decreased
Zhao et al., 2004[120]	Diet	C57BL/6	*Timp1*	Increased
Eskandari et al., 2005[121]	Elastase	C57BL/6	*Sell*	Decreased
Hannawa et al., 2005[122]	Elastase	129/SvJ	*Mmp12*	Decreased
Longo et al., 2005[123]	CaCl₂	NR	*Ncf1*[c]	Decreased
Thomas et al., 2006[124]	AngII	C57BL/6	*Timp2*	Decreased
Xiong et al., 2006[125]	CaCl₂	C57BL/6J	*Ltb4r1*[c]	Decreased
Ahluwalia et al., 2007[126]	AngII	C57BL/6	*Alox5*[c]	None
Cao et al., 2007[127]	AngII	C57BL/6	*Agtr1a*[c]	Decreased
Cassis et al., 2007[128]	AngII	C57BL/6Jx129/Ola	*Ptgs2*	Decreased
Gitlin et al., 2007[129]	AngII	129/Sv	*Ccr5*	None
			Cxcr3	None
MacTaggart et al., 2007[130]	CaCl₂	NR	*Ccr2*	Decreased
Pagano et al., 2007[131]	Elastase	C57BL/6	*Ctsc*	Decreased
Sun et al., 2007[132]	Elastase and CaCl₂	C57BL/6	*Kit*	Decreased

AAA abdominal aortic aneurysms, *NR* not reported

[a] Strain as reported in the original study

[b] MGI-approved gene symbols obtained from http://www.informatics.jax.org/mgihome/nomen/index.shtml

[c] Study performed in an *Apoe* knockout background

[d] Increased means that knockout animals developed AAAs more frequently than wild-type animals. Decreased means that knockout animals developed AAAs less frequently than wild-type animals

demonstrated the same results in the $CaCl_2$ model but also showed a decreased susceptibility in *Mmp2* knockout mice. However, the susceptibility was not restored in the *Mmp2* knockouts on reconstitution, suggesting that *Mmp9* is produced by cells migrating into the aorta but *Mmp2* is produced locally. Additionally, work has also been done suggesting roles for *Mmp12*, *Timp1*, and *Timp2* in aneurysms, although only one of two studies on *Mmp12* showed an effect from knockout of the gene.[112,121,123,125] Interestingly, studies on *Timp1* and *Timp2* showed divergent effects for the two genes. Knockout of *Timp1* resulted in increased susceptibility to aneurysms whereas knockout of *Timp2* resulted in the opposite, demonstrating that despite a gene's name or known biological roles, it may also have additional unexpected functions.

Characterization of the immune response in aneurysms has also been possible through mouse knockout models. MacTaggart et al.[130] found that *Ccr2* but not *Ccr5* or *Cxcr3* is involved in aneurysm formation in the $CaCl_2$ model. The importance of *Ccr2* was also confirmed in the angiotensin II model. Xiong et al.[119] found that *Cd4* and interferon-γ knockout decreased susceptibility to $CaCl_2$ aneurysm formation suggesting a role for T-cell signaling in AAA. Finally, Hannawa et al.[122] and Pagano et al.[131] have shown a role for neutrophils in elastase-induced aneurysm formation through knockouts of L-selectin (*Sell*) and dipeptidyl peptidase (*Ctsc*), respectively.

Since animal models of aneurysms can be used to study the importance of genes *in vivo*, this approach will be utilized long into the future. As new genes and pathways are identified through other methods such as linkage, association, microarray, and even pathology studies, animal models can be used to study their role in detail in aneurysms. Additionally, as our understanding of aneurysm pathophysiology increases, better animal models can be developed to assist in future studies such as developing new therapeutic modalities.

Conclusions: The Future of Aneurysm Genetics

AAA can be considered a complex genetic disorder with a so far unknown etiology and a poorly defined pathogenesis. Each of the techniques described above can be considered to have one goal in the study of AAA: the identification of candidate genes, either for genetic screening or for targeted therapies. Aside from familial syndromes, only one mutation, in the procollagen III gene, has been identified as contributing to AAA risk in a small number of patients.[133] Several genes have been identified as potential drug targets, such as *MMP9*, but no specific therapies have been developed. Therefore, there is still much to be learned about aneurysms from genetic studies. At least three of four methods described above have had significant developments in recent years, suggesting that they will contribute to our understanding of aneurysms (Fig. 2). However, the most important contributions may be from the combined approaches using more than one of these methods. For instance, expression profiling from microarray studies may identify candidate genes to be tested using either association studies or animal models. Alternatively, linked intervals could be used as a guide for selecting genes for association studies. Regardless of the specific approach, studying the genetics of AAA will hopefully solve unanswered questions and lead to better screening and treatment.

Acknowledgments The authors thank Dr. Gerard Tromp for preparing Fig. 1. The original work carried out in the Kuivaniemi laboratory was funded in part by the National Heart, Lung, and Blood Institute of the NIH (HL045996 and HL06410 to H.K.). J.H.L. is a recipient of a Predoctoral Fellowship from the National Institute on Aging, NIH (AG030900), and G.M.L. is a recipient of a Predoctoral Fellowship from the American Heart Association (0510063Z and 0710099Z).

References

1. Alcorn HG, Wolfson SK, Jr., Sutton-Tyrrell K, Kuller LH, O'Leary D. Risk factors for abdominal aortic aneurysms in older adults enrolled in The Cardiovascular Health Study. Arterioscler Thromb Vasc Biol 1996;16(8):963–970.
2. WISQARS Leading Causes of Death Reports, 1999–2004. 2007. (Accessed October 15, 2007, at http://webappa.cdc.gov/sasweb/ncipc/leadcaus10.html.)
3. Johansen K, Kohler TR, Nicholls SC, Zierler RE, Clowes AW, Kazmers A. Ruptured abdominal aortic aneurysm: the Harborview experience. J Vasc Surg 1991;13(2):240–245.
4. Krupski WC, Rutherford RB. Update on open repair of abdominal aortic aneurysms: the challenges for endovascular repair. J Am Coll Surg 2004;199(6):946–960.
5. Lederle FA, Johnson GR, Wilson SE, et al. The aneurysm detection and management study screening program: validation cohort and final results. Aneurysm Detection and Management Veterans Affairs Cooperative Study Investigators. Arch Intern Med 2000;160(10):1425–1430.
6. Kuivaniemi H, Tromp G, Prockop DJ. Genetic causes of aortic aneurysms. Unlearning at least part of what the textbooks say. J Clin Invest 1991;88(5): 1441–1444.
7. Bengtsson H, Sonesson B, Bergqvist D. Incidence and prevalence of abdominal aortic aneurysms, estimated by necropsy studies and population screening by ultrasound. Ann N Y Acad Sci 1996;800:1–24.
8. Kuivaniemi H, Marshall A, Ganguly A, Chu ML, Abbott WM, Tromp G. Fibulin-2 exhibits high degree of variability, but no structural changes concordant with abdominal aortic aneurysms. Eur J Hum Genet 1998;6(6):642–646.
9. Kuivaniemi H, Tromp G. Search for the aneurysm susceptibility gene(s). In: Keen RR, Dobrin PB, eds. Development of Aneurysms. Georgetown: Landes Bioscience; 2000:219–233.
10. Norrgard O, Rais O, Angquist KA. Familial occurrence of abdominal aortic aneurysms. Surgery 1984;95(6):650–656.
11. Johansen K, Koepsell T. Familial tendency for abdominal aortic aneurysms. JAMA 1986;256(14):1934–1936.
12. Powell JT, Greenhalgh RM. Multifactorial inheritance of abdominal aortic aneurysm. Eur J Vasc Surg 1987;1(1):29–31.
13. Johnston KW, Scobie TK. Multicenter prospective study of nonruptured abdominal aortic aneurysms. I. Population and operative management. J Vasc Surg 1988;7(1):69–81.
14. Cole CW, Barber GG, Bouchard AG, et al. Abdominal aortic aneurysm: consequences of a positive family history. Can J Surg 1989;32(2):117–120.
15. Darling RC, 3rd, Brewster DC, Darling RC, et al. Are familial abdominal aortic aneurysms different? J Vasc Surg 1989;10(1):39–43.
16. Majumder PP, St Jean PL, Ferrell RE, Webster MW, Steed DL. On the inheritance of abdominal aortic aneurysm. Am J Hum Genet 1991;48(1):164–170.
17. Verloes A, Sakalihasan N, Koulischer L, Limet R. Aneurysms of the abdominal aorta: familial and genetic aspects in three hundred thirteen pedigrees. J Vasc Surg 1995;21(4):646–655.

18. Lederle FA, Johnson GR, Wilson SE, et al. Prevalence and associations of abdominal aortic aneurysm detected through screening. Aneurysm Detection and Management (ADAM) Veterans Affairs Cooperative Study Group. Ann Intern Med 1997;126(6):441–449.

19. Lawrence PF, Wallis C, Dobrin PB, et al. Peripheral aneurysms and arteriomegaly: is there a familial pattern? J Vasc Surg 1998;28(4):599–605.

20. Salkowski A, Greb A, Al-Aouar R, et al. Familial incidence of abdominal aortic aneurysms. J Genet Couns 1999;8:407.

21. Rossaak JI, Hill TM, Jones GT, Phillips LV, Harris EL, van Rij AM. Familial abdominal aortic aneurysms in the Otago region of New Zealand. Cardiovasc Surg 2001;9(3):241–248.

22. Bengtsson H, Norrgard O, Angquist KA, Ekberg O, Oberg L, Bergqvist D. Ultrasonographic screening of the abdominal aorta among siblings of patients with abdominal aortic aneurysms. Br J Surg 1989;76(6):589–591.

23. Collin J, Walton J. Is abdominal aortic aneurysm familial? BMJ 1989; 299(6697):493.

24. Webster MW, St Jean PL, Steed DL, Ferrell RE, Majumder PP. Abdominal aortic aneurysm: results of a family study. J Vasc Surg 1991;13(3):366–372.

25. Adamson J, Powell JT, Greenhalgh RM. Selection for screening for familial aortic aneurysms. Br J Surg 1992;79(9):897–898.

26. Bengtsson H, Sonesson B, Lanne T, et al. Prevalence of abdominal aortic aneurysm in the offspring of patients dying from aneurysm rupture. Br J Surg 1992;79(11):1142–1143.

27. van der Lugt A, Kranendonk SE, Baars AM. Screening for familial occurrence of abdominal aortic aneurysm. Ned Tijdschr Geneeskd 1992;136(39):1910–1913.

28. Adams DC, Tulloh BR, Galloway SW, Shaw E, Tulloh AJ, Poskitt KR. Familial abdominal aortic aneurysm: prevalence and implications for screening. Eur J Vasc Surg 1993;7(6):709–712.

29. Moher D, Cole CW, Hill GB. Definition and management of abdominal aortic aneurysms: results from a Canadian survey. Can J Surg 1994;37(1):29–32.

30. Fitzgerald P, Ramsbottom D, Burke P, et al. Abdominal aortic aneurysm in the Irish population: a familial screening study. Br J Surg 1995;82(4):483–486.

31. Larcos G, Gruenewald SM, Fletcher JP. Ultrasound screening of families with abdominal aortic aneurysm. Australas Radiol 1995;39(3):254–256.

32. Baird PA, Sadovnick AD, Yee IM, Cole CW, Cole L. Sibling risks of abdominal aortic aneurysm. Lancet 1995;346(8975):601–604.

33. Jaakkola P, Kuivaniemi H, Partanen K, Tromp G, Liljestrom B, Ryynanen M. Familial abdominal aortic aneurysms: screening of 71 families. Eur J Surg 1996;162(8):611–617.

34. van der Graaf Y, Akkersdijk GJ, Hak E, Godaert GL, Eikelboom BC. Results of aortic screening in the brothers of patients who had elective aortic aneurysm repair. Br J Surg 1998;85(6):778–780.

35. Salo JA, Soisalon-Soininen S, Bondestam S, Mattila PS. Familial occurrence of abdominal aortic aneurysm. Ann Intern Med 1999;130(8):637–642.

36. Frydman G, Walker PJ, Summers K, et al. The value of screening in siblings of patients with abdominal aortic aneurysm. Eur J Vasc Endovasc Surg 2003;26(4):396–400.

37. Ogata T, MacKean GL, Cole CW, et al. The lifetime prevalence of abdominal aortic aneurysms among siblings of aneurysm patients is eightfold higher than among siblings of spouses: an analysis of 187 aneurysm families in Nova Scotia, Canada. J Vasc Surg 2005;42(5):891–897.

38. Badger SA, O'Donnell ME, Boyd CS, et al. The low prevalence of abdominal aortic aneurysm in relatives in northern Ireland. Eur J Vasc Endovasc Surg 2007;34(2):163–168.

39. Kuivaniemi H, Shibamura H, Arthur C, et al. Familial abdominal aortic aneurysms: collection of 233 multiplex families. J Vasc Surg 2003;37(2):340–345.

40. Thompson MW, E. MR, F. WH. Genetics in Medicine. 5th ed. Philadelphia: W.B. Saunders Company; Harcourt Brace Jovanovisch, Inc.; 1991.

41. Norman PE, Powell JT. Abdominal aortic aneurysm: the prognosis in women is worse than in men. Circulation 2007;115(22):2865–2869.

42. Katz DJ, Stanley JC, Zelenock GB. Operative mortality rates for intact and ruptured abdominal aortic aneurysms in Michigan: an eleven-year statewide experience. J Vasc Surg 1994;19(5):804–815.

43. Katz DJ, Stanley JC, Zelenock GB. Gender differences in abdominal aortic aneurysm prevalence, treatment, and outcome. J Vasc Surg 1997;25(3):561–568.

44. Limet R. Familial risk of abdominal aortic aneurysm and its consequences for organization of selective detection. J Mal Vasc 1995;20(4):285–287.

45. Nakka P, Chu J, Roake J, Lewis D. Variability in counselling patients regarding the hereditary nature of abdominal aortic aneurysm (AAA). Lack of evidence or resources? N Z Med J 2007;120(1251):U2460.

46. Harper PS. Practical Genetic Counseling. 6th ed. London: Arnold Publishers; 2004.

47. Brewster DC, Cronenwett JL, Hallett JW, Jr., Johnston KW, Krupski WC, Matsumura JS. Guidelines for the treatment of abdominal aortic aneurysms. Report of a subcommittee of the Joint Council of the American Association for Vascular Surgery and Society for Vascular Surgery. J Vasc Surg 2003;37(5):1106–1117.

48. Vande Geest JP, Wang DH, Wisniewski SR, Makaroun MS, Vorp DA. Towards a noninvasive method for determination of patient-specific wall strength distribution in abdominal aortic aneurysms. Ann Biomed Eng 2006;34(7):1098–1106.

49. Screening for Abdominal Aortic Aneurysm, Topic Page. US Preventative Services Task Force. Agency for Healthcare Research and Quality, 2005. (Accessed November 7th, 2007, at http://www.ahrq.gov/clinic/uspstf/uspsaneu.htm.)

50. Fleming C, Whitlock EP, Beil TL, Lederle FA. Screening for abdominal aortic aneurysm: a best-evidence systematic review for the US Preventive Services Task Force. Ann Intern Med 2005;142(3):203–211.

51. Kent KC, Zwolak RM, Jaff MR, et al. Screening for abdominal aortic aneurysm: a consensus statement. J Vasc Surg 2004;39(1):267–269.

52. Le Hello C, Koskas F, Cluzel P, et al. French women from multiplex abdominal aortic aneurysm families should be screened. Ann Surg 2005;242(5):739–744.

53. Olson JM, Witte JS, Elston RC. Genetic mapping of complex traits. Stat Med 1999;18(21):2961–2981.

54. Shibamura H, Olson JM, Van Vlijmen-Van Keulen CJ, et al. Genome scan for familial abdominal aortic aneurysm using sex and family history as covariates suggests genetic heterogeneity and identifies linkage to chromosome 19q13. Circulation 2004;109(17):2103–2108.

55. van Vlijmen-Van Keulen CJ, Rauwerda JA, Pals G. Genome-wide linkage in three Dutch families maps a locus for abdominal aortic aneurysms to chromosome 19q13.3. Eur J Vasc Endovasc Surg 2005;30(1):29–35.

56. Online Mendelian Inheritance in Man, OMIM (TM). (Accessed November 13, 2007, at http://www.ncbi.nlm.nih.gov/omim/.(

57. Pannu H, Avidan N, Tran-Fadulu V, Milewicz DM. Genetic basis of thoracic aortic aneurysms and dissections: potential relevance to abdominal aortic aneurysms. Ann N Y Acad Sci 2006;1085:242–255.

58 Beckman JA. Aortic aneurysms: pathophysiology, epidemiology, and prognosis. In: Creager MA, Dzau VJ, Loscalzo J, eds. Vascular Medicine. Philadelphia: Saunders Elsevier, Inc.; 2006:543–559.

59. Elston RC. Linkage and association. Genet Epidemiol 1998;15(6):565–576.

60. Devlin B, Roeder K. Genomic control for association studies. Biometrics 1999;55(4):997–1004.

61. Bamshad MJ, Wooding S, Watkins WS, Ostler CT, Batzer MA, Jorde LB. Human population genetic structure and inference of group membership. Am J Hum Genet 2003;72(3):578–589.

62. Chanock SJ, Manolio T, Boehnke M, et al. Replicating genotype-phenotype associations. Nature 2007;447(7145):655–660.

63. Powell JT, Bashir A, Dawson S, et al. Genetic variation on chromosome 16 is associated with abdominal aortic aneurysm. Clin Sci (Lond) 1990;78(1):13–16.

64. St Jean PL, Zhang XC, Hart BK, et al. Characterization of a dinucleotide repeat in the 92 kDa type IV collagenase gene (CLG4B), localization of CLG4B to chromosome 20 and the role of CLG4B in aortic aneurysmal disease. Ann Hum Genet 1995;59(Pt 1):17–24.

65. Hamano K, Ohishi M, Ueda M, et al. Deletion polymorphism in the gene for angiotensin-converting enzyme is not a risk factor predisposing to abdominal aortic aneurysm. Eur J Vasc Endovasc Surg 1999;18(2):158–161.

66. Wang X, Tromp G, Cole CW, et al. Analysis of coding sequences for tissue inhibitor of metalloproteinases 1 (TIMP1) and 2 (TIMP2) in patients with aneurysms. Matrix Biol 1999;18(2):121–124.

67. Yoon S, Tromp G, Vongpunsawad S, Ronkainen A, Juvonen T, Kuivaniemi H. Genetic analysis of MMP3, MMP9, and PAI-1 in Finnish patients with abdominal aortic or intracranial aneurysms. Biochem Biophys Res Commun 1999;265(2):563–568.

68. Brunelli T, Prisco D, Fedi S, et al. High prevalence of mild hyperhomocysteinemia in patients with abdominal aortic aneurysm. J Vasc Surg 2000;32(3):531–536.

69. Kotani K, Shimomura T, Murakami F, et al. Allele frequency of human endothelial nitric oxide synthase gene polymorphism in abdominal aortic aneurysm. Intern Med 2000;39(7):537–539.

70. Rossaak JI, Van Rij AM, Jones GT, Harris EL. Association of the 4G/5G polymorphism in the promoter region of plasminogen activator inhibitor-1 with abdominal aortic aneurysms. J Vasc Surg 2000;31(5):1026–1032.

71. Pola R, Gaetani E, Santoliquido A, et al. Abdominal aortic aneurysm in normotensive patients: association with angiotensin-converting enzyme gene polymorphism. Eur J Vasc Endovasc Surg 2001;21(5):445–449.

72. Schillinger M, Exner M, Mlekusch W, et al. Heme oxygenase-1 gene promoter polymorphism is associated with abdominal aortic aneurysm. Thromb Res 2002;106(2):131–136.

73. Unno N, Nakamura T, Mitsuoka H, et al. Association of a G994 T missense mutation in the plasma platelet-activating factor acetylhydrolase gene with risk of abdominal aortic aneurysm in Japanese. Ann Surg 2002;235(2):297–302.

74. Jones GT, Phillips VL, Harris EL, Rossaak JI, van Rij AM. Functional matrix metalloproteinase-9 polymorphism (C-1562T) associated with abdominal aortic aneurysm. J Vasc Surg 2003;38(6):1363–1367.

75. Bown MJ, Burton PR, Horsburgh T, Nicholson ML, Bell PR, Sayers RD. The role of cytokine gene polymorphisms in the pathogenesis of abdominal aortic aneurysms: a case-control study. J Vasc Surg 2003;37(5):999–1005.

76. Ghilardi G, Biondi ML, Battaglioli L, Zambon A, Guagnellini E, Scorza R. Genetic risk factor characterizes abdominal aortic aneurysm from arterial occlusive disease in human beings: CCR5 Delta 32 deletion. J Vasc Surg 2004;40(5):995–1000.

77. Massart F, Marini F, Menegato A, et al. Allelic genes involved in artery compliance and susceptibility to sporadic abdominal aortic aneurysm. J Steroid Biochem Mol Biol 2004;92(5):413–418.

78. Fatini C, Pratesi G, Sofi F, et al. ACE DD genotype: a predisposing factor for abdominal aortic aneurysm. Eur J Vasc Endovasc Surg 2005;29(3):227–232.

79. Fatini C, Sofi F, Sticchi E, et al. eNOS G894T polymorphism as a mild predisposing factor for abdominal aortic aneurysm. J Vasc Surg 2005;42(3):415–419.

80. Ogata T, Shibamura H, Tromp G, et al. Genetic analysis of polymorphisms in biologically relevant candidate genes in patients with abdominal aortic aneurysms. J Vasc Surg 2005;41(6):1036–1042.

81. Schulz V, Hendig D, Schillinger M, et al. Analysis of sequence variations in the ABCC6 gene among patients with abdominal aortic aneurysm and pseudoxanthoma elasticum. J Vasc Res 2005;42(5):424–432.

82. Golledge J, Muller J, Daugherty A, Norman P. Abdominal aortic aneurysm: pathogenesis and implications for management. Arterioscler Thromb Vasc Biol 2006;26(12):2605–2613.

83. Armani C, Curcio M, Barsotti MC, et al. Polymorphic analysis of the matrix metalloproteinase-9 gene and susceptibility to sporadic abdominal aortic aneurysm. Biomed Pharmacother 2007;61(5):268–271.

84. Bown MJ, Lloyd GM, Sandford RM, et al. The interleukin-10–1082 "A" allele and abdominal aortic aneurysms. J Vasc Surg 2007;46(4):687–693.

85. Smallwood L, Allcock R, van Bockxmeer F, et-al. Polymorphisms of the interleukin-6 gene promoter and abdominal aortic aneurysm. Eur J Vasc Endovasc Surg 2007.

86. Helgadottir A, Thorleifsson G, Magnusson KP, et al. The same sequence variant on 9p21 associates with myocardial infarction, abdominal aortic aneurysm and intracranial aneurysm. Nat Genet 2008;40(2):217–224.

87. Jones GT, Thompson AR, van Bockxmeer FM, et al. Angiotensin II type 1 receptor 1166C polymorphism is associated with abdominal aortic aneurysm in three independent cohorts. Arterioscler Thromb Vasc Biol 2008;28(4):764–770.

88. Gotting C, Prante C, Schillinger M, et al. Xylosyltransferase I variants and their impact on abdominal aortic aneurysms. Clin Chim Acta 2008;391(1–2):41–45.

89. Norrgard O, Cedergren B, Angquist KA, Beckman L. Blood groups and HLA antigens in patients with abdominal aortic aneurysms. Hum Hered 1984;34(1):9–13.

90. Rasmussen TE, Hallett JW, Jr., Metzger RL, et al. Genetic risk factors in inflammatory abdominal aortic aneurysms: polymorphic residue 70 in the HLA-DR B1 gene as a key genetic element. J Vasc Surg 1997;25(2):356–364.

91. Hirose H, Takagi M, Miyagawa N, et al. Genetic risk factor for abdominal aortic aneurysm: HLA-DR2(15), a Japanese study. J Vasc Surg 1998;27(3):500–503.

92. Hirose H, Tilson MD. Negative genetic risk factor for abdominal aortic aneurysm: HLA-DQ3, a Japanese study. J Vasc Surg 1999;30(5):959–960.

93. Rasmussen TE, Hallett JW, Jr., Schulte S, Harmsen WS, O'Fallon WM, Weyand CM. Genetic similarity in inflammatory and degenerative abdominal aortic aneurysms: a study of human leukocyte antigen class II disease risk genes. J Vasc Surg 2001;34(1):84–89.

94. Rasmussen TE, Hallett JW, Jr., Tazelaar HD, et al. Human leukocyte antigen class II immune response genes, female gender, and cigarette smoking as risk and modulating factors in abdominal aortic aneurysms. J Vasc Surg 2002;35(5):988–993.

95. Ogata T, Gregoire L, Goddard KA, et al. Evidence for association between the HLA-DQA locus and abdominal aortic aneurysms in the Belgian population: a case control study. BMC Med Genet 2006;7:67.

96. Badger SA, Soong CV, O'Donnell ME, Middleton D. The role of human leukocyte antigen genes in the formation of abdominal aortic aneurysms. J Vasc Surg 2007;45(3):475–480.

97. Ashburner M, Ball CA, Blake JA, et al. Gene ontology: tool for the unification of biology. The Gene Ontology Consortium. Nat Genet 2000;25(1):25–29.

98. Kanehisa M, Goto S. KEGG: kyoto encyclopedia of genes and genomes. Nucleic Acids Res 2000;28(1):27–30.

99. Allison DB, Cui X, Page GP, Sabripour M. Microarray data analysis: from disarray to consolidation and consensus. Nat Rev Genet 2006;7(1):55–65.

100. Tung WS, Lee JK, Thompson RW. Simultaneous analysis of 1176 gene products in normal human aorta and abdominal aortic aneurysms using a membrane-based complementary DNA expression array. J Vasc Surg 2001;34(1):143–150.

101. Armstrong PJ, Johanning JM, Calton WC, Jr., et al. Differential gene expression in human abdominal aorta: aneurysmal versus occlusive disease. J Vasc Surg 2002;35(2):346–355.

102. Absi TS, Sundt TM, 3rd, Tung WS, et al. Altered patterns of gene expression distinguishing ascending aortic aneurysms from abdominal aortic aneurysms: complementary DNA expression profiling in the molecular characterization of aortic disease. J Thorac Cardiovasc Surg 2003;126(2):344–357.

103. Yamagishi M, Higashikata T, Ishibashi-Ueda H, et al. Sustained upregulation of inflammatory chemokine and its receptor in aneurysmal and occlusive atherosclerotic disease: results form tissue analysis with cDNA macroarray and real-time reverse transcriptional polymerase chain reaction methods. Circ J 2005;69(12):1490–1495.

104. Lenk GM, Tromp G, Weinsheimer S, Gatalica Z, Berguer R, Kuivaniemi H. Whole genome expression profiling reveals a significant role for immune function in human abdominal aortic aneurysms. BMC Genomics 2007;8:237.

105. Daugherty A, Cassis LA. Mouse models of abdominal aortic aneurysms. Arterioscler Thromb Vasc Biol 2004;24(3):429–434.

106. Thompson RW, Curci JA, Ennis TL, Mao D, Pagano MB, Pham CT. Pathophysiology of abdominal aortic aneurysms: insights from the elastase-induced model in mice with different genetic backgrounds. Ann N Y Acad Sci 2006;1085:59–73.

107. Shimizu K, Shichiri M, Libby P, Lee RT, Mitchell RN. Th2-predominant inflammation and blockade of IFN-gamma signaling induce aneurysms in allografted aortas. J Clin Invest 2004;114(2):300–308.

108. Carmeliet P, Moons L, Lijnen R, et al. Urokinase-generated plasmin activates matrix metalloproteinases during aneurysm formation. Nat Genet 1997;17(4):439–444.

109. Silence J, Collen D, Lijnen HR. Reduced atherosclerotic plaque but enhanced aneurysm formation in mice with inactivation of the tissue inhibitor of metalloproteinase-1 (TIMP-1) gene. Circ Res 2002;90(8):897–903.

110. Sukhova GK, Wang B, Libby P, et al. Cystatin C deficiency increases elastic lamina degradation and aortic dilatation in apolipoprotein E-null mice. Circ Res 2005;96(3):368–375.

111. Daugherty A, Manning MW, Cassis LA. Angiotensin II promotes atherosclerotic lesions and aneurysms in apolipoprotein E-deficient mice. J Clin Invest 2000;105(11):1605–1612.

112. Pyo R, Lee JK, Shipley JM, et al. Targeted gene disruption of matrix metalloproteinase-9 (gelatinase B) suppresses development of experimental abdominal aortic aneurysms. J Clin Invest 2000;105(11):1641–1649.

113. Chen J, Kuhlencordt PJ, Astern J, Gyurko R, Huang PL. Hypertension does not account for the accelerated atherosclerosis and development of aneurysms in male apolipoprotein e/endothelial nitric oxide synthase double knockout mice. Circulation 2001;104(20):2391–2394.

114. Lee JK, Borhani M, Ennis TL, Upchurch GR, Jr., Thompson RW. Experimental abdominal aortic aneurysms in mice lacking expression of inducible nitric oxide synthase. Arterioscler Thromb Vasc Biol 2001;21(9):1393–1401.

115. Longo GM, Xiong W, Greiner TC, Zhao Y, Fiotti N, Baxter BT. Matrix metalloproteinases 2 and 9 work in concert to produce aortic aneurysms. J Clin Invest 2002;110(5):625–632.

116. Bruemmer D, Collins AR, Noh G, et al. Angiotensin II-accelerated atherosclerosis and aneurysm formation is attenuated in osteopontin-deficient mice. J Clin Invest 2003;112(9):1318–1331.

117. Deng GG, Martin-McNulty B, Sukovich DA, et al. Urokinase-type plasminogen activator plays a critical role in angiotensin II-induced abdominal aortic aneurysm. Circ Res 2003;92(5):510–517.
118. Ishibashi M, Egashira K, Zhao Q, et al. Bone marrow-derived monocyte chemoattractant protein-1 receptor CCR2 is critical in angiotensin II-induced acceleration of atherosclerosis and aneurysm formation in hypercholesterolemic mice. Arterioscler Thromb Vasc Biol 2004;24(11):e174–178.
119. Xiong W, Zhao Y, Prall A, Greiner TC, Baxter BT. Key roles of CD4 + T cells and IFN-gamma in the development of abdominal aortic aneurysms in a murine model. J Immunol 2004;172(4):2607–2612.
120. Zhao L, Moos MP, Grabner R, et al. The 5-lipoxygenase pathway promotes pathogenesis of hyperlipidemia-dependent aortic aneurysm. Nat Med 2004;10(9): 966–973.
121. Eskandari MK, Vijungco JD, Flores A, Borensztajn J, Shively V, Pearce WH. Enhanced abdominal aortic aneurysm in TIMP-1-deficient mice. J Surg Res 2005;123(2):289–293.
122. Hannawa KK, Eliason JL, Woodrum DT, et al. L-selectin-mediated neutrophil recruitment in experimental rodent aneurysm formation. Circulation 2005;112(2):241–247.
123. Longo GM, Buda SJ, Fiotta N, et al. MMP-12 has a role in abdominal aortic aneurysms in mice. Surgery 2005;137(4):457–462.
124. Thomas M, Gavrila D, McCormick ML, et al. Deletion of p47phox attenuates angiotensin II-induced abdominal aortic aneurysm formation in apolipoprotein E-deficient mice. Circulation 2006;114(5):404–413.
125. Xiong W, Knispel R, Mactaggart J, Baxter BT. Effects of tissue inhibitor of metalloproteinase 2 deficiency on aneurysm formation. J Vasc Surg 2006;44(5): 1061–1066.
126. Ahluwalia N, Lin AY, Tager AM, et al. Inhibited aortic aneurysm formation in BLT1-deficient mice. J Immunol 2007;179(1):691–697.
127. Cao RY, Adams MA, Habenicht AJ, Funk CD. Angiotensin II-induced abdominal aortic aneurysm occurs independently of the 5-lipoxygenase pathway in apolipoprotein E-deficient mice. Prostaglandins Other Lipid Mediat 2007;84(1–2):34–42.
128. Cassis LA, Rateri DL, Lu H, Daugherty A. Bone marrow transplantation reveals that recipient AT1a receptors are required to initiate angiotensin II-induced atherosclerosis and aneurysms. Arterioscler Thromb Vasc Biol 2007;27(2):380–386.
129. Gitlin JM, Trivedi DB, Langenbach R, Loftin CD. Genetic deficiency of cyclooxygenase-2 attenuates abdominal aortic aneurysm formation in mice. Cardiovasc Res 2007;73(1):227–236.
130. MacTaggart JN, Xiong W, Knispel R, Baxter BT. Deletion of CCR2 but not CCR5 or CXCR3 inhibits aortic aneurysm formation. Surgery 2007;142(2):284–288.
131. Pagano MB, Bartoli MA, Ennis TL, et al. Critical role of dipeptidyl peptidase I in neutrophil recruitment during the development of experimental abdominal aortic aneurysms. Proc Natl Acad Sci U S A 2007;104(8):2855–2860.
132. Sun J, Sukhova GK, Yang M, et al. Mast cells modulate the pathogenesis of elastase-induced abdominal aortic aneurysms in mice. J Clin Invest 2007;117(11): 3359–3368.
133. Tromp G, Wu Y, Prockop DJ, et al. Sequencing of cDNA from 50 unrelated patients reveals that mutations in the triple-helical domain of type III procollagen are an infrequent cause of aortic aneurysms. J Clin Invest 1993;91(6):2539–2545.

Chapter 2

Inflammatory Pathogenesis and Pathophysiology of Abdominal Aortic Aneurysms

William H. Pearce and Vera P. Shively

Abstract The aorta is a high-pressure conduit that also conserves the energy output of the heart (elastic recoil). The main structural proteins of the aorta – collagen and elastin – serve these functions. The aortic architecture is not uniform and varies from the thoracic aorta to the infrarenal aorta. With these basic understandings of the aortic structure and function in mind, it is clear that inflammation, genetics, and mechanical forces play important roles in the pathogenesis of abdominal aortic aneurysms. Additional research is needed to further understand the relationship between these factors.

Keywords Abdominal aortic aneurysm, Pathophysiology, Pathogenesis

Introduction

The aorta is a complex structure in which form follows function. The aorta is a high-pressure conduit that also conserves the energy output of the heart (elastic recoil). The main structural proteins of the aorta – collagen (strength) and elastin – serve these functions. In addition to these proteins, there are thousands of other proteins that make up the extracellular matrix (ECM) of the aorta. In recent years, it has been discovered that the ECM is not a passive structure but contains growth factors and encrypted protein fragments. The packaging of growth factors and the disregulation of transforming growth factor-beta (TGF-β) play a central role in the pathogenesis of Marfan's disease.[1,2] The ECM, therefore, may also play a central role in healing and disease.

Aortic architecture is not uniform and varies from the thoracic aorta to the infrarenal aorta.[3] This variation in aortic structure may be explained in part by differences in regional hemodynamics. The abdominal aorta is the source of visceral blood flow and, below the renal arteries, the muscles of the lower extremity. The infrarenal aorta, thus, experiences large oscillations in blood flow, depending on lower extremity activity.[4]

G. Upchurch and E. Criado (eds.) *Aortic Aneurysms, Contemporary Cardiology*
DOI: 10.1007/978-1-60327-204-9_2, © Humana Press, a part of
Springer Science + Business Media, LLC 2009

With these basic understandings of the aortic structure and function in mind, the role that inflammation plays in the pathogenesis of abdominal aortic aneurysms (AAAs) becomes more apparent. In 1950, Dubost reported the first repair of an AAA using a human homograft.[5] In his report, he also describes clearly the inflammation found in AAAs: "The main feature, together with the destruction of the elastic tissue is the presence throughout the outer half of the aorta of masses of lymphocytic cells accompanying the vaso vasorum; these cells form concentric sheets but are also seen sometimes to follow the vessels at right angles to all layers of the wall. … In summary … this endarteritis and periarteritis would suggest an inflammatory process without any specific indication as to its nature." This observation was not studied in detail until the mid-1980s. Rizzo et al. described an inflammatory infiltrate in the outer walls of the aorta in biochemical studies of patients with aneurysms and occlusive disease.[6] This inflammatory infiltrate was later characterized by Koch who found that the majority of cells within the median and adventitia of AAAs were CD3-positive T lymphocytes ranging from 67% to 80%.[7] In addition, CD19-positive B cells were also found within the arterial wall. Further, there was a spectrum of disease progressing from occlusive disease to AAA and to inflammatory AAA with increasing inflammation. This data suggested that aortic aneurysms may represent an immune-mediated event rather than simple degeneration of the arterial wall. Brophy et al. also described the presence of Russell bodies, which are the accumulation of large amounts of immunoglobulins in the arterial wall.[8] Tilson et al. purified these immunoglobulins and characterized a potential antigenic source, aneurysm-associated protein-40.[9]

The histological and cytokine profiles of the inflammatory infiltrate suggest both an adaptive and an innate immune response. Platsoucas et al.[10] examined whether the infiltrate represented a monoclonal or a polyclonal T-cell amplification. The β-chain T-cell receptor transcripts from patients with AAAs were amplified and characterized. In nine of the ten patients studied, there was an oligoclonal population of T cells. In addition, they found that many of the mononuclear cells found in AAAs expressed early, intermediate, and late activation antigens. They concluded that AAAs are a specific antigen-driven T-cell disease with evidence of an ongoing inflammation.

The relationship between inflammatory infiltrate and the subsequent damage to the arterial wall has been evaluated in many animal models.[11] Using an elastase-induced aneurysm model, Thompson et al. studied the progression of disease.[12] Three days following an acute response, a transitional inflammatory state exists. By days 10–14, the inflammation becomes chronic. (*See* Fig. 1.) During this period, there are alterations in the cytokine proteins as well as the expression of metalloproteinases and their inhibitors. However, experimental aneurysms may occur without an initial injury. APO E knockout mice when exposed to angiotensin II spontaneously develop aortic aneurysms without the sequence of events described above.[13] Thus, the role that inflammation plays in the initiation of AAA is uncertain.

Matrix metalloproteinases (MMPs) appear to play a critical role in the pathogenesis of aneurysms. Busuttil et al. first described collagenase-like activity in the wall of patients with AAAs in 1980.[14] Since then many investigators have described the role that MMPs play in aneurysm formation. The metalloproteinases are a subfamily of the metazincin superfamily of proteinases.[15] The majority of these proteins are secreted as a proenzyme,

	Early	Intermediate	Late
	1-7 days	**7-14 days**	**14+ days**
M E D I A T O R S	ECM fragments Oxygen radicals Angiotensin Chemokines Cytokines	MMPs TIMP ECM fragments Cytokines Chemokines	Dysregulation of healing Self-sustaining immune response
C E L L S	PMN Monocytes T-cells	Macrophages Th1-cells	Macrophages Th2-cells
	Progressive elastin degradation and AAA formation →		

Th= T helper, PMN= polymorphonuclear neutrophil, ECM= extracellular matrix

Fig. 1 Arterial response following injury. Modified from Thompson et al.[12]

requiring extracellular activation. However, several of the MMPs are membrane-bound. Aortic aneurysms have been associated with a variety of MMPs, including 2, 9, and 13.[16] The substrate specificity of each MMP is variable and, while at first it was thought to be only ECM proteins, other substrates have been identified. Enzyme substrates include both noncollagenase ECM proteins, such as fibronectin and laminen, as well as nonstructural components. The nonstructural components may be even more important to the pathogenesis of AAAs. Nonstructural substrates of the MMPs include interleukin-1 alpha (IL-1α), active MMP-9, chemokine (C-X-C motif) ligand 5 (CXCL-5), IL-1β, IL-2 receptor, TGF-β, and many of the pro-MMPs.[17] Thus, MMPs may regulate the inflammatory response.

The immune response is highly regulated to prevent injury to the host. In the majority of instances, the inflammatory process leads to a healing process and tissue repair. However, in some instances, this process becomes pathologic, leading to continued tissue damage secondary to the immune response. An infectious etiology is clear in many cases; however, the initiating event may be unknown. The key intersection of MMPs in the regulations of inflammation may be the central process in the pathogenesis of AAAs. The modification of proinflammatory cytokines, chemokines, and the shedding of the membrane receptors by the MMPs are critical. CXCL-7, CXCL-12, CXCL-5 (chemokine), and TGF-β are substrates of MMP-2, MMP-3, and MMP-9.[18] The lack of critical control of the immune response at multiple layers may, therefore, lead to the same phenotype (AAAs). Therefore, AAAs may arise from a variety of stimulators and the response (healing or destruction) is guided by subtle differences in the control of inflammation.

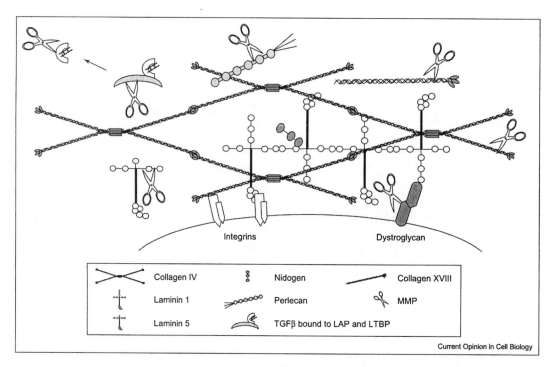

Fig. 2 A schematic diagram of some of the proteins that comprise the extracellular matrix (*ECM*) and the potential for matrix metalloproteinase (*MMP*) cleavage. The ECM is composed of both laminin and collagen networks. Within ECM network, many laminins and collagens are present as well as proteins such as nidogen, perlecan (i.e., heparin sulate proteoglycans), and fibronectin (not shown). Cell surface receptors such as integrins and dystroglycan interact with proteins of the basement membrane network. Cleavage of ECM molecules releases bioactive fragments that have been referred to as matricryptins or matrikines. Furthermore, growth factors, such as latent transforming growth factor-beta (*TGF-β*), are embedded with ECM, and proteolysis of binding proteins that keep the growth factors in a latent state is a major activation pathway. In addition, some of the cell surface receptors such as dystroglycan are targets for proteolysis. Cleavage of these types of molecules breaks cell–ECM contact. Reprinted from Mott and Werb.[19] Reproduced with permission from Elsevier

As MMPs digest the matrix, signals may be released to the surrounding vascular smooth muscle cells and inflammatory cells. Cryptic fragments include arrestin, deprellin, endostatin, restin, elastin degradation products, and the growth factors TGF-β and vascular endothelial growth factor.[19] Thus, a possible scenario for the progression of aneurysms is digestion of the ECM by the inflammatory infiltrate, which exposes encrypted fragments that continue to stimulate the immune response. A simple example may be elastin degradation products, which have been shown to be chemotactic for monocytes.[20] (Fig. 2.)

The Genetic Basis of the Inflammatory Response in AAA

The differential expression of genes involved in immune function in AAA versus control aortic tissue was recently described by Lenk et al.[21] They used Illumina and Affymetrix microarray platforms to obtain gene expression profiles, and Gene Ontology and Kyoto Encyclopedia of Genes and Genomes database tools to analyze biological pathways. The AAA tissues showed significantly more expression of genes involved in immune function, most notably in pathways regulating cell adhesion molecules, natural killer cell-mediated cytotoxicity, and leukocyte transendothelial migration. The authors acknowledged that a limitation of their study was sampling of AAA tissue from late-stage disease. However, their gene expression data provides valuable insight into the future development of immune-based treatment strategies, as well as direction to the search for underlying genetic factors in AAA.

Family history, or genetics, is a significant and independent risk factor for AAA.[22] Which genes predispose to AAA is yet to be determined, but several candidate gene polymorphism studies have shown an association between AAA and genes mediating inflammation. A recent review by Sandford et al. includes a comprehensive evaluation of genetic research in AAA, based on familial, segregation, and candidate gene studies.[23] In a case-control study of 100 AAA patients and age- and gender-matched controls, Bown et al. reported cytokine gene polymorphism data for the proinflammatory IL-1β + 3953, IL-6 – 174, and tumor necrosis factor-alpha (TNF-α) – 308, and the anti-inflammatory IL-10 promoter polymorphisms at positions −1082 and −592. The A allele for IL-10 – 1082 was found in association with AAA, while the others failed to reach statistical significance.[24] This allele is associated with low IL-10 secretion, and may contribute to the chronic inflammation that is characteristic of AAA. In another study, Ghilardi et al. reported the association of chemokine receptor CCR5 Δ32 deletion and AAA when compared to patients with peripheral arterial occlusive disease, carotid artery disease, and controls. Within the AAA subjects, CCR5 Δ32 was also more commonly found in patients with ruptured aneurysms.[25] The deletion results in the production of fewer receptors and, in theory, less cytokine activation through this receptor pathway. This would appear contrary to increased cytokine levels found in AAA tissue, although the mechanism of this receptor has not been fully described.

Our laboratory compared five inflammatory mediator gene polymorphisms in a population of 79 elderly male Caucasian AAA patients versus 71 case-matched healthy controls free of inflammatory conditions. Proinflammatory cytokine polymorphisms included IL-1β Taq I fragment in exon 5 and TNF-α – 308, and the anti-inflammatory cytotoxic T-lymphocyte antigen-4 (CTLA-4) at positions −318 and +49, and IL-1 receptor antagonist variable nucleotide tandem repeat in intron 2. The +49 CTLA-4 A/G allele frequencies differed significantly ($p < 0.01$) between the two groups, while the others did not reach significance. The healthy controls violated Hardy-Weinberg equilibrium (75% of the subjects were heterozygous), indicating a possible bias. This may have been due to the exclusion of subjects with emphysema, autoimmune disorders, arthritis, stroke, myocardial infarction, and diabetes. However, the controls were matched to AAA cases by age, gender, ethnicity, and smoking history, so it is possible that the data support the idea that the A/G genotype is associated with protection against inflammatory diseases in our study population.

Evidence of Inflammation in the Circulation of AAA Patients

The presence of inflammatory cells and a number of cytokines within AAA tissue has been well-documented through histology, immunohistochemistry, and in situ hybridization, although reports of elevated circulating levels of cytokines have been fewer. One exception is IL-6. In 1999, Rohde et al. reported increased plasma IL-6 concentrations with increasing abdominal aortic diameter in subjects without aortic dilatation.[26] Recently, Dawson et al. reported elevated levels of plasma IL-6 in AAA patients, and a positive correlation between aneurysm surface area and mean plasma IL-6 concentration.[27]

As our understanding of inflammation moves beyond proinflammatory cytokines, a number of interesting studies have emerged. A recent paper by Duftner et al. reviewed serological markers of inflammation in AAA, and also presented data supporting a T-cell-mediated pathophysiology of AAA.[28]

The authors review one of the most common, and controversial, serological markers to be analyzed in AAA, C-reactive protein (CRP). Data from studies of CRP levels in asymptomatic AAA have produced varying results, although data from subsets of patients have been more consistent. For example, elevations of serum CRP were found in symptomatic and ruptured AAA,[29] and hsCRP was positively associated with aneurysm size.[30] Duftner also described data from her own studies that showed an increased prevalence of circulating CD4+, CD8+, and CD28- T cells in AAA patients free of preexisting immune-mediated disease, cancer, or acute infection. This subgroup of T cells is known to produce large amounts of interferon-γ, and has been previously seen in patients with a variety of autoimmune diseases.

Our own work has recently focused on T-cell costimulatory factors in AAA. In collaboration with the laboratory of the late Ann Kari Lefvert of the Karolinska Hospital in Stockholm, Sweden, plasma samples from 100 of our AAA patients and 109 normal controls were analyzed for the soluble forms of the following T-cell costimulatory factors: sCD28, sCTLA-4, sCD86, and sCD80, as well as MMP-9. Compared to controls, plasma from AAA patients showed elevated levels of the T-cell-activating sCD28 and sCD86 ($p = 0.0001$), and a decrease in an inhibitor of T-cell activation, sCTLA-4 ($p = 0.0018$). We also found a significant inverse relationship between concentrations of sCTLA-4 and sCD80 with MMP-9.[31] Soluble costimulatory molecules of T-cell activation may provide a new set of markers of immune activation in AAA and possible therapeutic targets for future therapies.

Conclusions

Inflammation appears to play a central role in the pathogenesis of AAAs. The initiating factors that begin the inflammatory cascade are unknown. It is certainly possible that atherosclerosis may be the initiating event. However, smoking is an essential component to the progression of the disease. Once the inflammatory response has been initiated, it appears to be self-perpetuating. Possible explanations for this perpetuation of the inflammation is repeated exposures of cryptic protein fragments. However, what is interesting is that once these patients are treated with endovascular grafts, the aneurysm sac regresses and continued destruction of the aneurysm ceases. If it were true that the inflammatory process was self-sustained, why is it then that the aneurysm sac shrinks when an endograft is placed? Thus, mechanical forces must also play a role in sustaining the process. From the endovascular aneurysm repair experience, it is not pulsatility in as much as its continued pressure. Much additional research must be accomplished to further understand the relationship between mechanical forces, inflammatory disease, and genetics.

References

1. Neptune ER, Frischmeyer PA, Arking DE, Myers L, Bunton TE, Gayraud B, et al. Dysregulation of TGF-β activation contributes to pathogenesis in Marfan syndrome. Nat Genet 2003;33:407–411.

2. Pannu H, Fadulu VT, Chang J, Lafont A, Hasham SN, Sparks E, et al. Mutations in transforming growth factor-β receptor type II cause familial thoracic aortic aneurysms and dissections. Circulation 2005;112:513–520.

3. Glagov S. Hemodynamic risk factors: Mechanical stress, mural architecture, medial nutrition and the vulnerability of arteries to atherosclerosis. *In*: Wissler RW, Geer JC, eds. Pathogenesis of Atherosclerosis. Baltimore: Williams & Wilkins, chap 6, 1972.

4. Taylor CA, Hughes TJ, Zarins CK. Effect of exercise on hemodynamic conditions in the abdominal aorta. J Vasc Surg 1999;29:1077–1089.

5. Dubost C, Allary M, Oeconomos N. Resection of an aneurysm of the abdominal aorta. Reestablishment of the continuity by a preserved human arterial graft, with a result after five months. Arch Surg 1952;65:405–408.

6. Rizzo RJ, McCarthy WJ, Dixit SN, Lilly MP, Shively VP, Flinn WR, et al.. Collagen types and matrix protein content in human abdominal aortic aneurysms. J Vasc Surg 1989;10:365–373.

7. Koch AE, Haines GK, Rizzo RJ, Radosevich JA, Pope RM, Robinson PG, Pearce WH. Human abdominal aortic aneurysms: Immunophenotypic analysis suggesting an immune-mediated response. Am J Pathol 1990;137:1199–1213.

8. Brophy CM, Reilly JM, Smith GJ, Tilson MD. The role of inflammation in non-specific abdominal aortic aneurysm disease. Ann Vasc Surg 1991;5:229–233.

9. Tilson MD III, Kuivaniemi H, Upchurch GR Jr., eds. 2006;The abdominal aortic aneurysm: Genetics, pathophysiology, and molecular biology. Ann NY Acad Sci 1085.

10. Platsoucas CD, Lu S, Nwaneshiudu I, Solomides C, Agelan A, Ntaoula N, et al. Abdominal aortic aneurysm is a specific antigen-driven T cell disease. Ann NY Acad Sci 2006;1085:224–235.

11. Halpern VJ, Nackman GB, Gandhi RH, Irizarri E, Scholes JV, Ramey WG, Tilson MD. The elastase infusion model of experimental aortic aneurysms: Synchrony of induction of endogenous proteinases with matrix destruction and inflammatory cell response. J Vasc Surg 1994;20:51–60.

12. Thompson RW, Curci JA, Ennis TL, Mao D, Pagano MB, Pham CTN. Pathophysiology of abdominal aortic aneurysms: Insights from the elastase-induced model in mice with different genetic backgrounds. Ann NY Acad Sci 2006;1085:59–73.

13. Daugherty A, Rateri DL, Cassis LA. Role of the rennin-angiotensin system in the development of abdominal aortic aneurysms in animals and humans. Ann NY Acad Sci 2006;1085:82–91.

14. Busuttil RW, Abou-Zamzam AM, Machleder HI. Collagenase activity of the human aorta. A comparison of patients with and without abdominal aortic aneurysms. Arch Surg 1980;115:1373–1378.

15. Lee MH, Murphy G. Matrix metalloproteinases at a glance. J Cell Sci 2004;117: 4015–4016.

16. Pearce WH, Shively VP. Abdominal aortic aneurysm as a complex multifactorial disease: Interactions of polymorphisms of inflammatory genes, features of autoimmunity, and current status of MMPs. Ann NY Acad Sci 2006;1085:117–132.

17. Somerville RP, Oblander SA, Apte SS. Matrix metalloproteinases: old dogs with new tricks. Genome Biol 2003;4:216.1–216.11.

18. Parks WC, Wilson CL, Lopez-Boado YS. Matrix metalloproteinases as modulators of inflammation and innate immunity. Nat Rev Immunol 2004;4:617–629.

19. Mott JD, Werb Z. Regulation of matrix biology by matrix metalloproteinases. Cur Opin Cell Biol 2004;16:558–564.

20. Senior RM, Griffin GL, Mecham RP. Chemotactic activity of elastin-derived peptides. J Clin Invest 1980;66:859–862.
21. Lenk GM, Tromp G, Weinsheimer S, Gatalica Z, Bergeur R, Kuivaniemi H. Whole genome expression profiling reveals a significant role for immune function in human abdominal aortic aneurysms. BMC Genomics 2007;8:237.
22. Blanchard JF, Armenian HK, Friesen PP. Risk factors for abdominal aortic aneurysm: Results of a case-control study. Am J Epidemiol 2000;151:575–583.
23. Sandford RM, Bown MJ, London NJ, Sayers RD. The genetic basis of abdominal aortic aneurysms: A review. Eur J Vasc Endovasc Surg 2007;33:381–390.
24. Bown MJ, Burton PR, Horsburgh T, Nicholson ML, Bell PRF, Sayers RD. The role of cytokine gene polymorphisms in the pathogenesis of abdominal aortic aneurysms: A case-control study. J Vasc Surg 2003;37:999–1005.
25. Ghilardi G, Biondi ML, Battaglioli L, Zambon A, Guagnellini E, Scorza R. Genetic risk factor characterizes abdominal aortic aneurysm from arterial occlusive disease in human beings: CCR5 Delta 32 deletion. J Vasc Surg 2004;40:995–1000.
26. Rohde LEP, Arroyo LH, Rifai N, Creager MA, Libby P, Ridker RM, Lee RT. Plasma concentrations of interleukin-6 and abdominal aortic diameter among subjects without aortic dilatation. Arterioscler Thromb Vasc Biol 1999;19: 1695–1699.
27. Dawson J, Cockerill GW, Choke E, Belli AM, Loftus I, Thompson MM. Aortic aneurysms secrete interleukin-6 into the circulation. J Vasc Surg 2007;45:350–356.
28. Duftner C, Seiler R, Dejaco C, Fraidrich G, Schirmer M. Increasing evidence for immune-mediated processes and new therapeutic approaches in abdominal aortic aneurysms-A review. Ann NY Acad Sci 2006;1085:331–338.
29. Domanovits H, Schillinger M, Mullner M, Holzenbein K, Janata K, Bayegan K, Laggner AN. Acute phase reactants in patients with abdominal aortic aneurysm. Atherosclerosis 2002;163:297–302.
30. Vainas T, Lubbers T, Stassen FRM, Herngreen S, van Dieijen-Visser MP, Bruggeman CA, et al.. Serum C-reactive protein level is associated with abdominal aortic aneurysm size and may be produced by aneurysmal tissue. Circulation 2003;107:1103–1105.
31. Sakthivel P, Shively V, Kakoulidou M, Pearce W, Leffert AK. The soluble forms of CD28, CD86 and CTLA-4 constitute possible immunological markers in patients with abdominal aortic aneurysm. J Intern Med 2007;261:399–407.

Chapter 3

Contemporary Imaging of Aortic Disease

Peter S. Liu and David M. Williams

Abstract Recent advances in computed tomography angiography (CTA) and magnetic resonance angiography (MRA) have revolutionized the diagnostic work-up of aortic disease. Currently, catheter-based angiography is largely used as an adjunct during interventional procedures to treat aortic disease. This chapter reviews recent technical advances in CTA and MRA, and briefly discusses the roles of carbon dioxide angiography and intravascular ultrasound in aortic interventions.

Keywords Aortic disease imaging, CT of aortic disease, MR of aortic disease, Aortic aneurysms, Noninvasive aortic imaging, CTA of aortic disease, MRA of aortic disease, Catheter-based angiography

Introduction

The advent of modern computed tomography (CT) scanners and magnetic resonance imaging (MRI) devices has made noninvasive high-resolution evaluation of the vascular system a reality. Contemporary CT and MR techniques have revolutionized the diagnosis of vascular pathology, without the procedural risks of transarterial catheterization. In the evaluation of aneurysmal disease, cross-sectional imaging is particularly important for depiction of the length of diseased vessel, total aortic and arterial diameters, true vascular diameter, including the patent lumen and the extent of mural thrombus formation[1] (Fig. 1), and distance of diseased wall from critical aortic branches. Cross-sectional techniques also provide valuable information on extravascular pathology (Fig. 2a–c). Noninvasive cross-sectional imaging is now frequently used as a single examination for both diagnosis and preprocedural planning of aortic interventions, with demonstrable decrease in operative morbidity and mortality.[2] Furthermore, noninvasive imaging is also an excellent method for monitoring the postoperative patient for complication, including both traditional open repairs and endovascular therapies.[3,4] Three-dimensional reformatted and volume rendered images can be made to aid in clinical diagnosis and easily depict pathology (Fig. 3a and b). The basic principles of computed tomography angiography (CTA) and magnetic resonance angiography (MRA) will be discussed, as well as their specific relevance toward aneurysmal disease. Despite the advances in

G. Upchurch and E. Criado (eds.) *Aortic Aneurysms, Contemporary Cardiology*
DOI: 10.1007/978-1-60327-204-9_3, © Humana Press, a part of
Springer Science+Business Media, LLC 2009

Fig. 1 Axial contrast-enhanced computed tomography (*CT*) image demonstrates a 5.4-cm infrarenal abdominal aortic aneurysm. Cross-sectional imaging nicely depicts how the patent vascular lumen (*arrowhead*) comprises only a portion of the total aortic diameter (*arrow*).

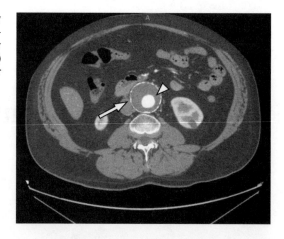

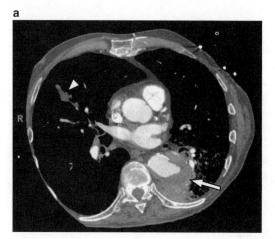

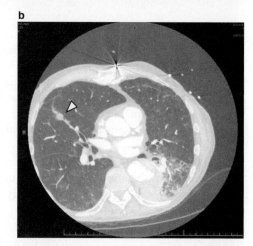

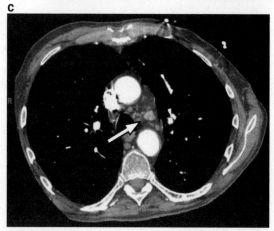

Fig. 2 (**a**) Axial contrast-enhanced computed tomography (*CT*) image (soft tissue windowing) demonstrates a focal saccular aneurysm involving the distal descending thoracic aorta (*arrow*). There is abnormal attenuation in the right middle lobe (arrowhead). (**b**) Axial contrast-enhanced CT image (lung windowing) reveals spiculation associated with the right middle lobe mass (*arrowhead*). Biopsy was positive for nonsmall cell lung carcinoma. (**c**) Axial contrast-enhanced CT image (soft tissue windowing) demonstrates mediastinal adenopathy (arrow) that was positive on subsequent PET scan

cross-sectional imaging, there remains a solid basis for catheter-based angiography. Although it has lost its primary importance as a diagnostic modality, catheter-based angiography must be discussed in the setting of its still irreplaceable role in the endovascular treatment of aortic disease. As it is currently integrated with contemporary cross-sectional imaging, catheter-based angiography entails the use of carbon dioxide angiography and intravascular ultrasound (IVUS).

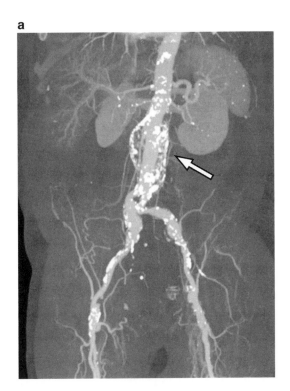
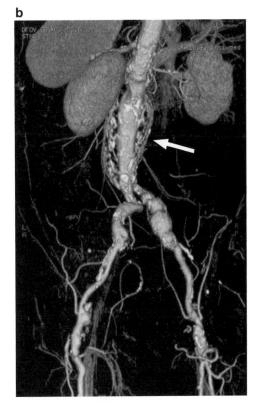

Fig. 3 (**a**) 3D Reformatted image demonstrates abdominal aortic aneurysm (*arrow*) with atherosclerotic calcification throughout the abdominal aorta and branch vessels. (**b**) Surface-shaded display of same data set redemonstrates the abdominal aortic aneurysm (*arrow*)

Computed Tomography

Computed tomography is an x-ray-based method of imaging which uses a rotating gantry including an x-ray tube and detector plate to generate tomographic images of the body. Early on, CT played only a minor role in clinical vascular imaging, as it was mostly used for stationary anatomic imaging due to slow acquisition speed. However, the development of helical scanning technique and multidetector row technology in the early 1990s revolutionized the role of CT in angiographic applications.[3,5] Slip-ring technology allows continuous rotation of the gantry without the need to unwind power/electricity cables, allowing modern gantry rotation speeds of approximately 0.33 s per rotation. When combined with a moving table, the data acquisition changes from axial 2D imaging to volumetric 3D imaging. The overall scan time is reduced and the acquired data can be reconstructed into traditional axial slices or other reformatted planes. In the early implementation of this technology, the anatomy recorded by detectors at the beginning of the gantry rotation was different than at the end of the gantry rotation (due to continuous table movement), leading to exaggerated volume-averaging effects and decreased through-plane resolution. The development of multiple detector rows on the circulating gantry addressed this problem, thereby allowing multiple rows of data to be acquired in a single rotation.[6] With advances in detector technology, thinner detector elements were developed with subsequent gains in through-plane resolution (individual detector size) as well as overall z-axis coverage (total number of rows on the gantry). Currently, detector element width is approximately 0.5–0.625 mm. The combination of helical scanning and multiple detector rows is the foundation for modern multidetector CT (MDCT) scanners, which can provide data sets with equal spatial and contrast resolution in all three planes and ultrafast imaging times (complete vascular interrogation from arch to toes in less than 30 s).[7]

CT studies focused on vascular disease often involve MDCT scanners with protocols consisting of multiple imaging phases, including a precontrast image series and at least one contrast-enhanced image series. Although the contrast-enhanced images provide exquisite luminal imaging, it is important to not overlook the precontrast images. Precontrast images are critical for the detection of blood, as acute hemorrhage/hematoma is usually hyperdense on noncontrast images (Fig. 4a and b). Although CT attenuation values are absolute numbers related to the constituents that make up a given voxel, subtle areas of acute hemorrhage can be less conspicuous when dense intraluminal contrast is present (Fig. 5a and b). From the standpoint of clinical management, the presence of extraluminal high attenuation in a patient suspected of ruptured aneurysm should obviate the need for further imaging and decrease the delay time to definitive treatment.[7] Additionally, atherosclerotic calcifications, calcified old hematomas, surgical grafts, and felt pledgets/rings are often more reliably seen on precontrast images than postcontrast images[8] (Fig. 6a and b). Identification of these components will aid in rendering a final opinion about the patient's disease status.

The contrast-enhanced portion of a CTA study is typically performed with mechanical dual-chamber power injectors. Given the potential coverage speed of MDCT, contrast bolus geometry and injection protocols have become areas of considerable research with the rapid evolution of MDCT technology; a detailed discussion of this research is beyond the scope of this chapter and

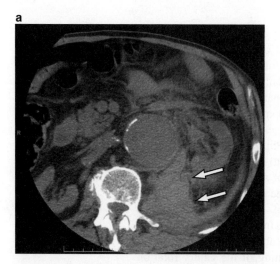
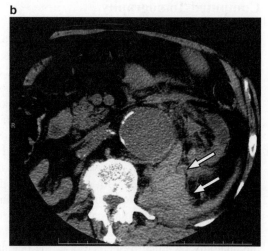

Fig. 4 (**a**) Axial noncontrast computed tomography (*CT*) image through the abdomen in standard abdominal soft tissue windowing (window = 400, level = 40) demonstrates retroperitoneal high attenuation (*arrows*) with concomitant fascial thickening around the anterolaterally displaced left kidney, indicating retroperitoneal hemorrhage. (**b**) Axial noncontrast CT image with narrow window settings (window = 100, level = 30) demonstrates increased conspicuity of high attenuation related to suspected retroperitoneal hemorrhage (*arrows*). The patient expired during attempted open repair of abdominal aortic aneurysm rupture

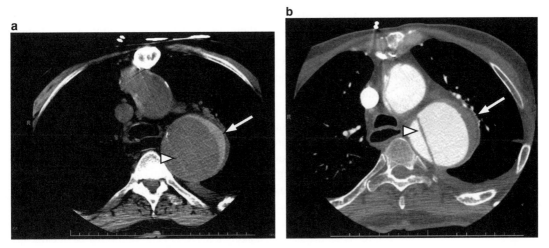

Fig. 5 (**a**) Axial noncontrast computed tomography (*CT*) image through the chest demonstrates crescentic high attenuation (*arrow*) associated with the left lateral aspect of the descending thoracic aorta, compatible with an intramural hematoma. There is also a suggestion of a dissection flap on the medial aspect of the aorta (*arrowhead*). (**b**) Axial contrast-enhanced CT image at the same level easily demonstrates the suspected dissection flap (*arrowhead*). However, the visual conspicuity of the intramural hematoma on the left-lateral aspect of the aorta is decreased (*arrow*) versus the dense contrast bolus in the aortic lumen

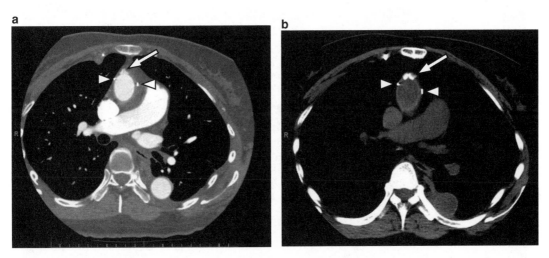

Fig. 6 (**a**) Axial contrast-enhanced computed tomography (*CT*) image of the chest demonstrates irregularity of the anterior aspect of the ascending aorta (*arrow*). The patient had prior surgical graft repair of the ascending aorta for aneurysm. Tiny clips are present (arrowheads) around the ascending aorta as well. (**b**) Axial noncontrast CT image at the same level demonstrates very high attenuation in the area of questioned abnormality on the contrast-enhanced CT image (*arrow*). This area was stable for over 5 years and had been present on every postoperative scan, probably representing felt pledgets buttressing closure of an aortotomy wound. Surgical clips are again demonstrated (*arrowheads*)

includes consideration of physiological and anatomical factors, injection rate, total volume, and iodine concentration.[9] Generally, CTA studies utilize contrast media with iodine concentrations of 300–400 mmol iodine/ml, injection rates of 3–5 ml/s, and a total volume of 70–150 ml. However, the fundamental challenge in CTA is optimal delivery of the appropriate amount of contrast to the volume of interest. This often requires some degree of protocol specificity particular to the scanner being used. The scan time to cover a certain distance can vary considerably depending on the number of detectors available on a given MDCT system, and therefore the contrast injection protocol must vary to meet the ability of the scanner. As an example, a 4-detector scanner may take 21 s to cover a 25 cm length with standard parameters, whereas a 64-detector scanner could achieve similar or better imaging parameters in 4 s.[10] Additionally, delayed postcontrast images can be valuable portions of a complete aortic protocol, especially in patients who have had prior endovascular therapy for aneurysms.[11] Therefore, it is critical to tailor scan protocols for the specific task toward the actual device being used for acquisition.

There are specific advantages and disadvantages of CTA when compared to other cross-sectional techniques such as MRA. In general, CTA requires less technical sophistication to achieve a diagnostic quality examination than does MRA, which leads to more generalized reproducibility among studies obtained at different institutions.[12] CTA is also superior to MRA in terms of spatial resolution and temporal acquisition, making it the test of choice for trauma or clinically unstable patients (Fig. 7). As opposed to the high degree of background suppression obtained in MRA, the extraluminal detail is retained during the angiographic/

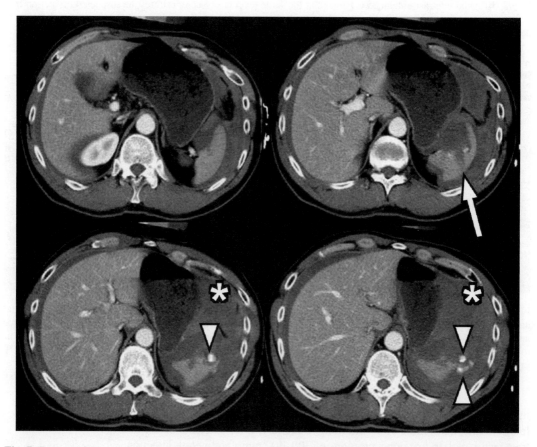

Fig. 7 Four contiguous axial contrast-enhanced computed tomography (*CT*) images through the upper abdomen in a patient after motor vehicle collision demonstrate a hypodense linear tract through the spleen (*arrow*), compatible with a splenic laceration. There are scattered foci of very high attenuation within the laceration bed (*arrowheads*) that represent active extravasation of iodinated contrast material into left upper quadrant, or hemoperitoneum (*). The patient was taken for emergent embolization of active hemorrhage in order to maintain splenic function. Because of its short scan times, CT is ideally suited for the initial imaging of trauma patients

contrast-enhanced portion of the CTA, which offers a single comprehensive evaluation of the vascular system[7] (Fig. 8). The major clinical disadvantages associated with CTA include the use of ionizing radiation (which limits dynamic or real-time imaging of contrast bolus propagation) and a nephrotoxic contrast agent, while other technical disadvantages include artifact related to the injected contrast material, indwelling metallic prostheses, or adjacent osseous structures.[13]

With respect to aneurysmal disease, CTA provides a fast, reproducible study that yields important clinical information. CTA is frequently the first-line tool for the emergent evaluation of patients with suspected aortic aneurysm rupture; noncontrast studies can be performed rapidly and can render a diagnosis that expedites definitive surgical treatment.[14] CTA can be used to follow patients with known aneurysms for rate of interval growth, to facilitate the preoperative management of such patients when their aneurysm reaches critical dimensions, and to follow up patients in the postoperative period for complication development[13] (Fig. 9a and b). In the era of endovascular repair, CTA has become even more valuable as the acquired data set from MDCT scanners

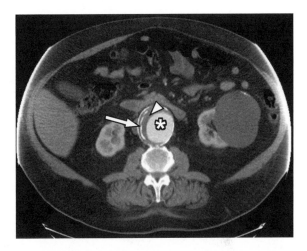

Fig. 8 Axial contrast-enhanced computed tomography (*CT*) image demonstrates a 6.8-cm abdominal aortic aneurysm. Note how CT demonstrates the luminal and extraluminal components of the vessel wall, including the patent lumen (*), incorporated mural thrombus (*arrowhead*), and intimal calcifications (*arrow*). The patient underwent subsequent successful endovascular repair

a
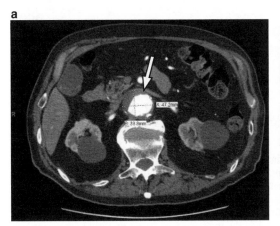

b
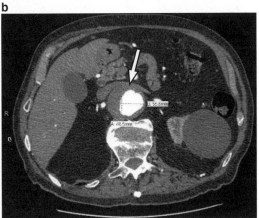

Fig. 9 (**a**) Axial contrast-enhanced computed tomography (*CT*) image demonstrates an abdominal aortic aneurysm (*arrow*) with maximal axial dimensions of 3.88 × 4.72 cm. (**b**) Axial contrast-enhanced CT image of the same patient in a similar location approximately 1 year later demonstrates interval growth of the aneurysm, now measuring 4.85 × 5.56 cm

can be loaded into postprocessing software to generate the salient preoperative parameters for stent-graft deployment (Fig. 10a–d). Additionally, CTA is a robust modality for following endograft patients in the postoperative period, as CT can directly visualize the intraluminal graft and look for stent graft complications such as endoleaks[15] (Fig. 11a and b). With the increasing use of endovascular systems for the aortic aneurysmal disease, CTA has become the definitive imaging modality used for both planning and follow-up of surgery.

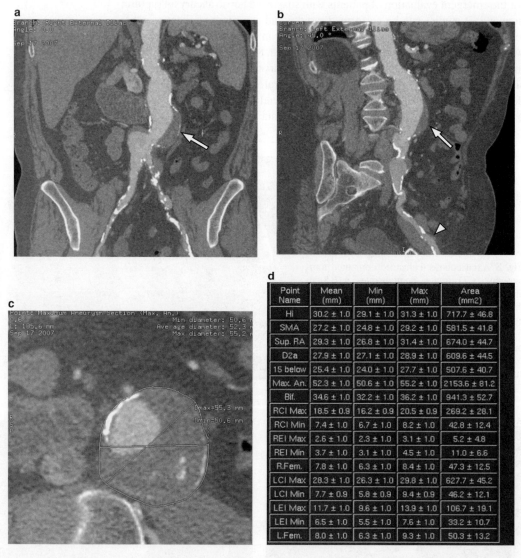

Point Name	Mean (mm)	Min (mm)	Max (mm)	Area (mm2)
Hi	30.2 ± 1.0	29.1 ± 1.0	31.3 ± 1.0	717.7 ± 46.8
SMA	27.2 ± 1.0	24.8 ± 1.0	29.2 ± 1.0	581.5 ± 41.8
Sup. RA	29.3 ± 1.0	26.8 ± 1.0	31.4 ± 1.0	674.0 ± 44.7
D2a	27.9 ± 1.0	27.1 ± 1.0	28.9 ± 1.0	609.6 ± 44.5
15 below	25.4 ± 1.0	24.0 ± 1.0	27.7 ± 1.0	507.6 ± 40.7
Max. An.	52.3 ± 1.0	50.6 ± 1.0	55.2 ± 1.0	2153.6 ± 81.2
Bif.	34.6 ± 1.0	32.2 ± 1.0	36.2 ± 1.0	941.3 ± 52.7
RCI Max	18.5 ± 0.9	16.2 ± 0.9	20.5 ± 0.9	269.2 ± 28.1
RCI Min	7.4 ± 1.0	6.7 ± 1.0	8.2 ± 1.0	42.8 ± 12.4
REI Max	2.6 ± 1.0	2.3 ± 1.0	3.1 ± 1.0	5.2 ± 4.8
REI Min	3.7 ± 1.0	3.1 ± 1.0	4.5 ± 1.0	11.0 ± 6.6
R.Fem.	7.8 ± 1.0	6.3 ± 1.0	8.4 ± 1.0	47.3 ± 12.5
LCI Max	28.3 ± 1.0	26.3 ± 1.0	29.8 ± 1.0	627.7 ± 45.2
LCI Min	7.7 ± 0.9	5.8 ± 0.9	9.4 ± 0.9	46.2 ± 12.1
LEI Max	11.7 ± 1.0	9.6 ± 1.0	13.9 ± 1.0	106.7 ± 19.1
LEI Min	6.5 ± 1.0	5.5 ± 1.0	7.6 ± 1.0	33.2 ± 10.7
L.Fem.	8.0 ± 1.0	6.3 ± 1.0	9.3 ± 1.0	50.3 ± 13.2

Fig. 10 (**a**) Coronal maximum intensity projection from contrast-enhanced computed tomography angiography (*CTA*) study demonstrates a 5.5-cm abdominal aortic aneurysm (*arrow*). (**b**) Curved reformatted image from the same CTA data set using a center-line automated approach allows continuous visualization of the arterial anatomy through the left external iliac artery (*arrowhead*) for endovascular treatment planning. Abdominal aortic aneurysm is again seen (*arrow*). (**c**) Single oblique image from postprocessing software package demonstrates how the vessel is sized at this specific level. The user may modify the included area based on visual inspection. (**d**) Final vessel analysis provides maximal and minimal luminal diameter at various levels to assist in planning the endovascular operative approach

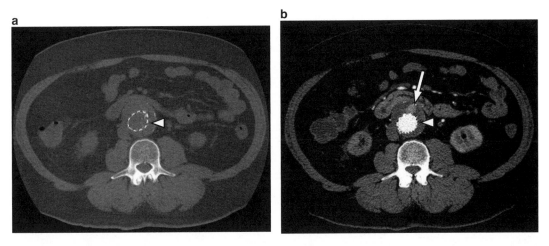

Fig. 11 (**a**) Axial noncontrast computed tomography (*CT*) image of the abdomen demonstrates an abdominal aortic aneurysm with indwelling endovascular stent graft (*arrowhead*). There is no abnormal high attenuation in the excluded aneurysm sac on these noncontrast images. (**b**) Axial contrast-enhanced CT image at the same level demonstrates a blush of contrast within the aneurysm sac (*arrow*), which is outside the stent graft itself (*arrow*). Since this was not present on the precontrast images, this area fills through an endoleak. Contrast angiography confirmed a type II endoleak from retrograde flow through the inferior mesenteric artery (*IMA*).

Magnetic Resonance Imaging

Magnetic resonance imaging allows imaging of the body utilizing a magnetic field and radiofrequency pulses. The patient is placed within a strong magnetic field (modern clinical scanners function at 1.5–3.0 T) that aligns the net magnetic field of the protons within a patient's body along the bore of the main magnetic field.[16] When a radiofrequency pulse is sent out from a transmitter, the net magnetization is deflected from its resting axis along the main magnetic field. As the protons relax back to their original state in the main magnetic field, a detectable signal – called an echo – is generated and localized by a receiver coil.[17] The frequency data ("k-space data") received by the coil is converted into an image via the Fourier transform.[18] Magnetic recovery after an RF pulse has been sent out by the transmitter actually has two discrete components: a longitudinal relaxation (parallel to the main magnetic field) and a transverse relaxation (perpendicular to the main magnetic field).[16] Tissue-specific parameters related to longitudinal and transverse recovery are called T1 and T2 relaxation times, respectively. Depending on the parameters of the imaging sequence, the acquired data set (and subsequent generated images) can demonstrate T1- or T2-weighting to highlight these characteristics.[18] Additionally, the imaging contrast can be altered either by changing the intrinsic contrast of an organ (the addition of Gadolinium-based intravenous contrast) or by selectively nullifying certain tissues based on known T1/T2 values (fat saturation techniques), particularly in evaluation of the vascular tree.[19] In general, the more specific lesion characterization that is offered by MRI relies on the integrated spectrum of tissue appearances on various types of T1- and T2-weighted sequences.

The use of magnetic resonance imaging in noninvasive vascular imaging has been termed MRA. Similar to other applications in MRI, angiographic applications require more than one sequence to generate a complete diagnosis. Precontrast T1-weighted images can be used to obtain information about anatomy, including delineation of the aortic wall and adjacent mediastinal or retroperitoneal pathology[20] (Fig. 12a). Fat-saturated T1-weighted images often increases the conspicuity of extracellular methemoglobin in hematomas, which is particularly important in angiographic applications (Fig. 13a and b). T2-weighted images are used less in angiographic applications than in other anatomic regions, mainly due to their lengthy time of acquisition, though these sequences remain useful in cases of vasculitis or suspected vascular malformation[20,21] (Fig. 14a and b). Black-blood vascular imaging technique is a technique based on fast spin-echo imaging that uses a set of two inversion pulses

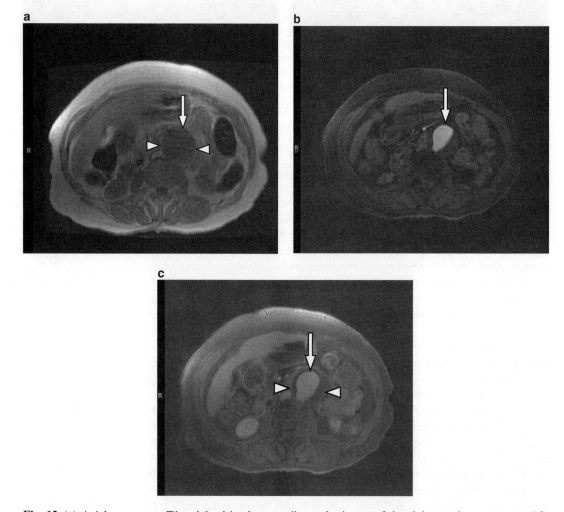

Fig. 12 (**a**) Axial precontrast T1-weighted in-phase gradient echo image of the abdomen demonstrates a 4.9-cm abdominal aortic aneurysm (*arrow*). Note that the complete/full diameter of the aneurysm (*arrowheads*) is depicted on this sequence. (**b**) Axial fat-suppressed postcontrast T1-weighted spoiled gradient echo image at the same level as panel **a** during the arterial phase of enhancement demonstrates that the aneurysm lumen (*arrow*) is most conspicuous with relative paucity of signal in the wall and background tissues. (**c**) Axial fat-suppressed postcontrast T1-weighted spoiled gradient echo image at same level as panel **a**, obtained 5 min after injection, demonstrates aneurysm (*arrow*) with increased conspicuity of the vascular wall (*arrowheads*). There is higher signal in the background tissues as well

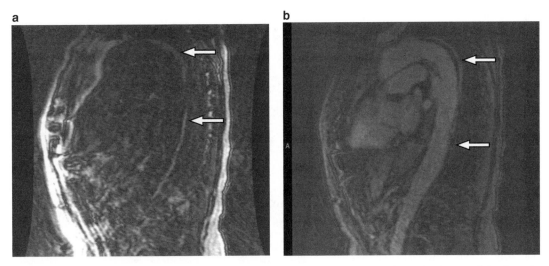

Fig. 13 (**a**) Oblique sagittal fat-suppressed precontrast T1-weighted spoiled gradient echo image of the thoracic aorta demonstrates curvilinear foci of high attenuation (*arrows*) which parallel the expected aortic channel, suspect for a thrombosed false lumen in a thoracic aortic dissection. The use of fat-suppression techniques allows greater conspicuity of the blood products versus the background tissues, as the mediastinal fat is nullified. (**b**) Oblique sagittal fat-suppressed postcontrast T1-weighted spoiled gradient echo image at the same location as panel **a** confirms suspected false lumen in aortic dissection. Note that the high signal intensity on the precontrast image is less conspicuous on this postcontrast image, which validates the need to look carefully at the precontrast image

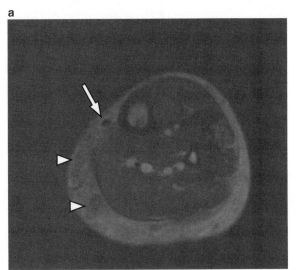

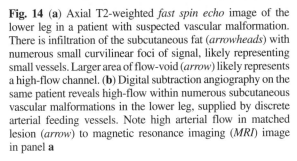

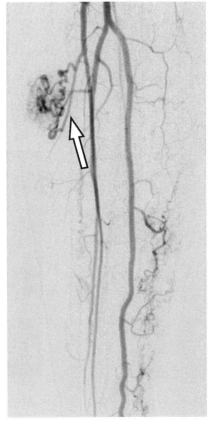

Fig. 14 (**a**) Axial T2-weighted *fast spin echo* image of the lower leg in a patient with suspected vascular malformation. There is infiltration of the subcutaneous fat (*arrowheads*) with numerous small curvilinear foci of signal, likely representing small vessels. Larger area of flow-void (*arrow*) likely represents a high-flow channel. (**b**) Digital subtraction angiography on the same patient reveals high-flow within numerous subcutaneous vascular malformations in the lower leg, supplied by discrete arterial feeding vessels. Note high arterial flow in matched lesion (*arrow*) to magnetic resonance imaging (*MRI*) image in panel **a**

Fig. 15 (**a**) Axial time-of-flight magnetic resonance angiography (*MRA*) image in the upper leg without any flow selection (*saturation band*) demonstrates flow in both arterial (*arrow*) and venous (*arrowheads*) directions with the superficial femoral arteries (*SFA*) and superficial femoral veins (*SFV*), respectively. No intravenous contrast was given. (**b**) Axial time-of-flight MRA image in the upper leg with inferior saturation band (arterial flow selection) demonstrates near complete nullification of venous signal and only flow-related enhancement in the arterial structures. Arrows = arterial flow in bilateral SFAs. (**c**) Axial time-of-flight MRA image in the upper leg with superior saturation band (venous flow selection) demonstrates reversal of panel **b**, with near complete nullification of arterial signal and only venous flow-related enhancement. Arrowheads = venous flow in bilateral SFVs

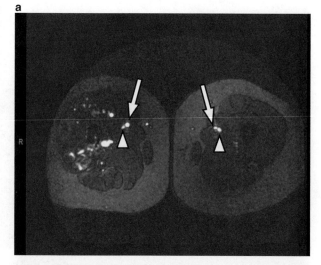

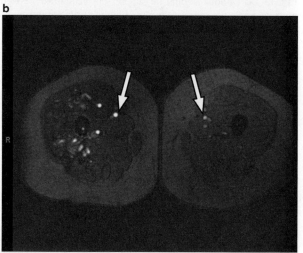

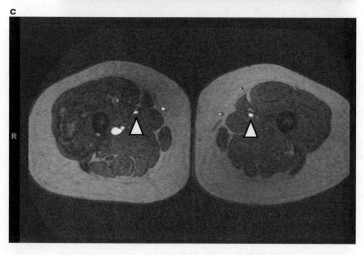

to "prepare" the imaging slice, ultimately leading to nullification of blood protons within the slice and yielding excellent depiction of intraluminal and mural abnormalities.[22] Contrast-enhanced MRA has become the predominant method of evaluating the vascular tree, as the injection of Gadolinium-based contrast agents allows accurate depiction of the luminal appearance on fast T1-weighted imaging[20,23] (Fig. 12b and c). Because MR techniques do not have ionizing radiation, similar images at multiple time points can be acquired without harm to the patient. Therefore, imaging techniques are frequently used in MRA which will demonstrate multiple phases of vascular contrast, including arterial, venous, and delayed phases of imaging. Contrast-enhanced MRA is particularly useful for aneurysmal disease of the aorta and iliac arteries, as the slow swirling flow in such aneurysms can degrade other MR sequences.[24] For aneurysm evaluation, both arterial and delayed images are critical to evaluate (Fig. 12b and c); the arterial images will accurately demonstrate the luminal contour while delayed images are useful for looking at the vascular wall and extent of mural thrombus formation.[20]

Prior to the use of contrast-enhanced MRA sequences, luminal flow information could be obtained on MRI from noncontrast techniques. With recent news that Gadolinium-based contrast agents may be linked to a skin and integument disorder called nephrogenic systemic fibrosis in patients with impaired renal function, there is a renewed interest in noncontrast MRA techniques.[25,26] Principal among these techniques is a variant T1-weighted gradient echo sequence called "time-of-flight" (TOF) imaging. TOF MRA relies on the difference in longitudinal magnetization of flowing protons in a bloodstream that enters into a slice of interest versus static protons within that slice of interest.[27] This signal difference can be manipulated by imaging parameters to provide luminal contrast. In fact, by using selective saturation bands adjacent to the slice of interest, isolated arterial or venous flow can be displayed[22,27] (Fig. 15a–c). Other techniques such as phase-contrast MRA and bright-blood steady-state free procession provide high signal intensity within vascular lumen without the addition of intravenous contrast[18,20,27] (Fig. 16). Given that many patients with aortic aneurysmal disease often have coexistent other medical comorbidities, including chronic renal

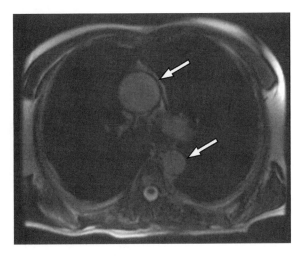

Fig. 16 Axial balanced steady-state free procession image through the chest demonstrates high signal intensity within the aortic lumen (*arrows*). No intravenous contrast was administered

insufficiency, such imaging techniques may become increasingly valuable as an alternative to both iodinated and Gadolinium-based contrast agents.

MRA has numerous benefits compared to other imaging modalities including native/direct multiplanar imaging, high soft tissue contrast, flow quantification, and the ability to evaluate both the vascular lumen and its wall.[20] As opposed to the rotating machinery involved in CT, MRI localizes signal in the body via the sophisticated interplay of magnetic gradients and radiofrequency pulses.[17] Therefore, it is not dependent on particular geometric constraints for acquiring images, and can image the body in any plane prescribed by the user. This is particularly useful in the thoracic aorta, where images can be obtained in the oblique sagittal plane to anatomically follow the oblique course of the thoracic aorta. The intrinsic difficulty in MRI of visualizing calcification can actually be useful for MRA applications – cortical bone structures are relatively inconspicuous on MRI versus CT where such structures can be quite confounding due to their high attenuation[7,20] (Fig. 17). With respect to CTA, there are some recognized disadvantages of MRA that must be considered, including decreased spatial resolution, increased examination length, contraindication with implantable electronically active hardware (such as pacemakers or defibrillator devices), interference with imaging by ferromagnetic components of vascular prostheses, and decreased equipment availability.[13] Additionally, the technical variability of

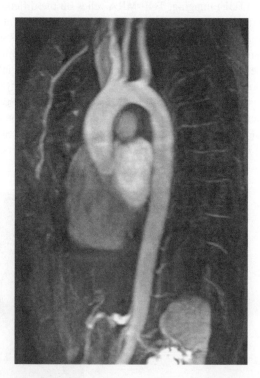

Fig. 17 Thick slab maximum intensity projection (*MIP*) from postgadolinium fat-suppressed T1-weighted oblique sagittal spoiled gradient echo data set demonstrates normal thoracic aorta. Note the lack of artifact related to osseous structures incorporated into the *MIP* image, as cortical bone is dark on magnetic resonance imaging (*MRI*)

MRA is higher than in CTA due to fluctuations in technologist skill level and inconsistency in available pulse sequences or gating techniques on different machines. Despite those limitations, MRA remains a useful vascular imaging tool whose future utility may continue to increase, given the recent increased concern about radiation doses in medical imaging and nephrotoxic effects of iodinated contrast material.[28]

MRA can be used effectively in the management of aneurysmal disease, particularly in detection and surveillance. MRA is indicated as a screening technique in patients with high risk of developing aneurysms, such as those with connective tissue disease or vasculitis.[13] A patient with known aneurysmal disease is well suited for noncontrast MRA surveillance, given that this technique has no ionizing radiation and does not use a nephrotoxic contrast agent (Fig. 18a and b). MRA provides excellent detail about the status of disease, including assessment of the true aneurysm diameter.[13,22] MRI is not frequently used in the emergent evaluation of patients with suspected aortic rupture due to examination time and generalized equipment availability. Because of slice thickness considerations, MRA has not been used as frequently as CTA for preoperative stent-graft measurements; nevertheless, studies have demonstrated that high spatial-resolution MRA can in fact be used as a sole preoperative test for endovascular planning, including integration with automated vessel analysis programs.[29–31] MRA can also be used in the postoperative period to follow patients with both open and endovascular repairs of aortic aneurysms. In patients with prior endovascular repair of aneurysm, the ability to visualize the stent graft itself is highly dependent on the graft material composition.[12] Nitinol-based devices cause only minor distortions on acquired images, while stainless steel devices create substantial artifact that often precludes any detailed evaluation.[32] As opposed to CTA, the device itself is usually seen

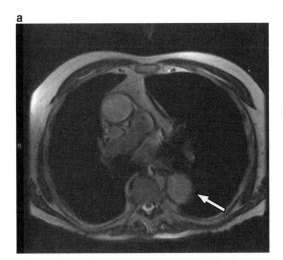
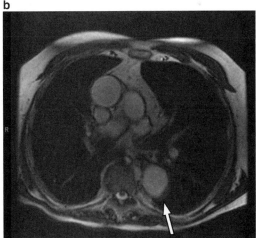

Fig. 18 (**a**) Axial balanced steady-state free procession image through the chest demonstrates a 4.2-cm thoracic aortic aneurysm of the descending thoracic aorta. (**b**) Axial balanced steady-state free procession image through a similar level 9 months later redemonstrates a 4.2-cm aortic aneurysm without interval change. This set of noncontrast images highlights how magnetic resonance angiography (*MRA*) can excel in following known aneurysmal disease without ionizing radiation or nephrotoxic iodinated contrast

a

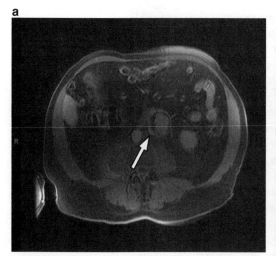

b

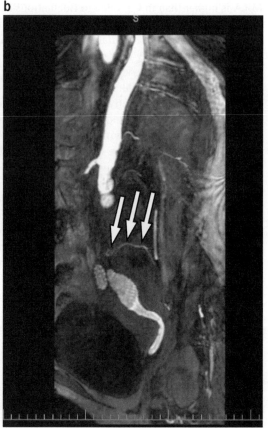

Fig. 19 (**a**) Axial fat-suppressed postcontrast T1-weighted spoiled gradient echo image of the abdomen demonstrates a 4.8-cm abdominal aortic aneurysm. There is also an indwelling stent graft. Along the right posterior aspect of the aorta, there is a small area of high signal intensity (*arrow*), outside the stent graft itself, suspect for an endoleak. (**b**) Reformatted maximum intensity projection image using arterial data set from an axial fat-suppressed postcontrast T1-weighted spoiled gradient echo sequence, demonstrating an enlarged lumbar artery leading into the aneurysm sac (*arrows*), thought to be responsible for the type II endoleak

in negative contrast versus the blood pool on T1-weighted gradient echo images. Endoleaks following endovascular repair with nonferromagnetic materials are also well delineated by MRA, with published studies demonstrating at least similar efficacy to CTA and perhaps superior detection of subtle type II endoleaks[33–35] (Fig. 19a and b). Newer techniques in MRA that allow blood pool and dynamic imaging may in fact improve endoleak detection even further and is an area of active investigation.[36,37] MRA is a robust tool for imaging both preoperative and postoperative patients with aneurysmal disease.

Catheter-Based Vascular Imaging

The technical improvements in CTA and MRA have almost completely eliminated the role of catheter-based angiography from diagnostic imaging of the aorta and its first-order branches. Limited roles for catheter-based angiography using vascular contrast agents remain in fine-adjusting final endograft placement with respect to renal or other critical branch artery origins, in monitoring branch artery interventions such as embolization of renal or internal iliac arteries, or in demonstrating and/or treating endoleaks. These are straightforward and fairly routine, and will not be discussed further.

Renal impairment has always been a relative contraindication to the use of iodinated contrast materials. The use of renal-protective strategies such as oral *N*-acetylcysteine or intravenous bicarbonate infusions appear to mitigate the renotoxicity of iodinated contrast agents, although unequivocal demonstration of their benefit has not yet been documented. Nevertheless, the safety margin of these agents is so broad that preimaging administration of one or both has won wide acceptance. Gadolinium-based contrast agents, the mainstay of contrast-enhanced MRI, were championed as renal-friendly contrast agents used in off-label applications as an x-ray contrast material, until the discovery of the nephrogenic systemic sclerosis specifically affecting patients in renal failure. In contrast, the use of intravascular carbon dioxide contrast, long championed by pioneers in the interventional radiology community, is gaining wide acceptance by all peripheral interventionalists. Safe use requires unflagging attention to numerous safety precautions and clinical rules of thumb, which have to be adopted in toto by the entire angiographic team.[38] For example, intra-arterial carbon dioxide cannot be considered safe if injected above the diaphragm. This and other precautions are based on the physical properties of carbon dioxide gas and idiosyncrasies of delivering a high-volume arterial bolus in a clinically tolerable fashion. For example, a patient with a previous right radical nephrectomy needed endograft treatment of an abdominal aortic aneurysm. This is an ideal application of carbon dioxide angiography. The goal is to display the renal and internal iliac artery origins, in order to guide endograft deployment; in this well-defined clinical scenario, carbon dioxide can reliably substitute for iodinated contrast agents. Subtraction angiography with carbon dioxide injections unequivocally localizes the solitary left renal artery and internal iliac arteries (Fig. 20a and b). The inferior mesenteric artery (IMA) is also filled because of its anterior origin off the aneurysm sac and preferential filling of nondependent structures by the buoyant gas (Fig. 20b, arrow). The IMA continues to fill after endograft deployment, both from iliac artery injection and from suprarenal aortic injection (Fig. 20c–e). This case illustrates a limit in our current understanding of carbon dioxide angiography, which has been encountered in the context of TIPS construction, diagnosis of gastrointestinal or traumatic hemorrhage, or arteriovenous shunting, namely, that carbon dioxide angiography may be too sensitive. The reliability of carbon dioxide in demonstrating clinically significant endoleaks requires further systematic study.

IVUS imaging of the aorta is based on 8–9 Fr catheter systems; imaging of arteries such as the superior mesenteric or renal arteries is best accomplished with 5–6 Fr systems. The former allows visualization of a 60-mm-diameter field of view, the latter an 8- to 20-mm-diameter field of view. IVUS is best for high-resolution clarification of specific localized anatomical questions. For example, in treating aortic aneurysmal disease, it is sometimes useful to place an IVUS catheter at the celiac or left common carotid origin, to allow absolute localization of the vessel origin independent of beam divergence, center of the fluoroscopic field, magnification, or other confounding geometrical distortion. IVUS imaging is even more generally useful during interventions to treat aortic dissection. IVUS allows unequivocal distinction between true and false lumens at any given level and permits immediate localization of a catheter or guidewire with respect to the aortic true and false lumens, without contrast injection. As such, it can guide interventions

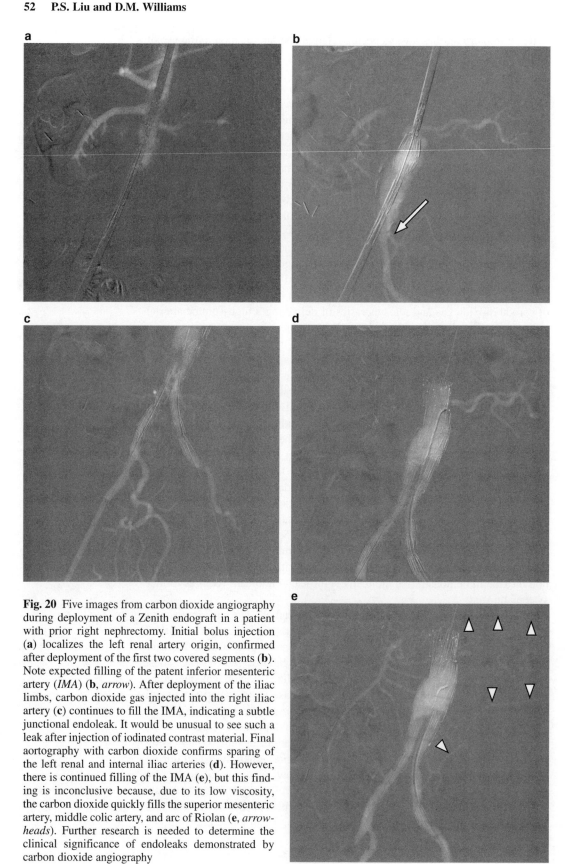

Fig. 20 Five images from carbon dioxide angiography during deployment of a Zenith endograft in a patient with prior right nephrectomy. Initial bolus injection (**a**) localizes the left renal artery origin, confirmed after deployment of the first two covered segments (**b**). Note expected filling of the patent inferior mesenteric artery (*IMA*) (**b**, *arrow*). After deployment of the iliac limbs, carbon dioxide gas injected into the right iliac artery (**c**) continues to fill the IMA, indicating a subtle junctional endoleak. It would be unusual to see such a leak after injection of iodinated contrast material. Final aortography with carbon dioxide confirms sparing of the left renal and internal iliac arteries (**d**). However, there is continued filling of the IMA (**e**), but this finding is inconclusive because, due to its low viscosity, the carbon dioxide quickly fills the superior mesenteric artery, middle colic artery, and arc of Riolan (**e**, *arrowheads*). Further research is needed to determine the clinical significance of endoleaks demonstrated by carbon dioxide angiography

in the dissected aorta as well as the superior mesenteric or other branch artery. Passing the IVUS over a guidewire allows positive identification of the entire course of the wire, which can inconspicuously traverse from one lumen across the flap into another. Lack of appreciation of an errant guidewire pathway, when implanting an aortic stent or endograft, can lead to anatomical blunders which can be disastrous at worst and time-consuming to correct at best. IVUS may be used to guide creation of fenestration tears and assess the response of the true lumen to creation of a fenestration tear or implantation of an endograft IVUS catheters. The guidewire lumen of the IVUS catheter can be attached to an electronic manometer for direct correlation of pressure drops with anatomical features of the aortic lumen. These and other applications make IVUS an indispensable tool in any high-volume aortic practice.

References

1. Costello P, Ecker CP, Tello R, Hartnell GG. Assessment of the thoracic aorta by spiral CT. Am J Roentgenol. 1992 May;158(5):1127–30.
2. Shapira OM, Aldea GS, Cutter SM, Fitzgerald CA, Lazar HL, Shemin RJ. Improved clinical outcomes after operation of the proximal aorta: a 10-year experience. Ann Thorac Surg. 1999 Apr;67(4):1030–7.
3. Tatli S, Yucel EK, Lipton MJ. CT and MR imaging of the thoracic aorta: current techniques and clinical applications. Radiol Clin North Am. 2004 May;42(3): 565–85.
4. Armerding MD, et al. Aortic aneurysmal disease: assessment of stent-graft treatment-CT versus conventional angiography. Radiology. 2000;215:138–46.
5. Dillon EH, van Leeuwen MS, Fernandez MA, Mali WP. Spiral CT angiography. Am J Roentgenol. 1993 Jun;160(6):1273–8.
6. Weg N, Scheer MR, Gabor MP. Liver lesions: improved detection with dual-detector-array CT and routine 2.5-mm thin collimation. Radiology. 1998 Nov;209(2): 417–26.
7. Kaufman, JA. Noninvasive vascular imaging. In: Vascular and Interventional Radiology: The Requisites, 1st Ed, Philadelphia: Mosby, 2004:71–82.
8. Sundaram B, Quint LE, Patel HJ, Deeb GM. CT findings following thoracic aortic surgery. Radiographics. 2007 Nov–Dec;27(6):1583–94.
9. Napoli A, et-al.. Computed tomography angiography: state-of-the-art imaging using multidetector-row technology. J Comput Assist Tomogr. 2004;28:S32–45.
10. Lell MM, et-al. New techniques in CT angiography. Radiographics. 2006; 26:S45–62.
11. Rozenblit AM, et-al.. Detection of endoleaks after endovascular repair of abdominal aortic aneurysm: value of unenhanced and delayed helical CT acquisitions. Radiology. 2003 May;227(2):426–33.
12. Stavropoulos SW, Charagundla SR. Imaging techniques for detection and management of endoleaks after endovascular aortic aneurysm repair. Radiology. 2007 Jun;243(3):641–55.
13. Olin JW, et-al.. Atherosclerotic Vascular Disease Conference: Writing Group IV: Imaging. Circulation. 2004 June 1;109(21):2626–33.
14. Federle MP, Pan KT, Pealer KM. CT criteria for differentiating abdominal hemorrhage: anticoagulation or aortic aneurysm rupture? Am J Roentgenol. 2007 May;188(5):1324–30.
15. Rozenblit A, Marin ML, Veith FJ, Cynamon J, Wahl SI, Bakal CW. Endovascular repair of abdominal aortic aneurysm: value of postoperative follow-up with helical CT. Am J Roentgenol. 1995 Dec;165(6):1473–9.

16. Pooley RA. AAPM/RSNA physics tutorial for residents: fundamental physics of MR imaging. Radiographics. 2005 Jul–Aug;25(4):1087–99.

17. Jacobs MA, Ibrahim TS, Ouwerkerk R. AAPM/RSNA physics tutorials for residents: MR imaging: brief overview and emerging applications. Radiographics. 2007 Jul–Aug;27(4):1213–29.

18. Bitar R, et-al. MR pulse sequences: what every radiologist wants to know but is afraid to ask. Radiographics. 2006 Mar–Apr;26(2):513–37.

19. Creasy JL, Price RR, Presbrey T, Goins D, Partain CL, Kessler RM. Gadolinium-enhanced MR angiography. Radiology. 1990;175:280–83.

20. Roberts D, Siegelman ES. Imaging and MR arteriography of the aorta. In: Body MRI, 1st Ed, Philadelphia: Elsevier, 2005:481–507.

21. Dobson MJ, Hartley RW, Ashleigh R, Watson Y, Hawnaur JM. MR angiography and MR imaging of symptomatic vascular malformations. Clin Radiol. 1997 Aug;52(8):595–602.

22. Tatli S, Lipton MJ, Davison BD, Skorstad RB, Yucel EK. From the RSNA refresher courses: MR imaging of aortic and peripheral vascular disease. Radiographics. 2003 Oct;23 Spec No:S59–78.

23. Zhang H, Maki JH, Prince MR. 3D contrast-enhanced MR angiography. J Magn Reson Imaging. 2007 Jan;25(1):13–25.

24. Prince MR. Gadolinium-enhanced MR aortography. Radiology. 1994 Apr;191(1):155–64.

25. Marckmann P, et-al. Nephrogenic systemic fibrosis: suspected causative role of gadodiamide used for contrast-enhanced magnetic resonance imaging. J Am Soc Nephrol. 2006; 17:2359–62.

26. Stafford RB, Sabati M, Mahallati H, Frayne R. 3D non-contrast-enhanced MR angiography with balanced steady-state free precession dixon method. Magn Reson Med. 2008 Feb;59(2):430–3.

27. Saloner D. The AAPM/RSNA physics tutorial for residents. An introduction to MR angiography. Radiographics. 1995 Mar;15(2):453–65.

28. Brenner DJ, Hall EJ. Computed tomography – an increasing source of radiation exposure. N Engl J Med. 2007 Nov 29;357(22):2277–84.

29. Thurnher SA, et-al.. Evaluation of abdominal aortic aneurysm for stent-graft placement: comparison of gadolinium-enhanced MR angiography versus helical CT angiography and digital subtraction angiography. Radiology. 1997 Nov;205 (2):341–52.

30. Lutz AM, et al. Evaluation of aortoiliac aneurysm before endovascular repair: comparison of contrast-enhanced magnetic resonance angiography with multidetector row computed tomographic angiography with an automated analysis software tool. J Vasc Surg. 2003 Mar;37(3):619–27.

31. Ludman CN, et al.. Feasibility of using dynamic contrast-enhanced magnetic resonance angiography as the sole imaging modality prior to endovascular repair of abdominal aortic aneurysms. Eur J Vasc Endovasc Surg. 2000 May;19(5): 524–30.

32. Thurnher S, Cejna M. Imaging of aortic stent-grafts and endoleaks. Radiol Clin North Am. 2002 Jul;40(4):799–833.

33. Cejna M, et al.. MR angiography vs CT angiography in the follow-up of nitinol stent grafts in endoluminally treated aortic aneurysms. Eur Radiol. 2002 Oct;12(10):2443–50.

34. Engellau L, et al. Magnetic resonance imaging and MR angiography of endoluminally treated abdominal aortic aneurysms. Eur J Vasc Endovasc Surg. 1998 Mar;15(3):212–9.

35. Haulon S, et al. Prospective evaluation of magnetic resonance imaging after endovascular treatment of infrarenal aortic aneurysms. Eur J Vasc Endovasc Surg. 2001 Jul;22(1):62–9.

36. Stavropoulos SW, Baum RA. Imaging modalities for the detection and management of endoleaks. Semin Vasc Surg. 2004 Jun;17(2):154–60.
37. Cohen EI, et al. Time-resolved MR angiography for the classification of endoleaks after endovascular aneurysm repair. J Magn Reson Imaging. 2008 Mar;27(3): 500–3.
38. Cho KJ, Hawkins IR, eds. Carbon Dioxide Angiography: Principles, Techniques, and Practice. New York: Informa Healthcare USA, Inc., 2007.

Chapter 4

Medical Management of Small Aortic Abdominal Aortic Aneurysms

B. Timothy Baxter

Abstract Aneurysmal degeneration of the abdominal aortic and iliac arteries (referred to as AAA) is a common and potentially lethal age-related disease process. Advanced age, history of cigarette smoking, male gender, and family history have been the most frequently recognized AAA risk factors identified in prior screening studies. At this point in time, the best predictor of rupture risk is aneurysm diameter. Typically when the aneurysm enlarges beyond 5–5.5 cm, progressive degenerative changes predominate, leading, in some cases, to mechanical failure. Currently mechanical intervention is shown to be the only treatment effective in preventing AAA rupture and aneurysm-related death; however, in the last decade, endovascular aneurysm repair has gained acceptance as an alternative to open surgical repair with reduced periprocedural risks. Recently, there is evidence from a number of studies suggesting that statins may influence aneurysm growth rate, presumably via pleiotropic effects. Additionally, β-blockers, ACE inhibitors, macrolides, and tetracyclines have all been proposed as a treatment for AAA with varying rationales and degrees of success.

Keywords Abdominal aortic aneurysms, AAA risk factors, Aneurysm diameter, AAA expansion/progression, AAA biomarkers, AAA metabolic imaging, mechanical AAA intervention, EVAR, Initial preventative physical examination, Smoking as AAA risk factor, Statins and AAA, b-blockers and AAA, ACE inhibitors, ARBs and AAA, macrolides and AAA, Tetracyclines and AAA

Clinical Problem of AAA

Aneurysmal degeneration of the abdominal aortic and iliac arteries (referred to as AAA) is a common and potentially lethal age-related disease process. The prevalence of asymptomatic and often unsuspected AAA in men and women over the age of 60 are 4–8% and 0.5–1.5%, respectively.[1]–[7] Advanced age, history of cigarette smoking, male gender, and family history have been the most frequently recognized AAA risk factors identified in prior screening studies.[8,9]

G. Upchurch and E. Criado (eds.) *Aortic Aneurysms, Contemporary Cardiology*
DOI: 10.1007/978-1-60327-204-9_4, © Humana Press, a part of
Springer Science+Business Media, LLC 2009

Of these, smoking may be the most important.[10] In a recent cohort study of over 1,00,000 Healtcare Maintenance Organization participants, after a median 13-year follow-up, additional factors associated with AAA development include treated and untreated hypertension, high total serum cholesterol, known coronary artery disease, and intermittent claudication.[11] African-American and Asian races were inversely associated with AAA risk in men.[3,11]

Ruptured AAA and complications following surgical treatment are responsible for at least 15,000 deaths per year in the United States.[12] The low autopsy rate and synchronous presence of Coronary Artery Disease, to which sudden death is most often ascribed, has led some to believe that the actual AAA mortality rate may be as high as 30,000 deaths/year, a mortality rate similar to prostate cancer and approaching that of breast cancer.[13] Open surgical repair for larger aneurysms is effective in preventing rupture but its morbidity is relatively high; newer endovascular exclusion strategies are less morbid but require continued surveillance, occasional late intervention, and do not always prevent aneurysm rupture.[14,15] Most investigators agree that AAA disease, in its initial stage, is an inflammatory condition associated with benign dilatation. At some point, typically when the aneurysm enlarges beyond 5 –5.5 cm, progressive degenerative changes predominate, leading, in some cases, to mechanical failure. The best predictor of rupture risk at this point in time is aneurysm diameter.

The natural history of an untreated AAA is one of progressive, exponential expansion. Two large prospective studies have found expansion rates between 2.6 and 3.3 mm/year.[16,17] A 3.5-cm AAA growing at 3.0 mm/year will exceed 5.5 cm in less than 7 years (Fig. 1). Pharmacological therapy that inhibited growth by only 40% would extend the time from detection at 3.5 cm to consideration for repair (>5.5 cm) to 12 years. AAAs typically occur in the sixth through eighth decade of life in a patient population with significant coexistent cardiovascular and cerebrovascular disease. Thus, an effective medical therapy could eliminate the need for mechanical repair.

Using mice with targeted gene deletions in models of AAA has identified a number of key proteins involved in aneurysm formation. Even with these sophisticated molecular tools, a complete understanding of human disease is

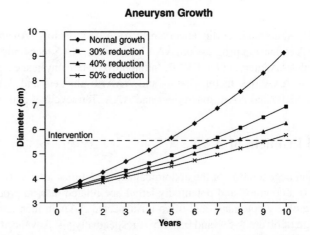

Fig. 1 Average change in aneurysm diameter as a function of time is indicated by the diamond markers. The other growth rates show the effects of a medical therapy that inhibited growth by 30% (square markers), 40% (triangle markers), and 50% (x markers)

still incomplete. This new information learned from models of AAA must now be evaluated prospectively looking at two important clinical parameters. Are any of the aneurysm-associated proteins useful biomarkers for (i) identification of occult AAA or (ii) predicting disease progression? Aneurysm expansion is gradual so that detecting growth suppression will require long-term serial imaging. Biomarkers or metabolic imaging studies could provide more dynamic information to identify responders and optimize drug dosage.

The abdominal aorta between the renal arteries and the iliac bifurcation is the most common extracranial site of aneurysm formation. Although aneurysms are generally defined by a 50% increase in native vessel diameter, aortic diameter increases with age even in the absence of overt disease and is related to body mass index.[18,19] Consequently, controversy exists as to when a large infrarenal aorta becomes an AAA. Some investigators have used an absolute aortic diameter of 3 cm.[3,18,20] This distinction has limitations, however, since it may fall within the upper limits of the normal aortic diameter in a large elderly man.[19] Because of these limitations, others have used relative measures compared with nondiseased aortic segments or adjacent vertebral bodies. Relative aortic indices (e.g., 1.5 or 2.0×) are, however, less useful in the setting of diffuse arteriomegaly or generalized aortic enlargement. An absolute diameter of 3.5 cm represents a practical compromise, separating the large aorta with age-related changes that will not progress to frank aneurysmal disease.

Current Treatment Modalities

Mechanical intervention is currently the only treatment shown to be effective in preventing AAA rupture and aneurysm-related death; it is reserved for AAA ³ 5.5 cm in diameter for men and ³ 5.0 in women. Although smaller aneurysms do rupture, the likelihood of aneurysm-related death only exceeds treatment risks above these thresholds. This conclusion in men is based on data from two large-scale randomized clinical trials (RCTs).[17,21] These studies did not have a sufficient number of women to precisely identify the size threshold for repair. The threshold of 5 cm, used by most clinicians for women, is based on a higher rate of rupture of 5 –5.5 cm aneurysms in women.[21,22] In the United States, elective AAA repairs, generally performed for asymptomatic or medically stable patients, averaged 87.7 per 100,000 Medicare patients between 2000 and 2003.[23] In the last decade, endovascular aneurysm repair (EVAR) has gained acceptance as an alternative to open surgical repair with reduced periprocedural risks.[14,15] Several FDA-approved commercial EVAR devices are currently available and in use. Reflecting the impact of EVAR strategies and devices, perioperative (30-day) mortality for all elective AAA repairs declined from 5.0% to 3.7% ($p < .001$) between 2000 and 2003 with no change in outcome for open repairs alone. By 2003, endovascular repair accounted for 41% of elective AAA repairs.[23] Alt hough treatment outcomes have clearly improved for surgical patients in the EVAR era, evidence from prospective screening studies on three continents suggests that a substantial window of opportunity exists for earlier intervention in AAA disease.[5]

Following congressional passage of the Screening for Abdominal Aortic Aneurysms Very Efficiently (SAAAVE) Amendment in 2006, the Centers for Medicare and Medicaid Services in the United States added a screening

AAA ultrasound examination to the i nitial preventative physical examination (IPPE) for new program enrollees as they turn 65. This benefit is extended to men between the ages of 65 and 75, who have smoked at least 100 cigarettes in their lifetime, and men and women in this age range with a family history of AAA disease. The IPPE must be completed within 6 months of Medicare eligibility. This benefit was justified based on a review by the US Preventive Services Task Force that concluded that ultrasound screening may reduce AAA mortality by 43% in men aged 65–75.[24] The potentia l utility of intervention in smaller (<5.5 cm) AAA was considered, but the risks of surgical repair greatly outweighed the potential benefit of reduced AAA rupture, even taking into account the likelihood that widespread screening will identify thousands of new patients with smaller AAA.[22] In the largest previous US screening study, 90% of AAAs identified were less than 5.5 cm in diameter.[8] In the next several years, increasing awareness of AAA disease driven by provider and patient education related to this new screening benefit could dramatically increase the pool of small AAA patients seeking treatment options for early stage disease.

Prospective screening studies using abdominal ultrasound indicate that AAAs occur in 4–9% of the population over the age of 65, as defined by an infrarenal aortic diameter greater than 3.0 cm.[25] Extrapolation of these figures to US census data indicates that aneurysm disease currently affects at least 1.7 million individuals. Several factors help explain the discrepancy between the true incidence of AAAs and the limited number of patients who are currently treated for this disease (40–55,000). AAAs are usually asymptomatic until rupture and routine physical examination is insensitive in their detection. Deaths from ruptured AAAs may be underrepresented in mortality data, as sudden death is typically attributed to other cardiopulmonary disease in the absence of autopsies, which are rarely performed. Historically, most AAAs requiring treatment are found by serendipity during studies performed for unrelated reasons. Smaller AAAs identified in this fashion may not be reported since specific treatment is not carried out.

For these patients with AAA < 5–5.5 cm, watchful waiting with surveillance for growth is the accepted practice. There is, however, good evidence that this approach is not satisfactory to most individuals. Quality of life surveys done by the validated SF-36 Health Survey show a decline in perceived health after diagnosis of AAA during this period of watchful waiting. This improves to baseline levels following definitive repair. While these survey tools cannot delineate the cause of this change, it is logical to assume that being diagnosed with a potentially life-threatening problem that is not immediately addressed in some fashion causes this perceived decline in health. Endograft treatment reduced but does not entirely eliminate the risk of aneurysm rupture and yet it has a salutary effect. It seems logical that an effective medical treatment initiated at the time of AAA diagnosis could have a similar beneficial effect.

Measuring Aneurysm Progression

Traditionally, aneurysm diameter has been used as the principle surrogate marker for disease progression. For purposes of population-based disease screening studies as well as determining the timing of surgical intervention, abdominal ultrasound imaging has proven accurate and reproducible.[26,27] While more is being learned about AAA biology and progression, aneurysm diameter remains the most important clinical determinant for risk of rupture.[28,29] Interpretation of ultrasonic diameter data is frequently complicated by lengthening and increased angulation from the axial plane during disease progression.

This variability may be overcome partially in the course of serial examinations.[23] Computed tomographic (CT) imaging protocols may be reproducible to within a millimeter when a standardized technique is used in their interpretation. The computerized reconstruction available with CT images provides accurate three-dimensional images that allow for planning of operative repair but the cost, risk, and inconvenience associated with CT imaging do not lend themselves to screening and surveillance applications.

Factors Influencing Aneurysm Progression

The most common method of AAA detection is an abdominal imaging study obtained for an unrelated problem. The mean growth rate for small AAAs (£5.5 cm) is 2.6–3.2 mm/year, increasing with aneurysm diameter.[16,17] Studies of AAA expansion, and the factors associated with expansion, have been limited by sample size or a limited number of serial observations. In the UK SAT, AAA expansion in 1743 patients followed for up to 7 years was most strongly associated with diameter at baseline.[30] No association with growth rate was noted between age and gender. Self-reported cigarette smoking status was associated with an incrementally increased growth rate of 0.4 mm/year which persisted after adjustment for potential confounding variables. Of other potential risk factors considered in the UK SAT, including hypertension, peripheral arterial occlusive disease (PAD), total or HDL plasma cholesterol concentration and diabetes, only the presence of PAD or diabetes influenced aneurysm growth; PAD decreasing it by 0.2 mm/year for each 0.2 change in ankle brachial index (95% CI –0.03 to 0.25), and diabetes reducing the growth rate by 0.79 mm/year (95% CI 0.27 to 1.33). On the basis of these data, investigators calculated that screening intervals of 36, 24, 12, and 3 months for patients with AAA diameter of 35, 40, 45, and 50 mm, respectively, yield less than a 1% chance of patients unexpectedly exceeding 55 mm in diameter between examinations.[30] In clinical practice, examination intervals vary but rarely exceed more than 12 months with increasing frequency associated with progressive enlargement. Part of the reason for the more frequent studies is reassurance for both the patient and the physician. Quality of life surveys indicate that diagnosis without treatment of AAA can be associated with significant anxiety.[31]

Although not considered in the analyses of most AAA trials, lifelong patterns of lower extremity exercise may provide some protection from AAA. Computational flow modeling studies of hemodynamic conditions in the distal aorta suggest that the decreased flow from prolonged sedentary existence may promote aneurysmal disease.[32] Indirect clinical evidence in support of this concept include the fact that above knee traumatic amputation[33] and chronic spinal cord injury[32] are associated with increased AAA risk independent of other risk factors including cigarette smoking.

Tobacco

Tobacco smoking as a specific risk factor for AAA disease prevalence, incidence, and progression deserves special mention. The relative risk of AAA in individuals who have ever smoked is 2.5 times greater than the relative risk for coronary heart disease.

AAA is more closely associated with cigarette smoking than any other tobacco-related disease except lung cancer.[10] Nearly all (>90%) AAA patients relate a history of smoking; however, only about half of those continue to smoke at the time of diagnosis.[1] Several small studies have associated continued cigarette smoking with more rapid aneurysm expansion. Chang and associates found a significant correlation with continued smoking and aneurysm expansion.[1] MacSweeney et al. followed 43 patients with small (median size < 4.0 cm) AAA assessing active smoking (serum co tinine levels), blood pressure, cholesterol, and triglycerides.[34] Only active smoking was associated with a small but significant increase in growth rate. Lindholt et al. evaluated and prospectively followed 117 AAA patients. He found a positive correlation between continued smoking and the rate of expansion.[35] In the UK SAT itself, smoking and initial aneurysm size were the only two factors positively associated with aneurysm growth, although they did not find a dose response between self-reported smoking habits or serum cotinine levels and aneurysm growth rate.[30] Animal studies have confirmed accelerated aneurysm growth with smoking, although the mechanism for this effect does not appear to be related to a direct increase in MMP-9 levels.[36] When the studies are considered together, continued smoking appears to be associated with a relatively small (15%) increase in growth rate that, when compounded over several years, has important implications. At the present time, smoking cessation should be considered one of the most certain approaches to decreasing the rate of aneurysm expansion.

Statins

Statin therapy reduces the progression of atherosclerosis and improves clinical outcomes in cardiovascular diseases. Although effective in reducing atherogenic lipoproteins, statins also demonstrate additional biological effects (i.e., pleiotropic effects), including reduction of C-reactive protein (CRP) levels, that may be relevant to the pathogenesis of AAA disease.[37] Several studies have found an association between the presence of AAA and total cholesterol.[8,11] There is, however, no clear relationship between total cholesterol and AAA expansion rate.[30,34,35] Despite the absence of a relationship between cholesterol and growth rate, there is evidence from a number of studies suggesting that statins may influence aneurysm growth rate, presumably via these pleiotropic effects. Simvastatin therapy at 2 mg/kg/day reduces both aortic diameter and the percentage of mice with aneurysms after elastase infusion.[38] No changes in effect size were noted by repeating these experiments in hypercholesterolemic apoE-deficient mice. MMP-9 expression is closely linked to aneurysm formation in animal models of abdominal aortic aneurysm. In human AAA specimens explanted for organ culture, addition of cervistatin (0.001 to 0.1 mm/liter) significantly reduces tissue levels of both total and active MMP-9 in a concentration-dependent manner.[39] Cervistatin did not reduce the number of macrophages or neutrophils presents in cultured aneurysms, suggesting that statin therapy inhibited inflammatory cell activation. In a prospective study by Evans et al., patients were randomized to a 3-week preoperative course of simvastatin versus placebo prior to open aneurysm repair. MMP-9 levels, in excised aneurysm tissue, were decreased in the simvastatin group.[40] In one observational study of 130 patients followed for 2 years, no aneurysm expansion was observed in the 75 patients taking statins, while the mean aneurysm size in the group not taking statins increased from 4.5 to 5.3 cm.[41] Schouten et al. followed 150 patients for a minimum of 12 months with at least three measurements. Aneurysm expansion rate was decreased in the patients taking statins (2.0 mm/year) compared with those not taking statins (3.6 mm/year).

Although these associative data are intriguing, there are many potential biases in these uncontrolled observational studies. They are reminiscent of similar analyses suggesting that b-blockers would inhibit aneurysm expansion, while RCTs showed propranolol to be ineffective. Because AAA, CAD, and PVD share common risk factors such as tobacco use, there will be clear indications for statin use in many AAA patients related to CAD and PVD. The use of statins will become more common with efforts to meet the National Heart, Lung, and Blood Institutes (NHLBI) increasingly stringent Adult Treatment Protocol (ATP) guidelines. A high prevalence of statin use among AAA patients will make it challenging to design trials to assess the specific role of statin therapy as an inhibitor of aneurysm expansion. Such studies will be important, however, because some guidelines such as those for the Women's Health Initiative have made the leap to categorizing AAA as a PVD equivalent.[42] At the present time, there does not appear to be sufficient evidence to recommend that statin therapy be initiated for the diagnosis of AAA alone.

β-blockers

Several animal studies have indicated that propranolol might have beneficial effects on aneurysmal disease based on both its hemodynamic properties and its biochemical effects on matrix proteins.[43,44] Two clinical studies used retrospective analysis to assess the impact of β-blockers in aneurysm growth rates.[45,46] Both identified a significant inhibitory effect of β-blockers. These studies provided the underpinning for two multicenter randomized trials testing propranolol in aneurysm patients. Propranolol did not inhibit aneurysm expansion in a trial reported by Lindholt et al.[47] These results were compromised by low compliance in the propranolol arm since only 22% of patients continued the medication for 2 years. The mean growth rate was slightly (but not significantly) higher in the propranolol group. A Canadian trial that recruited 552 patients suffered similarly from compliance problems in that 42% of propranolol-treated participants discontinued the drug during the trial.[48] The growth rate in the placebo group and the propranolol group did not differ although there was a slight trend in favor of propranolol. Quality of life, assessed by the SF-36 questionnaire, showed that propranolol had a significant negative effect as one would anticipate from the low compliance rate. [48]

ACE Inhibitors and Angiotensin Receptor Blockers

A number of animal experiments using different models of aneurysmal disease have suggested an important role for the angiotensin/renin axis in aneurysm development. Captopril, but not losartan, an angiotensin receptor blocker, prevents aneurysm formation in the rat elastase model of AAA.[49] This m odel relies on infusion of elastase into the infrarenal aorta resulting in initial mechanical dilatation followed by progressive enlargement. Another commonly studied aneurysm model is based on chronic infusion of angiotensin II into apoE-deficient mice resulting initially in midaortic dilatation and eventual rupture.[50] Losartan prevents aneurysm formation in this model. This effect of losartan is consistent with observations in genetically engineered mice with Marfan syndrome (MFS). Work done in these mice has suggested that the inability of mutated fibrillin to sequester TGF-b plays a role in the progression of tissue changes associated with MFS.[51] In a series of studies, TGF-b antagonism by losartan was effective in preventing progressive matrix degradation.[50] The reason for the discrepant effects of losartan – ineffective in the elastase aneurysm model and effective in the angiotensin and Marfan models – may relate to differences among the models. In the angiotension infusion model, initial dissection of the upper abdominal aorta is followed by dilatation. This process may have more similarities to the MFS models where the thoracic aorta is affected. Clinical trials of losartan in MFS have recently begun enrollment.[52]

Hackam et al. recently published results of an analysis of a linked administrative database from Ontario, Canada analyzing ruptured ($n = 3379$) and nonruptured aortic aneurysms ($n = 11,947$) from 1992–2002.[53] ACE inhibitor use within the prior 3–12 months was less frequent among those admitted for aneurysm rupture (OR 0.82; CI 0.74 –0.90). b-blockers, lipid-lowering agents , and angiotensin receptor blockers showed no relationship to rupture. In a published response to the paper, Lederle and Taylor note that among those patients who discontinued ACE inhibitors within the last 3 –12 months, there is a harmful effect in favor of aneurysm rupture.[54] The case control study by Schouten et al. and post hoc analysis of the UK aneurysm trial data did not find a relationship between ACE inhibitors and aneurysm expansion rates.[30,55] Most patients presenting with aneurysm rupture have large, undetected aneurysms, while patients with known aneurysms typically undergo repair long before their rupture risk becomes significant. Thus, this information regarding ACE inhibitors and rupture risk might find its most practical application among the small number of patients deemed unfit for repair.

Macrolides

A number of antibiotics have been proposed as a treatment for AAA with varying rationales. One line of reasoning is that AAA progression is enhanced by secondary infection within the aortic wall. Chlamydia pneumonia has been found in atherosclerotic plaque and the wall of AAA.[56,57] There was once great enthusiasm for the hypothesis that treatment of the secondary Chlamydial infection could slow progression of atherosclerosis. This has been diminished by subsequent prospective randomized trials showing no cardiovascular benefit to a year of a treatment with azithromycin in patients with stable CAD.[58] Similar negative results were fou nd by Burkhardt et al.[59] A small study by Lindholt et al. suggested that serological evidence of a *Chlamydia pneumonia* infection was associated with an increased rate of aneurysm expansion.[57] This led to an RCT in which 43 patients received a 1- month course of roxithromycin while 49 patients received placebo.[60] Patients in the treatment arm had an expansion rate at the end of the study of 1.56 mm/year compared with a rate of 2.75 mm/year in the placebo group. The inhibition was greater in the first year than the second year. The study did not clarify the mechanism of effect since there was no correlation between Chlamydia titers and roxithromycin ability to inhibit aneurysm expansion.

Tetracyclines

The tetracycline antibiotics have been studied because of their known inhibition of matrix metalloproteinases (MMP). Petrinic et al. were the first to demonstrate that doxycycline could suppress aortic wall MMP activity, elastin degradation, and aneurysm development in the elastase-induced rat model.[61]

They achieved similar results using nonantimicrobial (chemically modified) tetracyclines and nonselective hydroxamic acid derivatives as MMP inhibitors, indicating that the aneurysm-suppressing effects of doxycycline are most likely related to its activity as an MMP inhibitor.[62] Longo et al. characterized a second murine aneurysm model using calcium chloride applied to the ablumenal surface to induce the aneurysm.[63] In this model, doxycycline demonstrates the same dose-dependent inhibition of aneurysm expansion.[64] The plasma doxycycline levels achieved in these animal studies were in the same range as those seen in AAA patients receiving doxycycline (100 mg bid).[65] These murine studies suggest that inhibition can still be achieved at plasma levels in the 1–2 mg/ml range. A number of studies in patients have suggested that doxycycline can inhibit MMPs in aneurysm tissue. Curci et al. treated a series of patients with a 3-week course of doxycycline prior to open aneurysm repair.[66] Tissue levels of MMP-9 were significantly reduced by doxycycline in comparison to untreated patients. Baxter et al. showed in a small series of 36 patients on a 6-month course of doxycycline plasma that MMP-9 levels decreased significantly in comparison to baseline levels.[65] This work has been followed by a small prospective randomized trial of doxycycline in which 32 patients were randomized with 17 receiving doxycycline (150 mg/day) for 3 months. Patients were followed for 18 months.[67] Chlamydia pneumonia titers were assessed but found not to be affected by doxycycline treatment. The calculated growth rate at the end of the 18-month period of observation was 1.5 mm/year in the doxycycline-treated group versus 3.0 mm/year in the placebo group. This difference did not achieve statistical significance but the 6- and 12-month time periods did show a significant difference in favor of doxycycline treatment. Level B evidence (small randomized trials) suggests that roxithromycin or doxycycline will decrease the rate of aneurysm expansion.

Considerations for Evaluating Medical Therapies

There are three important features of AAA that lend themselves to medical treatment.

Inexpensive and accurate methods for detection
Long period of surveillance prior to intervention
Life expectancy of the affected population

Increased public awareness and the availability of screening will lead to increased aneurysm detection in the next decade. Ninety percent of aneurysms detected at screening are below the threshold for immediate repair, and aneurysm expansion is gradual. Reducing the expansion rate of 4.0 AAA by 50% potentially increases the time before surgical intervention is required to greater than 10 years, exceeding the life expectancy of many aneurysm patients. The current standard of care for these small AAA is "watchful waiting." The provision of a relatively benign and efficacious medical therapy to these patients may reverse the diminished quality of life associated with detection of a potentially life-threatening condition for which no immediate treatment is offered. In the format of the American College of Cardiology/American Heart Association Clinical Practice Guidelines,[68] level A evidence (large randomized trials) is available to indicate that observation of aneurysms in men

Table 1 AAA Growth: effects of medical therapy.

Intervention	References	Effect on AAA growth	Level of evidence	Class of recommen-dation
Propranolol	49, 69AU: Reference 69 is not present in the Ref. list, please check.</AQ>	No effect	A	III
Macrolides	60	Inhibition	B	IIA
Tetracycline	67	Inhibition	B	IIA
Statins	38, 39	Inhibition	B	IIA
ACE inhibi-tors	27, 39, 52, 53	No effect	B and C	IIB
AR blockers	48, 50	Animal data	C	IIB

ªInhibition at 6 and 12 months after 3 months of treatment

is safe up to a size of 5.5 cm and that propranolol doses not inhibit aneurysm expansion (Table 1).

References

1. Powell JT, Worrell P, MacSweeney ST, et al. Smoking as a risk factor for abdominal aortic aneurysm. Ann N Y Acad Sci. Nov 18 1996;800:246–248.
2. Wilmink TB, Quick CR, Hubbard CS, et al. The influence of screening on the incidence of ruptured abdominal aortic aneurysms. J Vasc Surg. Aug 1999;30(2):203–208.
3. Lederle FA, Johnson GR, Wilson SE, et al. The aneurysm detection and management study screening program: validation cohort and final results. Aneurysm Detection and Management Veterans Affairs Cooperative Study Investigators. Arch Intern Med. May 22 2000;160(10):1425–1430.
4. Ashton HA, Buxton MJ, Day NE, et al. The Multicentre Aneurysm Screening Study (MASS) into the effect of abdominal aortic aneurysm screening on mortality in men: a randomised controlled trial. Lancet. Nov 16 2002;360(9345):1531–1539.
5. Wilmink AB, Quick CR. Epidemiology and potential for prevention of abdominal aortic aneurysm. Br J Surg. Feb 1998;85(2):155–162.
6. Lindholt JS, Juul S, Fasting H, et al. Hospital costs and benefits of screening for abdominal aortic aneurysms. Results from a randomised population screening trial. Eur J Vasc Endovasc Surg. Jan 2002;23(1):55–60.
7. Kent KC, Zwolak RM, Jaff MR, et al. Screening for abdominal aortic aneurysm: a consensus statement. J Vasc Surg. Jan 2004;39(1):267–269.
8. Lederle FA, Johnson GR, Wilson SE, et al. Prevalence and associations of abdominal aortic aneurysm detected through screening. Aneurysm Detection and Management (ADAM) Veterans Affairs Cooperative Study Group. Ann Intern Med. Mar 15 1997;126(6):441–449.
9. Chang JB, Stein TA, Liu JP, et al. Risk factors associated with rapid growth of small abdominal aortic aneurysms. Surgery. Feb 1997;121(2):117–122.
10. Lederle FA, Nelson DB, Joseph AM. Smokers' relative risk for aortic aneurysm compared with other smoking-related diseases: a systematic review. J Vasc Surg. Aug 2003;38(2):329–334.
11. Iribarren C, Darvinian JA, Go AS, et al. Traditional and novel risk factors for clinically diagnosed abdominal aortic aneurysm: The Kaiser multiphasic health checkup cohort study.. Ann Epidemiol May 16 2007:E pub ahead of print.
12. Deaths, percent of total deaths, and death rates for the 15 leading causes of death Accessed March 30, 2008.
13. Cancer Prevention and Control. Available at: http://www.cdc.gov/cancer/

14. Matsumura JS, Brewster DC, Makaroun MS, et al. A multicenter controlled clinical trial of open versus endovascular treatment of abdominal aortic aneurysm. J Vasc Surg. Feb 2003;37(2):262–271.

15. Blankensteijn JD, de Jong SE, Prinssen M, et al. Two-year outcomes after conventional or endovascular repair of abdominal aortic aneurysms. N Engl J Med. Jun 9 2005; 352(23):2398–2405.

16. The United Kingdom Small Aneurysm Trial Participants. Long-term outcomes of immediate repair compared with surveillance of small abdominal aortic aneurysms. N Engl J Med. May 9 2002;346(19):1445–1452.

17. Lederle FA, Wilson SE, Johnson GR, et al. Immediate repair compared with surveillance of small abdominal aortic aneurysms. N Engl J Med. May 9 2002;346(19): 1437–1444.

18. O'Rourke MF, Nichols WW. Aortic diameter, aortic stiffness, and wave reflection increase with age and isolated systolic hypertension. Hypertension. Apr 2005; 45(4):652–658.

19. Lederle FA, Johnson GR, Wilson SE, et al. Relationship of age, gender, race, and body size to infrarenal aortic diameter. The Aneurysm Detection and Management (ADAM) Veterans Affairs Cooperative Study Investigators. J Vasc Surg. Oct 1997; 26(4):595–601.

20. Lawrence-Brown MM, Norman PE, Jamrozik K, et al. Initial results of ultrasound screening for aneurysm of the abdominal aorta in Western Australia: relevance for endoluminal treatment of aneurysm disease. Cardiovasc Surg. Jun 2001;9(3):234–240.

21. Mortality results for randomised controlled trial of early elective surgery or ultrasonographic surveillance for small abdominal aortic aneurysms. The UK Small Aneurysm Trial Participants. Lancet. Nov 21 1998;352(9141):1649–1655.

22. Norman PE, Powell JT. Abdominal aortic aneurysm: the prognosis in women is worse than in men. Circulation. Jun 5 2007;115(22):2865–2869.

23. Dillavou ED, Muluk SC, Makaroun MS. Improving aneurysm-related outcomes: nationwide benefits of endovascular repair. J Vasc Surg. Mar 2006;43(3):446–451; discussion 451–442.

24. Fleming C, Whitlock EP, Beil TL, et al. Screening for abdominal aortic aneurysm: a best-evidence systematic review for the U.S. Preventive Services Task Force. Ann Intern Med. Feb 1 2005;142(3):203–211.

25. Alcorn HG, Wolfson SK, Jr., Sutton-Tyrrell K, et al. Risk factors for abdominal aortic aneurysms in older adults enrolled in The Cardiovascular Health Study. Arterioscler Thromb Vasc Biol. Aug 1996;16(8):963–970.

26. Wilmink AB, Forshaw M, Quick CR, et al. Accuracy of serial screening for abdominal aortic aneurysms by ultrasound. J Med Screen. 2002;9(3):125–127.

27. Wilmink AB, Hubbard CS, Quick CR. Quality of the measurement of the infrarenal aortic diameter by ultrasound. J Med Screen. 1997;4(1):49–53.

28. Wassef M, Baxter BT, Chisholm RL, et al. Pathogenesis of abdominal aortic aneurysms: a multidisciplinary research program supported by the National Heart, Lung, and Blood Institute. J Vasc Surg. Oct 2001;34(4):730–738.

29. Wassef M, Upchurch GR, Jr., Kuivaniemi H, et al. Challenges and opportunities in abdominal aortic aneurysm research. J Vasc Surg. Jan 2007;45(1):192–198.

30. Brady AR, Thompson SG, Fowkes FG, et al. Abdominal aortic aneurysm expansion: risk factors and time intervals for surveillance. Circulation. Jul 6 2004; 110(1):16–21.

31. Lederle FA, Johnson GR, Wilson SE, et al. Quality of life, impotence, and activity level in a randomized trial of immediate repair versus surveillance of small abdominal aortic aneurysm. J Vasc Surg. Oct 2003;38(4):745–752.

32. Yeung JJ, Kim HJ, Abbruzzese TA, et al. Aortoiliac hemodynamic and morphologic adaptation to chronic spinal cord injury. J Vasc Surg. Dec 2006;44(6):1254–1265.

33. Vollmar JF, Paes E, Pauschinger P, et al. Aortic aneurysms as late sequelae of above-knee amputation. Lancet. Oct 7 1989;2(8667):834–835.

34. MacSweeney ST, Ellis M, Worrell PC, et al. Smoking and growth rate of small abdominal aortic aneurysms. Lancet. Sep 3 1994;344(8923):651–652.

35. Lindholt JS, Heegaard NH, Vammen S, et al. Smoking, but not lipids, lipoprotein(a) and antibodies against oxidised LDL, is correlated to the expansion of abdominal aortic aneurysms. Eur J Vasc Endovasc Surg. Jan 2001;21(1):51–56.

36. Bergoeing MP, Arif B, Hackmann AE, et al. Cigarette smoking increases aortic dilatation without affecting matrix metalloproteinase-9 and -12 expression in a modified mouse model of aneurysm formation. J Vasc Surg. Jun 2007;45(6):1217–1227.

37. Gotto AM, Jr. Role of C-reactive protein in coronary risk reduction: focus on primary prevention. Am J Cardiol. Mar 1 2007;99(5):718–725.

38. Steinmetz EF, Buckley C, Shames ML, et al. Treatment with simvastatin suppresses the development of experimental abdominal aortic aneurysms in normal and hypercholesterolemic mice. Ann Surg. Jan 2005;241(1):92–101.

39. Nagashima H, Aoka Y, Sakomura Y, et al. A 3-hydroxy-3-methylglutaryl coenzyme A reductase inhibitor, cerivastatin, suppresses production of matrix metalloproteinase-9 in human abdominal aortic aneurysm wall. J Vasc Surg. 2002;36(1):158–163.

40. Evans J, Powell JT, Schwalbe E, et al. Simvastatin attenuates the activity of matrix metalloprotease-9 in aneurysmal aortic tissue. Eur J Vasc Endovasc Surg. Jun 15 2007.

41. Sukhija R, Aronow WS, Sandhu R, et al. Mortality and size of abdominal aortic aneurysm at long-term follow-up of patients not treated surgically and treated with and without statins. Am J Cardiol. Jan 15 2006;97(2):279–280.

42. Hsia J, Langer RD, Manson JE, et al. Conjugated equine estrogens and coronary heart disease: the Women's Health Initiative. Arch Intern Med. Feb 13 2006; 166(3):357–365.

43. Boucek RJ, Gunja-Smith Z, Noble NL, et al. Modulation by propranolol of the lysyl cross-links in aortic elastin and collagen of the aneurysm-prone turkey. Biochem Pharmacol. Jan 15 1983;32(2):275–280.

44. Brophy C, Tilson JE, Tilson MD. Propranolol delays the formation of aneurysms in the male blotchy mouse. J Surg Res. Jun 1988;44(6):687–689.

45. Gadowski GR, Pilcher DB, Ricci MA. Abdominal aortic aneurysm expansion rate: effect of size and beta-adrenergic blockade. J Vasc Surg. Apr 1994;19(4):727–731.

46. Leach SD, Toole AL, Stern H, et al. Effect of beta-adrenergic blockade on the growth rate of abdominal aortic aneurysms. Arch Surg. May 1988;123(5):606–609.

47. Lindholt JS, Henneberg EW, Juul S, et al. Impaired results of a randomised double blinded clinical trial of propranolol versus placebo on the expansion rate of small abdominal aortic aneurysms. Int Angiol. Mar 1999;18(1):52–57.

48. Propranolol Aneurysm Trial Investigators. Propranolol for small abdominal aortic aneurysms: results of a randomized trial. J Vasc Surg. Jan 2002;35(1):72–79.

49. Liao S, Miralles M, Kelley BJ, et al. Suppression of experimental abdominal aortic aneurysms in the rat by treatment with angiotensin-converting enzyme inhibitors. J Vasc Surg. May 2001;33(5):1057–1064.

50. Daugherty A, Manning MW, Cassis LA. Angiotensin II promotes atherosclerotic lesions and aneurysms in apolipoprotein E-deficient mice. J Clin Invest. Jun 2000;105(11):1605–1612.

51. Neptune ER, Frischmeyer PA, Arking DE, et al. Dysregulation of TGF-beta activation contributes to pathogenesis in Marfan syndrome. Nat Genet. Mar 2003; 33(3):407–411.

52. Comparison of two medications aimed at slowing aortic root enlargement in individuals with Marfan sndrome.

53. Hackam DG, Thiruchelvam D, Redelmeier DA. Angiotensin-converting enzyme inhibitors and aortic rupture: a population-based case-control study. Lancet. Aug 19 2006; 368(9536):659–665.

54. Lederle FA, Taylor BC. ACE inhibitors and aortic rupture. Lancet. Nov 4 2006; 368(9547):1571; author reply 1572.

55. Schouten O, van Laanen JH, Boersma E, et al. Statins are associated with a reduced infrarenal abdominal aortic aneurysm growth. Eur J Vasc Endovasc Surg. Jul 2006; 32(1):21–26.

56. Nieto FJ. Infective agents and cardiovascular disease. Semin Vasc Med. Nov 2002; 2(4):401–415.

57. Lindholt JS, Ashton HA, Scott RA. Indicators of infection with Chlamydia pneumoniae are associated with expansion of abdominal aortic aneurysms. J Vasc Surg. Aug 2001;34(2):212–215.

58. Grayston JT, Kronmal RA, Jackson LA, et al. Azithromycin for the secondary prevention of coronary events. N Engl J Med. Apr 21 2005;352(16):1637–1645.

59. Burkhardt U, Zahn R, Hoffler U, et al. Antibody levels against Chlamydia pneumoniae and outcome of roxithromycin therapy in patients with acute myocardial infarction. Results from a sub-study of the randomised Antibiotic Therapy in Acute Myocardial Infarction (ANTIBIO) trial. Z Kardiol. Sep 2004;93(9):671–678.

60. Vammen S, Lindholt JS, Ostergaard L, et al. Randomized double-blind controlled trial of roxithromycin for prevention of abdominal aortic aneurysm expansion. Br J Surg. Aug 2001;88(8):1066–1072.

61. Petrinec D, Liao S, Holmes DR, et al. Doxycycline inhibition of aneurysmal degeneration in an elastase-induced rat model of abdominal aortic aneurysm: preservation of aortic elastin associated with suppressed production of 92 kD gelatinase. J Vasc Surg. Feb 1996;23(2):336–346.

62. Petrinec D, Holmes DR, Liao S, et al. Suppression of experimental aneurysmal degeneration with chemically modified tetracycline derivatives. Ann N Y Acad Sci. Nov 18 1996;800:263–265.

63. Longo GM, Xiong W, Greiner TC, et al. Matrix metalloproteinases 2 and 9 work in concert to produce aortic aneurysms. J Clin Invest. Sep 2002;110(5):625–632.

64. Prall AK, Longo GM, Mayhan WG, et al. Doxycycline in patients with abdominal aortic aneurysms and in mice: comparison of serum levels and effect on aneurysm growth in mice. J Vasc Surg. May 2002;35(5):923–929.

65. Baxter BT, Pearce WH, Waltke EA, et al. Prolonged administration of doxycycline in patients with small asymptomatic abdominal aortic aneurysms: report of a prospective (Phase II) multicenter study. J Vasc Surg. Jul 2002;36(1):1–12.

66. Curci JA, Mao D, Bohner DG, et al. Preoperative treatment with doxycycline reduces aortic wall expression and activation of matrix metalloproteinases in patients with abdominal aortic aneurysms. J Vasc Surg. Feb 2000;31(2):325–342.

67. Mosorin M, Juvonen J, Biancari F, et al. Use of doxycycline to decrease the growth rate of abdominal aortic aneurysms: a randomized, double-blind, placebo-controlled pilot study. J Vasc Surg. Oct 2001;34(4):606–610.

68. Gibbons RJ, Smith SC, Jr., Antman E. American College of Cardiology/American Heart Association clinical practice guidelines: Part II: evolutionary changes in a continuous quality improvement project. Circulation. Jun 24 2003;107(24):3101–3107.

Chapter 5

Surgical Treatment of Nonruptured Infrarenal Abdominal Aortic Aneurysms

Michael Wilderman and Gregorio Sicard

Abstract Abdominal aortic aneurysm (AAA) rupture carries a 90% overall mortality, and a 40–50% mortality for those patients who reach a hospital alive. Because of this, the primary goal of AAA therapy is to avoid rupture. Treatment of ruptured AAAs is very costly to the health care system. To date, there are two effective methods to treat AAA, and thus exclude the AAA from pressurized blood flow. The first is an open surgical exclusion of the AAA, along with an interposition synthetic graft, while the second is an endoluminally placed covered stent graft (endovascular aortic aneurysm repair, EVAR) that can be inserted either via the femoral artery or the iliac artery. The most important factors that increase the risk of open aneurysm repair are renal dysfunction with a creatinine level greater than 1.8 mg, congestive heart failure, jugular venous distention, ischemic electrocardiographic changes with ST depression greater than 2 mm, history of a prior myocardial infarction, pulmonary dysfunction including chronic obstructive pulmonary disease, dyspnea on exertion or prior lung surgery, old age, and female gender. In the absence of risk factors, elective open AAA carries an operative mortality of 3–5%, but the risk rises as high as 40% if several of the aforementioned risk factors are present.

Keywords Infrarenal AAA, Preoperative risk, AAA, Operative mortality AAA, endoluminal AAA repair, Retroperitoneal approach AAA, Postoperative complications, AAA

Definition

Most medical dictionaries define an aneurysm as a localized widening or ballooning of a portion of an artery, greater than 50% of the normal caliber of the artery, commonly related to weakness in the wall of the blood vessel.[1] The most common location of an extracranial aneurysm is the infrarenal abdominal aorta. Using the above definition, an aorta with a diameter greater than 3 cm can therefore be considered aneurysmal, although normal aortic diameters vary with age, sex, and body habitus. Histologically, an abdominal aortic

G. Upchurch and E. Criado (eds.) *Aortic Aneurysms, Contemporary Cardiology*
DOI: 10.1007/978-1-60327-204-9_5, © Humana Press, a part of
Springer Science + Business Media, LLC 2009

aneurysm (AAA) is characterized by macrophage degradation of the medial elastin lamellar architecture by metalloproteinases.[2–5]

Historical Perspectives

Aneurysms have been recognized for thousands of years, in fact the Ebers Papyrus in 2000 BC discusses traumatic aneurysms of the peripheral arteries.[6] In the second century AD, Antyllus wrote of the first elective procedure to treat an aneurysm by proximal and distal ligation of the artery feeding the aneurysm, along with opening the sac and evacuation of its contents.[7] Andreas Vesalius, the sixteenth century Flemish anatomist, was the first to describe an AAA.[8] Antyllus's technique remained the principal treatment method for at least the next fifteen hundred years until Rudolph Matas, in 1923, performed the successful technical ligation of a ruptured syphilitic infrarenal AAA.[9] Because of the high mortality associated with aneurysm ligation, surgeons devised other therapies such as inducing thrombosis of the aneurysm with wires, also with poor results.[10] In the early 1940s, surgeons utilized wrapping of the aneurysm with various materials such as fascia lata, skin grafts, polyvinyl sponge, and even cellophane, in an attempt to prevent aneurysmal rupture.[11–13] The results of this method were not good and the mortality and rupture rate of aneurysms remained quite high. The current technique for AAA repair was conceptually devised in the early twentieth century by the 1912 Nobel laureate Alexis Carrel.[14–17] His method, which he performed only in animals, consisted of replacing a segment of aorta with a segment from another artery or vein. In 1951, Charles DuBost reported retroperitoneal approach to replace the aneurysmal infrarenal aorta with an aortic homograft.[18] In 1953, Michael DeBakey and Denton Cooley reported success using a similar technique.[19] In the same year, Henry Bahnson described the technique described by DuBost to repair a ruptured AAA.[20] The use of homografts was short-lived due to graft degeneration and subsequent graft rupture. The next major breakthrough for AAA repair was the use of arterial protetics made of Vinyon-N, originated in the work of Arthur Voorhees.[21] Blakemore placed the first Vinyon-N graft in a patient with a ruptured AAA.[22] In 1954, Voorhees and Blakemore described their results in 16 patients with AAA repaired using Vinyon-N grafts with a 56% survival.[23,24] These advances stimulated industry to evaluate and develop arterial conduits. In 1958, Michael DeBakey's group in Houston reported excellent results on a large group of patients undergoing AAA repair with knitted Dacron grafts.[25] Over the next two decades, many series were reported with operative mortalities in the 10–15% range, using polyester grafts.

Prevalence and Incidence

AAA is typically a disease of elderly males, with increasing prevalence after the sixth decade of life. AAA is two to six times more common in men than women, and two to three times more common in white than African-American population. The incidence of AAA varies from 3 to 117 per one hundred thousand person years.[26–29] Lederle et al.[30] reported that 2.6% of screened patients with a normal ultrasound 4 years prior developed an AAA. They also reported an incidence of AAA of 6.5 per thousand person years. In men, AAAs typically appear after age 50 and reach a peak incidence at age 80. In women, it is usually later, around age 60, with a steady increase after that.[31–33] Although

AAAs fail to demonstrate a clear genetic predisposition or transmission pattern, numerous reports suggest that 15–20% of first-order relatives of patients with AAAs will have also have an aneurysm.[34-36]

Aortic aneurysm rupture is among the tenth leading causes of death in elderly males. Most AAAs are found incidentally and only rarely cause symptoms such as abdominal or back pain. Therefore, ruptured AAA may be the initial form of presentation. Aortic aneurysm rupture carries a 90% overall mortality, and a 40–50% mortality for those patients who reach a hospital alive. The primary goal of AAA therapy is to avoid rupture. Treatment of ruptured AAAs is very costly to the health care system. A study from Great Britain found that about 2000 lives and nearly $50 million dollars could be saved if AAAs were repaired prior to rupture.[37] Breckwoldt et al. suggested that emergent interventions for patients with ruptured AAAs led to hospital losses of $24,655 per patient.[38] Another study from the United Kingdom found that the total costs of emergency AAA repair was 96,700 pounds, with a cost per life saved of 24,175 pounds. The total cost of elective AAA repair was 76,583 with a cost per life saved of 5470 pounds. The cost of emergency intervention was found to be fivefold that of elective repair, per life saved, per year.[39]

Diagnosis and Risk of Rupture

Since most AAAs are asymptomatic and patients may not present until their AAA has ruptured, targeted screening of high risk population is recommended. A study by Schermerhorn et al. showed that ultrasound screening for AAA was cost effective and beneficial for men 65–74 years of age with known risk factors such as coronary artery disease (CAD), smoking, or a family history of AAA.[40] A report by Derubertis et al. suggested a high incidence of AAA among women older than 65, with a history of smoking or heart disease. Women with such risk factors, therefore, should also be considered for AAA screening.[41] Aneurysm screening programs have been introduced in some countries.[42-50] A large randomized trial in the United Kingdom demonstrated an early mortality benefit of screening ultrasonography for AAA.[51] Since January 2007, Medicare has offered coverage of a one-time, ultrasound screening for senior males with a smoking history of at least 100 cigarettes in their lifetime and for individuals with a family history of AAA. In the Multicentre Aneurysm Screening Study, 70,495 men age 65–74 were randomized to ultrasound screening versus no screening for AAA. Of the 33,839 patients randomized to ultrasound screening, 80% were screened and 5% had AAAs greater than 3 cm. At 4 years, there were 113 AAA-related deaths in the nonscreened control group compared with 65 in the screened group. This trial suggested a 32% reduction in AAA-related mortality in the screened group.[50]

Currently, AAAs are more commonly found incidentally when patients are imaged, either with ultrasound, CT scan, or MRI for other diseases or symptomatology.

The Department of Veterans Affairs Aneurysm Detection and Management (ADAM) study was designed to compare long-term AAA survival following either surveillance or surgical treatment when aneurysm reached 5.5 cm versus immediate open surgical repair for managing AAAs less than 5.5 cm. A total of 1136 patients were enrolled and followed for a mean time of 4.8 years. No significant difference was found between the two groups in terms of long-term mortality, and the study concluded that there was no long-term survival advantage by repairing AAA smaller than 5.5 cm. They thus recommended surveillance of small AAAs until they reach a 5.5 cm diameter.[52]

The UK Small Aneurysm Trial followed over 1000 patients for 10 years. This study found no long-term survival benefit for early elective open repair of small aneurysm between 4 and 5.4 cm of maximal diameter.[53]

The refinement in the preoperative evaluation of patients undergoing AAA repair during the last two decades has significantly decreased the mortality rate of open AAA repair (Table 1).[54–64]

The risk of rupture of an AAA is estimated based on its maximal diameter. Aneurysms between 3 and 5 cm have less than 1% per year risk of rupture. A progressive risk of aneurysm rupture occurs with increasing aneurysm diameter. An aneurysm growth rate greater than 0.5 cm in a 6-month period also appears to increase the risk of rupture. Therefore, it is generally accepted that aneurysms less than 5.5 cm can be safely followed with yearly ultrasound.

Most aneurysms, especially smaller ones, tend to grow at a rate of 0.3–0.5 cm per year.[65–67]

Other factors that have been associated with increased expansion or rupture rate are uncontrolled hypertension, chronic obstructive pulmonary disease (COPD), female gender, severe CAD, a large volume of luminal thrombus, and advanced age.

Fillinger et al. have reported that aortic wall stress is a key predictor of rupture risk for AAA. A mathematical analysis of AAA geometry, known as finite element analysis, has been suggested to be a better way to estimate wall stress and the risk of rupture. Using this model, Fillinger's group looked at three groups of patients: those who presented with a ruptured AAA, those who were symptomatic and required urgent surgery, and those who underwent elective AAA repair. They found that peak wall stress was significantly higher in ruptured AAA and symptomatic groups compared with that of the elective repair group for diameter-matched subjects. They also found that the location of maximal wall stress in their series was not at the site of maximal AAA diameter but rather in the posterolateral location where most ruptures do occur.[68,69]

Table 1 Operative mortality following elective infrarenal abdominal aortic aneurysm (*AAA*).

Authors	n	30-Day mortality (%)
Bush et al.[61]	1580 (high risk)	5.2
Sicard et al.[64]	61 (high risk)	5.1
Hua et al.[55]	582	3.95
Lifeline Registry[82]	334	1.4
Blankensteijn et al.[62] (randomized)	178	4.6
Anderson et al.[60]	783 (2002)	4.21 (2002)
	1043 (2001)	3.55 (2001)
	1238 (2000)	4.12 (2000)
Greenhalgh et al.[63] (randomized)	539	4.7
Akkersdijk et al.[59]	16,466	7.3
Lee et al.[58]	4607	3.8
Hertzer et al.[57]	1135	1.2
Huber et al.[56]	16,450	4.2
Heller et al.[54]	358,521	5.6

Preoperative Risk Assessment

The principle behind surgical intervention for AAA is to prevent aneurysmal rupture. To date, there are two effective methods to treat AAA, and thus exclude the AAA from pressurized blood flow. The first is an open surgical exclusion of the AAA, along with an interposition synthetic graft. The second is an endoluminally placed covered stent graft (EVAR) that can be inserted via either the femoral or the iliac artery. Each method has advantages and disadvantages, and therefore every situation must be assessed independently, based on a patient's age, infrarenal aortic anatomy, and comorbidities.

If a patient is discovered to have a symptomatic AAA (i.e., back or abdominal pain or hypotension), urgent or expedient surgical intervention is indicated. Stable patients can undergo laboratory testing and cross-sectional imaging to assess their potential for an endoluminal approach. If the patient is unstable, then the patient should be taken to the operating room for an open repair.

Asymptomatic male patients with aneurysms greater than 5.5 cm or asymptomatic female patients with aneurysms greater than 5.0 cm should undergo aneurysm repair. Based on preoperative assessments such as aneurysmal anatomy, along with the patient's age and other comorbidities, the treatment strategy is selected. The most important factors that increase the risk of open aneurysm repair are renal dysfunction with a creatinine level greater than 1.8 mg, congestive heart failure, jugular venous distention, ischemic electrocardiographic changes with ST depression greater than 2 mm, history of a prior myocardial infarction, pulmonary dysfunction including COPD, dyspnea on exertion or prior lung surgery, old age, and female gender. In the absence of risk factors, elective open AAA carries an operative mortality of 3–5%, but the risk rises as high as 40% if several of the aforementioned risk factors are present.[70] Renal failure alone is the strongest predictor of mortality with a 4- to 9-fold increase in risk, whereas CAD carries a 2.5- to 5-fold increase in mortality.[71]

Mortality is also affected by the given surgeon or hospital experience with AAA repair. Larger centers with higher volumes have better outcomes than less-experienced surgeons or small-volume centers.[72] Dimick et al. reported that hospitals that perform more than 35 open AAA per year have a 30 day mortality of 3%, as compared with lower volume centers that have a 30 day mortality of 5.5%. In general, they found that high-volume surgeons with vascular surgery specialty training working at high-volume hospitals have the best outcomes.[73]

To reduce overall operative mortality, perioperative cardiac optimization is vital, especially since CAD is the principle cause of early and late mortality after AAA.[74] The American College of Cardiology has standardized preoperative cardiac evaluation for noncardiac surgery, and created categories for the risk of the procedure and the clinical risk to the patient. Patients with unstable coronary syndromes such as acute or recent MI (less than 30 days) or unstable angina, decompensated CHF, significant arrhythmias such as high-grade AV block or symptomatic ventricular arrhythmias, or severe valvular disease are considered to have major cardiac risks. Intermediate-risk patients are those with stable angina, prior MI by history or the presence of Q waves on an ECG, compensated CHF, insulin-dependent diabetes mellitus, or renal insufficiency. Patients with minor risk include those of advanced age, have an abnormal ECG (left ventricular hypertrophy, left bundle branch block), have a history of a prior stroke, or have uncontrolled hypertension.[75]

Van Damme et al. found that in patients without clinical markers of CAD, noninvasive cardiac testing did not predict cardiac complications. In patients with definite clinical or ECG evidence of CAD, a negative stress test had a high negative predictive value.[76] Poldermans et al. reported that in intermediate-risk patients, cardiac testing can be safely omitted, provided that patients are treated with β-blockers to keep their heart rates until tight control.[77] In one of the high-risk patients, it was found that coronary revascularization prior to major vascular surgery did not improve overall 30-day outcomes.[78]

The indication for cardiac testing and treatment prior to AAA repair are the same as in the nonoperative setting, but the timing of such evaluations is dependent upon the urgency of the surgery, patient risk factors, and surgery-specific considerations. The preoperative evaluation aims at cardiac risk stratification and treatment strategies to reduce the patient's risk of cardiac events.[75]

Patients with a history of pulmonary insufficiency require preoperative pulmonary function testing, and those who smoke should be encouraged to stop smoking before surgery. Some patients with severe bronchospastic pulmonary disease should be optimized with bronchodilator therapy or steroids prior to open AAA repair.

In patients with a history of stroke or transient ischemic attack or in the presence of a carotid bruit, a carotid duplex scan should be performed. If a high-grade stenosis is found in the internal carotid artery, carotid revascularization should precede elective AAA repair.

Procedural Considerations

Juan Parodi reported the first endoluminal repair of an AAA in 1991.[79] Since then, numerous endoluminal devices have been tested in clinical trials.[55,59,61–64,80–83] Endovascular repair of AAA has been shown to reduce operative morbidity, mortality, length of hospital stay, and postprocedure disability. Two randomized trials, EVAR-1 and DREAM trials, demonstrated a significantly lower mortality for EVAR when compared to open repair, but a higher reintervention requirement for EVAR.[62,63] To date, open repair has proven to be more durable and requires less follow-up than endoluminal repair. Conrad et al. reported on a large series of patients undergoing open AAA repair, with an excellent 10 year survival for patients less than 75 years of age. In addition, the freedom from graft-related reintervention is superior to EVAR.[84] A large series published by Hertzer et al. also showed a low 30-day mortality and excellent long-term survival with open AAA repair.[57]

One issue for today's vascular surgeons is the fact that with better endovascular devices, fewer open infrarenal AAAs are being performed each year. From 2001 to 2005, the mean volume of elective open infrarenal AAA repairs declined by 27%. During that same period, EVAR procedures increased by 212% for vascular surgery trainees. Dillavou et al. reviewed a sample of Medicare's inpatient database from 2000 to 2003 and found a significant increase nationwide in EVAR for elective repair of AAA and during that same period, a concomitant decrease in operative mortality from 5.0% to 3.7%.[85] In a review of the New York statewide discharge database, Anderson et al. found a similar dramatic increase in EVAR for elective AAA repair and an associated decrease in operative mortality.[60] Similarly, large referral centers report

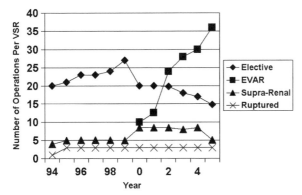

Modified from Cronenwett J. Sem Vasc Surg 2006; 187-190.

Fig. 1 Treatment of abdominal aortic experience of vascular surgery residents in the United States from 1994 to 2005

over 80% use of EVAR in elective AAA repair. In 2005, 70% of all elective infrarenal AAAs performed by vascular surgery trainees were endovascular techniques. During the same period, the number of open ruptured repairs and elective suprarenal AAA repairs has remained constant, although the numbers have been low (Fig. 1). This has created a challenge for vascular surgery residents to achieve the necessary skills to perform complex aortic surgery.[86]

Technical Considerations

Once a patient has been deemed medically suitable for open surgery, the specific approach and operation is individualized based on several factors. The most critical is the CT scan evaluation of the shape and configuration of the aneurysm. The infrarenal neck, the portion of the aorta immediately below the renal arteries, along with the iliac arteries must be assessed. If the iliac arteries have significant occlusive disease, the graft may have to be anastomosed to the femoral arteries. The presence of severe COPD is important because a laparotomy may not be well tolerated in these patients. The history of previous abdominal surgeries will also determine which approach is utilized. The two most frequently used approaches for AAA repair are the left retroperitoneal and the midline transperitoneal. A transverse incision has also been described, especially for patients with multiple upper abdominal surgeries (Fig. 2).

For a transperitoneal exposure, the patient is placed in a supine position and prepped and draped from his nipples to his knees. A long midline incision is made extending from a patient's xiphoid to pubis to provide maximal exposure for an infrarenal repair. After entering the abdominal cavity, a full exploration of the abdominal contents should occur to rule out other intra-abdominal pathology that might have not been visible in the CT scan. If an unexpected lesion is discovered, it must be evaluated and a surgeon must make a judgment as to how best to proceed. Our group and others strongly discourage combining a sterile vascular case with a potentially contaminated gastrointestinal case.

The next step is to retract superiorly the greater omentum and transverse colon. The small bowel is eviscerated to the right side of the abdomen. This exposes the base of the mesenteries of the left colon and the small intestine (Fig. 3).

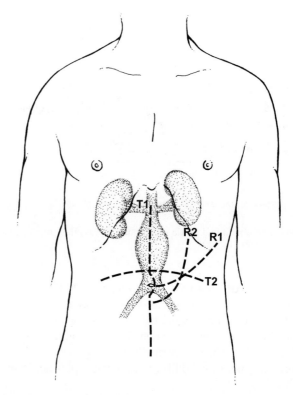

Fig. 2 Three most commonly used incisions for open repair of infrarenal abdominal aortic aneurysm: transabdominal midline (T1), transabdominal transverse (T2), and retroperitoneal (R1)

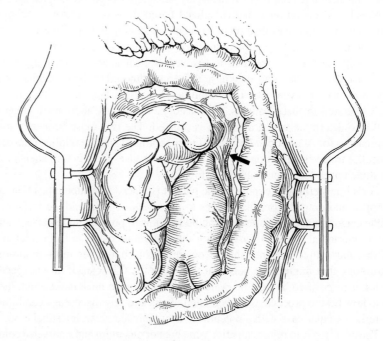

Fig. 3 Midline transabdominal exposure of infrarenal abdominal aortic aneurysm (*AAA*). Note inferior mesenteric vein (*arrow*)

The posterior peritoneum is then incised from the ligament of Treitz to the aortic bifurcation, thus exposing the infrarenal aorta (Fig. 4). The posterior peritoneum should be incised just to the right of the inferior mesenteric vein until the left renal vein crossing over the neck of the AAA is identified (Fig. 5a). In rare occasions of juxtarenal aneurysm, the left renal vein can be divided close to the IVC and ligated or reanastomosed if indicated. If the left renal vein is divided, it is important to preserve the left gonadal and adrenal vein to preserve left renal function. In cases in which the CT scan demonstrates a wide infrarenal neck, our group prefers the left retroperitoneal approach with elevation of the left kidney which provides excellent exposure of the juxta- and suprarenal aorta for appropriate cross-clamping without the need to divide the left renal vein (Fig. 6). The use of self-retaining retractors should be employed to aid in the exposure of the operative field. Distally, the iliac arteries must be exposed for cross-clamping. If

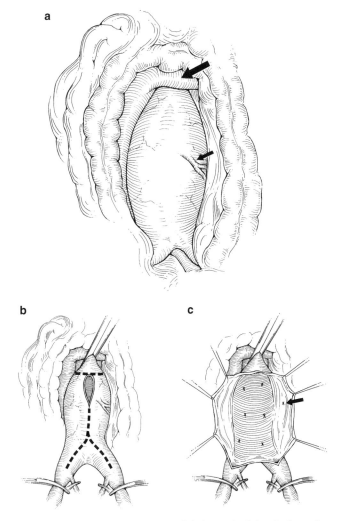

Fig. 4 Midline transabdominal exposure of infrarenal abdominal aortic aneurysm (*AAA*); (**a**) note left renal vein (*large arrow*) and inferior mesenteric artery (*small arrow*), (**b**) opening aortic aneurysm sac postdistal and proximal clamp, (**c**) endoluminal oversewing of bleeding lumbar arteries and inferior mesenteric artery (*arrow*)

a

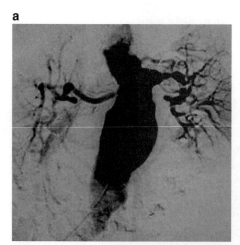

b

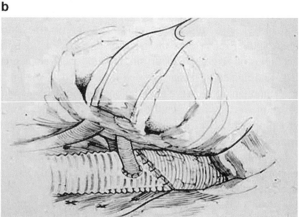

c

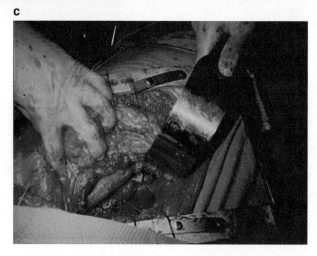

Fig. 5 (**a**) Abdominal aortic aneurysm (*AAA*) involving left renal artery treated via retroperitoneal approach. (**b**) Retroperitoneal exposure with superior displacement, left kidney, and renal artery reimplantation. (**c**) Intraoperative picture demonstrating retroperitoneal exposure with completed aortic graft and reimplantation of left renal artery (*See Color Plates*)

the aneurysm involves one or both iliacs, the dissection must be extended to the bifurcation of the common iliac(s), assuring identification of ureters and parasympathetic pudendal fibers. Usually circumferential aortic or iliac dissection is not necessary and may avoid venous injuries.

Throughout the operation, active communication should take place between the surgical and the anesthesia teams. Once the dissection is complete, the anesthesia team should give 60–80 U/kg of intravenous heparin and then be notified that aortic and iliac clamps will be applied shortly. Clamp placement should begin with the distal vessels and then the aorta, to prevent or reduce the risk of distal embolization. The aneurysm sac is then opened longitudinally and the mural thrombus should be removed. Any back bleeding from lumbar arteries or the IMA can be controlled with silk suture ligatures from within the aneurysm sac (Fig. 5b and c). If extraluminal control of the IMA is attempted,

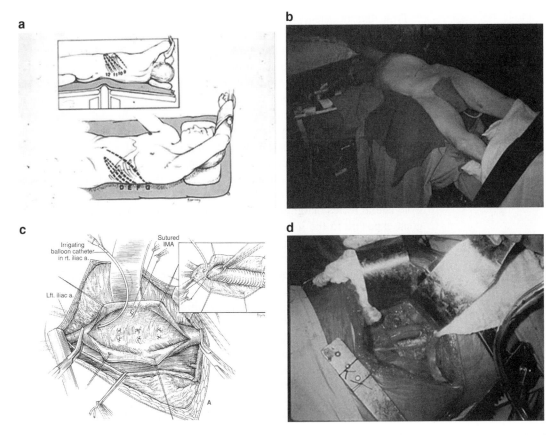

Fig. 6 Retroperitoneal approach to aortic pathology. (**a**) Various incisions based on body habitus and proximal extent of aortic pathology. (**b**) Patient position for retroperitoneal aortic exposure. (**c**) Drawing of retroperitoneal exposure for infrarenal AAA repair. (**d**) Intraoperative view of infrarenal AAA repair with tube graft (*See Color Plates*)

inadvertent ligation of marginal or sacral branches may also be divided, thus decreasing sigmoid perfusion.

If the aneurysm has an adequate infrarenal neck and no involvement of the iliac vessels, a tube graft can be used. If, however, the iliac arteries are aneurysmal, a bifurcated graft should be used and the distal limbs should be anastomosed end-to-end to the distal common iliac arteries preserving hypogastric flow. If more extensive iliac disease is present, one of the limbs can be anastomosed end-to-side to the external iliac artery and the common iliac artery can be oversewn at the level of the iliac bifurcation, attempting to preserve hypogastric perfusion. If severe bilateral iliac disease is present, the limbs of the graft can be sewn to the common femoral arteries, oversewing the distal common iliac artery/ies to preserve hypogastric flow. The femoral arteries should be preferably avoided as the distal anastomotic sites to decrease the risk of wound and graft infection.

Prior to removing all the clamps, it is important to back bleed the iliac system and flush any residual or remaining debris out of the graft. The graft should then be filled with diluted heparinized saline solution. After hemostasis is achieved, distal pulses should be assessed prior to beginning the closure.

Typically, the aneurysm sac and then separately the posterior peritoneum are closed over the graft in an effort to prevent intestinal contact with the aortic graft. The abdomen wall is then closed.

The transperitoneal approach affords the most flexibility for exposure of the aneurysm, the renal arteries, both iliac arteries, and both femoral arteries. This approach can be challenging in a patient who has undergone multiple prior abdominal surgeries and has a great deal of adhesions. In addition, juxta- or suprarenal extension, the presence of ascities, or inflammatory aneurysm can be challenging with the transabdominal approach.

Some surgeons prefer a retroperitoneal approach for repairing AAAs. The aorta is a retroperitoneal structure and avoiding the intraperitoneal contents is preferable in certain circumstances. A left-sided retroperitoneal incision from lateral rectus margin through the 11th or 12th intercostal space provides great exposure to the infrarenal juxta- and suprarenal portions of the aorta. A surgeon using this approach is limited in the exposure to the right renal artery, the right distal common iliac artery, and partially the right femoral artery. In addition, intra-abdominal pathology may be missed because the peritoneum is not entered, although the preoperative evaluation and imaging should detect the greatest majority of significant intra-abdominal pathology. The relative indications for a retroperitoneal approach are a "hostile" abdomen secondary to multiple previous abdominal surgeries and adhesions, previous radiation therapy, abdominal wall stoma, a horseshoe kidney, or the need to extend the repair above the renal arteries.

For a retroperitoneal incision, a vacuum-assisted beanbag is placed on the operating room table. After induction of general anesthesia and placement of all of the required monitors, the patient is positioned in the right decubitus position with the kidney rest of the bed between the top of the iliac crest and the costal margin. The patient is the placed in approximately 45° of right lateral decubitus with his left arm padded on an arm support. Slightly more tilt of the upper portion of the patient and slightly less rotation of the hips allow for easier access to the right groin if it is needed. The kidney rest is elevated, the bed is flexed, and the suction is applied to the beanbag to maintain this desired position. Positioning is key, and improper positioning will lead to less than ideal exposure.

The precise location of the incision depends on what procedure is planned. For an infrarenal or aortoiliac exposure, the surgeon should make an incision medial but at the level on the umbilicus just lateral to the medial border of the rectus abdominus muscle. Based on the patient's size and body habitus, the incision should be extended in a curvilinear fashion superiorly and posteriorly to either the 12th rib or the interspace between the 11th and 12th ribs. The abdominal wall muscles can be divided using electrocautery, although every effort should be made to preserve the left rectus. The retroperitoneal space is entered at the junction of the left rectus abdominus muscle and the lateral abdominal wall muscles by dividing the transversalis fascia and mobilizing the peritoneum medially and superiorly. These moves allow for the exposure of the aorta from the renal arteries to the left external iliac artery and the right common iliac artery (Fig. 7).

The peritoneum is mobilized even further anteriorly until the left ureter and left gonadal vein are identified. The left ureter is then dissected and mobilized from the level of the renal pelvis down to the iliac artery bifurcation,

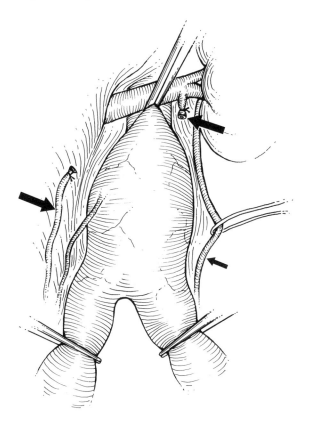

Fig. 7 Drawing of retroperitoneal exposure of large infrarenal abdominal aortic aneurysm (*AAA*). Note lateral mobilization of left ureter (*small arrow*) and ligation of left gonadal vein (*large arrow*)

looped with a vessel loop, and gently retracted medially to avoid an avulsion or traction injury. Care must also be taken not to devascularize the ureter, which can also lead to an ischemic injury. The gonadal vein is then dissected up to its insertion into the left renal vein. The gonadal vein is ligated and divided at the level of the left renal vein to allow for needed infrarenal exposure of the neck of the AAA (Fig. 8). Failure to ligate the gonadal vein can lead to avulsion injuries and further bleeding. Another step that is crucial is entering the avascular space between the peritoneum and the left kidney, which allows better exposure of the juxtarenal aorta and the left renal vein. Mobilization of Gerota's fascia circumferentially is indicated if suprarenal cross-clamping is needed since the left kidney will descend after circumferential mobilization, exposing the left diaphragmatic crus, which if divided gives full access to the suprarenal aorta.

In most cases, both common iliac arteries can be dissected to allow for clamp placement. If the right common iliac artery is involved with aneurysmal dilatation with a balloon catheter, intraluminal control of the right iliac system can be accomplished (Fig. 9).

The use of self-retaining retractors facilitates exposure and avoids unnecessary trauma to intra-abdominal organs, especially the spleen that may occur with hand retraction.

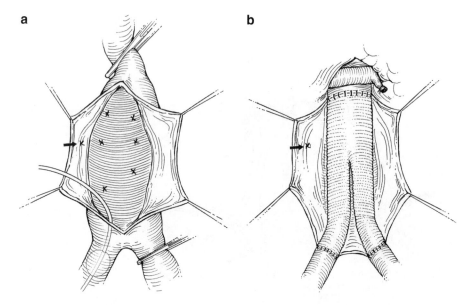

Fig. 8 Retroperitoneal exposure of abdominal aortic aneurysm (*AAA*) with balloon occlusion of right iliac artery. Note inferior mesenteric artery sutured from within the AAA sac (*arrow*)

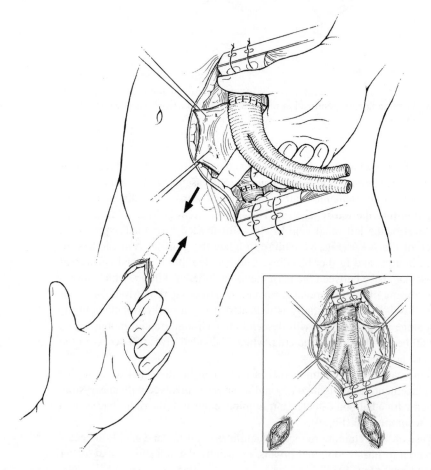

Fig. 9 Retroperitoneal exposure for AAA repair requiring aortobifemoral bypass. Tunnel to pass right limb must be posterior to ureter (*arrows*)

The clamping sequence is the same as for a transperitoneal approach, the iliac arteries first, and then the proximal aortic clamp is applied. The aneurysm sac is opened and the intramural thrombus is removed. Any back bleeding lumbar vessel, along with the IMA, is oversewn. If the right iliac system cannot be controlled with a clamp, a number 6 or 9 Pruitt-type balloon occlusion–irrigation catheter can be inserted into the right common iliac orifice. Based on a patient's AAA, either a tube graft or a bifurcated aortobi-iliac graft can be sewn into place. If an aortobifemoral bypass is required, we prefer to suture the common iliac arteries from within the aneurysm sac. We complete the aortic anastomosis and then rotate the table to provide better access to both groins. A careful tunnel is made with blunt finger dissection right on top of the iliac arteries and ureters from above and on top of the femoral arteries from below. It is critical to ensure that both femoral limbs are passed posterior to the patient's ureters to avoid ureteral injury or compression (Fig. 10). The femoral anastomoses are usually performed in a standard end-to-side fashion.

Once hemostasis has been achieved, the aneurysm sac is closed over the graft, if possible, and the abdominal lateral wall muscle and fascia are closed in two layers.

The two principal complications from this approach are wound bulges or hernias and chronic incisional pain. Our group did not find a significant difference in bulges or hernias when we looked at transperitoneal versus retroperitoneal approaches for AAA repair. Others have found differences, however. La Croix reported on a large series and found that only 5% had an incisional hernia, but 28% had a 2 cm or larger incision bulge.[87] Our group looked at more than 1000 patients who underwent retroperitoneal approaches for AAA. Many described some level of incisional pain that ultimately resolved after 12 to 24 months, but fewer than 1% required nerve blocks to relieve the pain.[88]

Is one approach better than the other? Many have advocated that a left retroperitoneal approach is more advantageous in patients with a gastrointestinal or urological stoma. There have also been studies that have shown that ileus, pulmonary complications, and fluid requirements are decreased with this approach.[88] Our group reported lower incidence of small bowel obstruction or prolonged ileus, along with overall better outcomes with retroperitoneal approaches to AAA repairs as compared with transperitoneal techniques.[88] Cambria et al. found no statistical difference in pulmonary complications, fluid or blood requirements, or other postoperative complications, except a slightly prolonged return to oral intake after the transperitoneal approach.[89] This study relied significantly on epidural analgesia that may decrease postoperative pulmonary complication. Another study by Quinones-Baldrich et al. in 1999 found no statistical difference in mortality between transperitoneal and retroperitoneal approaches. The study did find more pulmonary complications with the transperitoneal approach but more wound problems with the retroperitoneal approach.[90] One other study by Sieunarine et al. found no difference in operating time, cross-clamp time, blood loss, fluid replacement, analgesia requirement, gastrointestinal function, intensive care, or hospital stay looking at both approaches. In their long-term follow-up, there were significantly more wound problems such as hernias or pain in the retroperitoneal group.[91] The bottom line is that there is no clear-cut approach that is superior and thus, it is a matter of personal preference and experience.

Postoperative Complications

The open repair regardless of the approach does have its share of associated complications. Most patients are followed immediately postoperatively in a surgical intensive care unit, with dedicated intensivists. Some patients will require some period of continued mechanical ventilation while they are rewarmed and associated coagulopathies are corrected. Close monitoring is also vital to monitor hemodynamic responses, fluid shifts, and pain control. Patients should have full-laboratory values checked immediately postoperatively. In addition, they should have a chest x-ray and an ECG performed, and the patients should be maintained on their β-blockers. The perioperative complications from open AAA repairs can be either due to graft problems, such as bleeding, embolization. thrombosis, or kinking, or due to organ system problems.

The most common organ complication is cardiac, in nature, and have been reported to as high as 15%, including arrhythmia, infarction, and congestive heart failure. In one series by Ali et al. looking at 43 consecutive patients who underwent elective open AAA repairs found that 47% had troponin elevations postoperative, although only 26% met the criteria for a myocardial infarction.[92] Another study by Elkouri et al. reported on a large series of patients undergoing elective AAA repair and found cardiac complications in 22%.[93]

Pulmonary complications have also been observed and chronic ventilator dependence or pneumonias have also been seen. Elkouri et al. also reported that 16% of their patients had pulmonary complications.[93] A large series by Hertzer et al. at the Cleveland Clinic reported only 4.2% of their patients developing pulmonary complications, with the majority having pneumonia, although 1% developed adult respiratory distress syndrome.[57] Early extubation and aggressive pulmonary toilet and early ambulation can aid in preventing pulmonary complications.

Perioperative renal failure also predicts a worse outcome. Preoperative renal dysfunction is the greatest predictor of perioperative or postoperative renal complications.[94,95] Care must be taken to ensure adequate kidney perfusion to reduce this complication. Intraoperative techniques, such as careful clamp placement to avoid renal embolization and flushing the proximal anastomosis, will help. If flow to a kidney is halted for more than 30 min, iced heparinized saline can be flushed in the renal artery, but more practically, topical packing of the kidney with ice can help preserve renal function.

Perioperative procedure-related complications include renal and lower extremity embolization, iatrogenic injuries, hemorrhage, and colonic ischemia. Aggressive correction of a patient's coagulation parameters along with rewarming and maintenance of normothermia are key moves early in the postoperative period. Intraoperative or postoperative hemorrhage usually results from technical problems with the proximal anastomosis or a missed arterial or venous injury. Proximal suture line bleeding, especially along the back wall of the aorta, can be difficult to deal with. Interrupted sutures with felted pledgets can sometimes be useful. Others empirically use an entire piece of felted pledget for the back wall of suture line. Venous bleeding is usually due to an iliac or renal vein injury during the initial exposure or clamp injury. In fact, some advocate that there is no need for circumferential dissection of the iliac vessels because the arteries can be adherent to the veins.

Injuries to adjacent organs have also been described. Ureteral injury is rare, although if it occurs, it should be repaired at the time of discovery, over a double J stent using interrupted absorbable sutures. The spleen is another organ that is often injured, usually because of retraction. The treatment for a fractured spleen, especially in the face of an ongoing coagulopathy, is a splenectomy. Inadvertent enterotomies during the initial opening should be repaired and the AAA portion should be aborted. Another problem that can occur, as with any wound closure, is the inadvertent capture of a piece of small or large intestine in the closure. This could lead to a fistula, an obstruction, or a bowel ischemia.

Colonic ischemia after AAA repair is rare, but it can be deadly and a high index of suspicion is required. A patient with an unexplained leukocytosis, fever, and or left lower quadrant pain as well as one with bloody rectal discharge should be urgently evaluated for colonic ischemia with a flexible sigmoidoscopy or colonoscopy. A study by Brandt et al. in 1997 reported that flexible sigmoidoscopy reliably predicts full-thickness colonic ischemia for AAA repair. Patients with nonconfluent ischemia limited to the mucosa can be safely followed by serial endoscopic examinations.[96] Boley and coworkers have described three forms of ischemic colitis. In the mild version, which affects about 50% of the patients who underwent AAA repair, the ischemia is limited to the colonic mucosa and submucosa. Patients may have symptoms of abdominal pain, ileus, distention, or bloody diarrhea, but the disease process is self-limited and resolves with adequate resuscitation. A more progressive form involves ischemia of the muscularis and may lead to stricture formation. The most catastrophic and concerning form of colonic ischemia affects less than 20% of the patients. Transmural ischemia and colonic infarction are present with free or contained colonic perforation being present. This necessitates a return to the operating room for a washout of the contamination, along with a Hartmann's procedure and a colostomy. Concern here is also for graft infection.[97,98] The overall incidence of clinically relevant ischemia has been reported to be 1–3% after elective AAA repairs, and much higher after ruptured AAA repairs.[99–104] Another study of 105 patients undergoing flexible sigmoidoscopy found colonic ischemia in 11.4% of the patients.[105] The classic presentation of bloody diarrhea in the early postoperative period only occurs in about 30% of cases.[100]

AAA repair can alter sigmoid blood flow because ligation of the IMA or internal iliac artery, embolization of debris from the AAA, prolonged hypotension, or a retractor injury can affect the collateral branches to the colon. In patients undergoing an AAA repair, 50% have a patent IMA, which could be reimplanted or bypassed.[106] Most surgeons evaluate collateral colonic circulation by assessing the back bleeding of the IMA. Brisk back bleeding along with a normal looking colon typically would indicate to a surgeon that it is safe to ligate the IMA. Several studies have shown that IMA reimplantation did not influence postoperative colonic ischemia[103,104,107,108] but certainly was safe and may be advantageous in selected patients. Preoperative imaging by CT angiography can be useful in assessing the potential need to reimplant the IMA, especially if evidence of chronic mesenteric arterial obstruction is present.

One other complication, although usually more delayed, is sexual dysfunction as a result of injury to the autonomic nerves during the iliac dissection. It usually presents as erectile dysfunction or more frequently as retrograde ejaculation. Most men undergoing elective AAA repair have some component of this preoperatively. In the ADAM trial, 40% of men had impotence before AAA repair.[109] Being cautious when dissecting around the distal left side of the aorta, especially around the region of the IMA and the left common iliac artery, has been shown to reduce this complication substantially, which has been reported as high as 25%.[110,111] Another important component to preserved sexual function is preservation of at least one internal iliac artery with antegrade blood flow.

One other dreaded complication with a very high postoperative morbidity and mortality is spinal cord ischemia and paralysis. This is much more common after thoracoabdominal or suprarenal AAA repairs, rather than infrarenal AAA repairs, because the accessory spinal artery normally takes off the aorta in the chest or proximal abdominal aorta, although it has been reported. These reports have stressed the value of preserving pelvic collaterals and internal iliac arteries if at all possible. Occlusion or division of these vessels combined with periods of severe hypotension can lead to spinal cord ischemia and paralysis.[112]

Open infrarenal AAA repairs have been performed for over 50 years with significant improvement in clinical outcomes. This operation has proven to be extremely durable and safe, especially in centers that perform a high volume of these cases each year. Even with the increasing popularity, success, and durability of endovascular repairs, some patients will not have the correct anatomy for a stent graft and thus require an open operation. The knowledge and skill to perform an open infrarenal AAA is vital for today's vascular surgeon, regardless of which approach is used. Moreover, the knowledge about preoperative patient selection and optimization along with some of the pitfalls that can occur intraoperatively will further cut down a patient's perioperative morbidity and mortality. In addition, a keen eye to postoperative warning signs can potentially stave off major complications and improve long-term survival.

References

1. Johnston, K.W., et al. Suggested standards for reporting on arterial aneurysms. Subcommittee on Reporting Standards for Arterial Aneurysms, Ad Hoc Committee on Reporting Standards, Society for Vascular Surgery and North American Chapter, International Society for Cardiovascular Surgery. J Vasc Surg, 1991. 13(3):452–8.
2. Thompson, R.W., Basic science of abdominal aortic aneurysms: emerging therapeutic strategies for an unresolved clinical problem. Curr Opin Cardiol, 1996. 11(5): 504–18.
3. Thompson, R.W., et al. Production and localization of 92-kilodalton gelatinase in abdominal aortic aneurysms. An elastolytic metalloproteinase expressed by aneurysm-infiltrating macrophages. J Clin Invest, 1995. 96(1):318–26.
4. Thompson, R.W. and W.C. Parks, Role of matrix metalloproteinases in abdominal aortic aneurysms. Ann N Y Acad Sci, 1996. 800:157–74.
5. Curci, J.A., et al. Expression and localization of macrophage elastase (matrix metalloproteinase-12) in abdominal aortic aneurysms. J Clin Invest, 1998. 102(11): 1900–10.
6. Osler, W., Aneurysm of the Abdominal Aorta. Lancet, 1905. 2:1089.
7. Osler, W., Remarks on arterio-venous aneurysm. Lancet, 1915. 2(949).
8. Leonardo, R., History of Surgery. 1943, New York: Froben Press.

9. Matas, R., Aneurysm of the abdominal aorta at its bifurcation into the common iliac arteries: A pictorial supplement illustrating the history of corinne D. Previously reported as the first recorded instance of cure of an aneurysm of the abdominal aorta by ligation. Ann Surg, 1940. 112(5):909–22.

10. Power, D., The palliative treatment of aneurysms by wiring with Colt's apparatus. Br J Surg, 1921. 9(27).

11. Pearse, H.E., Experimental studies on the gradual occlusion of large arteries. Ann Surg, 1940. 112(5):923–37.

12. Harrison, P.W. and J. Chandy, A subclavian aneurysm cured by cellophane fibrosis. Ann Surg, 1943. 118(3):478–81.

13. Abbott, O.A., Clinical experiences with the application of polythene cellophane upon the aneurysms of the thoracic vessels. J Thorac Surg, 1949. 18(4):435–61.

14. Dente, C.J. and D.V. Feliciano, Alexis Carrel (1873–1944): Nobel Laureate, 1912. Arch Surg, 2005. 140(6):609–10.

15. Edwards, W., Alexis Carrel 1873–1944. Contemp Surg, 1979. 14:65–79.

16. Carrel, A., La technique operatoire des anastomoses vascularies et la transplation de viscere. Lyon Med, 1902. 98(859).

17. Carrel, A., Suture of blood vessels and transplantation of organs. Nobel Lecture, 1912, in Nobel Lectures in Physiology-Medicine. 1967, New York: Elsevier Publishing Company.

18. Dubost, C., M. Allary, and N. Oeconomos, Resection of an aneurysm of the abdominal aorta: reestablishment of the continuity by a preserved human arterial graft, with result after five months. AMA Arch Surg, 1952. 64(3):405–8.

19. DeBakey, M.E. and D.A. Cooley, Surgical treatment of aneurysm of abdominal aorta by resection and restoration of continuity with homograft. Surg Gynecol Obstet, 1953. 97:257–266.

20. Brock, R.C., C.G. Rob, and F. Forty, Discussion on reconstructive arterial surgery. Proc R Soc Med, 1953. 46(2):115–30.

21. Voorhees, A.B., Jr., A. Jaretzki, 3rd, and A.H. Blakemore, The use of tubes constructed from vinyon "N" cloth in bridging arterial defects. Ann Surg, 1952. 135(3):332–6.

22. Friedman, S., A History of Vascular Surgery. 1989, Mt Kisco, NY: Futura.

23. Levin, S.M., Reminiscences and ruminations: vascular surgery then and now. Am J Surg, 1987. 154(2):158–62.

24. Blakemore, A.H. and A.B. Voorhees, Jr., The use of tubes constructed from vinyon N cloth in bridging arterial defects; experimental and clinical. Ann Surg, 1954. 140(3):324–34.

25. De Bakey, M.E., et al. Clinical application of a new flexible knitted dacron arterial substitute. AMA Arch Surg, 1958. 77(5):713–24.

26. Katz, D.J., J.C. Stanley, and G.B. Zelenock, Operative mortality rates for intact and ruptured abdominal aortic aneurysms in Michigan: an eleven-year statewide experience. J Vasc Surg, 1994. 19(5):804–15; discussion 816–7.

27. LaMorte, W.W., T.E. Scott, and J.O. Menzoian, Racial differences in the incidence of femoral bypass and abdominal aortic aneurysmectomy in Massachusetts: relationship to cardiovascular risk factors. J Vasc Surg, 1995. 21(3):422–31.

28. Blanchard, J.F., Epidemiology of abdominal aortic aneurysms. Epidemiol Rev, 1999. 21(2):207–21.

29. Wilmink, A.B., et al. The incidence of small abdominal aortic aneurysms and the change in normal infrarenal aortic diameter: implications for screening. Eur J Vasc Endovasc Surg, 2001. 21(2):165–70.

30. Lederle, F.A., et al. Yield of repeated screening for abdominal aortic aneurysm after a 4-year interval. Aneurysm Detection and Management Veterans Affairs Cooperative Study Investigators. Arch Intern Med, 2000. 160(8):1117–21.

31. Melton, L.J., 3rd, et al. *Changing incidence of abdominal aortic aneurysms: a population-based study.* Am J Epidemiol, 1984. 120(3):379–86.

32. McFarlane, M.J., The epidemiologic necropsy for abdominal aortic aneurysm. JAMA, 1991. 265(16):2085–8.

33. Bengtsson, H., D. Bergqvist, and N.H. Sternby, Increasing prevalence of abdominal aortic aneurysms. A necropsy study. Eur J Surg, 1992. 158(1):19–23.

34. Verloes, A., et al. Aneurysms of the abdominal aorta: familial and genetic aspects in three hundred thirteen pedigrees. J Vasc Surg, 1995. 21(4):646–55.

35. Johansen, K. and T. Koepsell, Familial tendency for abdominal aortic aneurysms. JAMA, 1986. 256(14):1934–6.

36. Darling, R.C., 3rd, et al. Are familial abdominal aortic aneurysms different? J Vasc Surg, 1989. 10(1):39–43.

37. Pasch, A.R., et al. Abdominal aortic aneurysm: the case for elective resection. Circulation, 1984. 70(3 Pt 2):I1–4.

38. Breckwoldt, W.L., W.C. Mackey, and T.F. O'Donnell, Jr., The economic implications of high-risk abdominal aortic aneurysms. J Vasc Surg, 1991. 13(6):798–803; discussion 803–4.

39. Cota, A.M., et al. Elective versus ruptured abdominal aortic aneurysm repair: a 1-year cost-effectiveness analysis. Ann Vasc Surg, 2005. 19(6):858–61.

40. Schermerhorn, M., et al. Ultrasound screening for abdominal aortic aneurysm in medicare beneficiaries. Ann Vasc Surg, 2008. 22(1):16–24.

41. Derubertis, B.G., et al. Abdominal aortic aneurysm in women: prevalence, risk factors, and implications for screening. J Vasc Surg, 2007. 46(4):630–635.

42. Bengtsson, H., et al. A population based screening of abdominal aortic aneurysms (AAA). Eur J Vasc Surg, 1991. 5(1):53–7.

43. Lindholt, J.S., et al. Mass or high-risk screening for abdominal aortic aneurysm. Br J Surg, 1997. 84(1):40–2.

44. Morris, G.E., C.S. Hubbard, and C.R. Quick, An abdominal aortic aneurysm screening programme for all males over the age of 50 years. Eur J Vasc Surg, 1994. 8(2):156–60.

45. Scott, R.A., H.A. Ashton, and D.N. Kay, Abdominal aortic aneurysm in 4237 screened patients: prevalence, development and management over 6 years. Br J Surg, 1991. 78(9):1122–5.

46. Scott, R.A., S.G. Bridgewater, and H.A. Ashton, Randomized clinical trial of screening for abdominal aortic aneurysm in women. Br J Surg, 2002. 89(3):283–5.

47. Vardulaki, K.A., et al. Late results concerning feasibility and compliance from a randomized trial of ultrasonographic screening for abdominal aortic aneurysm. Br J Surg, 2002. 89(7):861–4.

48. Lindholt, J.S., et al. Hospital costs and benefits of screening for abdominal aortic aneurysms. Results from a randomised population screening trial. Eur J Vasc Endovasc Surg, 2002. 23(1):55–60.

49. Heather, B.P., et al. Population screening reduces mortality rate from aortic aneurysm in men. Br J Surg, 2000. 87(6):750–3.

50. Ashton, H.A., et al. The Multicentre Aneurysm Screening Study (MASS) into the effect of abdominal aortic aneurysm screening on mortality in men: a randomised controlled trial. Lancet, 2002. 360(9345):1531–9.

51. Kim, L.G., et al. A sustained mortality benefit from screening for abdominal aortic aneurysm. Ann Intern Med, 2007. 146(10):699–706.

52. Lederle, F.A., et al. Immediate repair compared with surveillance of small abdominal aortic aneurysms. N Engl J Med, 2002. 346(19):1437–44.

53. Powell, J.T., et al. Final 12-year follow-up of surgery versus surveillance in the UK Small Aneurysm Trial. Br J Surg, 2007. 94(6):702–8.

54. Heller, J.A., et al. Two decades of abdominal aortic aneurysm repair: have we made any progress? J Vasc Surg, 2000. 32(6):1091–100.

55. Hua, H.T., et al. Early outcomes of endovascular versus open abdominal aortic aneurysm repair in the National Surgical Quality Improvement Program-Private Sector (NSQIP-PS). J Vasc Surg, 2005. 41(3):382–9.

56. Huber, T.S., et al. Experience in the United States with intact abdominal aortic aneurysm repair. J Vasc Surg, 2001. 33(2):304–10; discussion 310–1.

57. Hertzer, N.R., et al. Open infrarenal abdominal aortic aneurysm repair: the Cleveland Clinic experience from 1989 to 1998. J Vasc Surg, 2002. 35(6):1145–54.

58. Lee, W.A., et al. Perioperative outcomes after open and endovascular repair of intact abdominal aortic aneurysms in the United States during 2001. J Vasc Surg, 2004. 39(3):491–6.

59. Akkersdijk, G.J., M. Prinssen, and J.D. Blankensteijn, The impact of endovascular treatment on in-hospital mortality following non-ruptured AAA repair over a decade: a population based study of 16,446 patients. Eur J Vasc Endovasc Surg, 2004. 28(1):41–6.

60. Anderson, P.L., et al. A statewide experience with endovascular abdominal aortic aneurysm repair: rapid diffusion with excellent early results. J Vasc Surg, 2004. 39(1):10–9.

61. Bush, R.L., et al. Performance of endovascular aortic aneurysm repair in high-risk patients: results from the Veterans Affairs National Surgical Quality Improvement Program. J Vasc Surg, 2007. 45(2):227–233; discussion 233–5.

62. Blankensteijn, J.D., et al. Two-year outcomes after conventional or endovascular repair of abdominal aortic aneurysms. N Engl J Med, 2005. 352(23):2398–405.

63. Greenhalgh, R.M., et al. Comparison of endovascular aneurysm repair with open repair in patients with abdominal aortic aneurysm (EVAR trial 1), 30-day operative mortality results: randomised controlled trial. Lancet, 2004. 364(9437):843–8.

64. Sicard, G.A., et al. Endovascular abdominal aortic aneurysm repair: long-term outcome measures in patients at high-risk for open surgery. J Vasc Surg, 2006. 44(2):229–36.

65. Hirose, Y., S. Hamada, and M. Takamiya, Predicting the growth of aortic aneurysms: a comparison of linear vs exponential models. Angiology, 1995. 46(5):413–9.

66. Englund, R., et al. Expansion rates of small abdominal aortic aneurysms. Aust N Z J Surg, 1998. 68(1):21–4.

67. Bengtsson, H., et al. Ultrasound screening of the abdominal aorta in patients with intermittent claudication. Eur J Vasc Surg, 1989. 3(6):497–502.

68. Fillinger, M.F., et al. In vivo analysis of mechanical wall stress and abdominal aortic aneurysm rupture risk. J Vasc Surg, 2002. 36(3):589–97.

69. Fillinger, M.F., et al. Prediction of rupture risk in abdominal aortic aneurysm during observation: wall stress versus diameter. J Vasc Surg, 2003. 37(4):724–32.

70. Steyerberg, E.W., et al. Perioperative mortality of elective abdominal aortic aneurysm surgery. A clinical prediction rule based on literature and individual patient data. Arch Intern Med, 1995. 155(18):1998–2004.

71. Hallin, A., D. Bergqvist, and L. Holmberg, Literature review of surgical management of abdominal aortic aneurysm. Eur J Vasc Endovasc Surg, 2001. 22(3):197–204.

72. Dardik, A., et al. Results of elective abdominal aortic aneurysm repair in the 1990s: A population-based analysis of 2335 cases. J Vasc Surg, 1999. 30(6):985–95.

73. Dimick, J.B., et al. Surgeon specialty and provider volumes are related to outcome of intact abdominal aortic aneurysm repair in the United States. J Vasc Surg, 2003. 38(4):739–44.

74. Roger, V.L., et al. Influence of coronary artery disease on morbidity and mortality after abdominal aortic aneurysmectomy: a population-based study, 1971–1987. J Am Coll Cardiol, 1989. 14(5):1245–52.

75. Fleisher, L.A., et al. ACC/AHA 2007 guidelines on perioperative cardiovascular evaluation and care for noncardiac surgery: a report of the American College of Cardiology/American Heart Association Task Force on Practice Guidelines (Writing Committee to Revise the 2002 Guidelines on Perioperative Cardiovascular Evaluation for Noncardiac Surgery): developed in collaboration with the American Society of

Echocardiography, American Society of Nuclear Cardiology, Heart Rhythm Society, Society of Cardiovascular Anesthesiologists, Society for Cardiovascular Angiography and Interventions, Society for Vascular Medicine and Biology, and Society for Vascular Surgery. Circulation, 2007. 116(17):e418–99.

76. Van Damme, H., et al. Cardiac risk assessment before vascular surgery: a prospective study comparing clinical evaluation, dobutamine stress echocardiography, and dobutamine Tc-99m sestamibi tomoscintigraphy. Cardiovasc Surg, 1997. 5(1):54–64.

77. Poldermans, D., et al. Should major vascular surgery be delayed because of preoperative cardiac testing in intermediate-risk patients receiving beta-blocker therapy with tight heart rate control? J Am Coll Cardiol, 2006. 48(5):964–9.

78. Poldermans, D., et al. A clinical randomized trial to evaluate the safety of a noninvasive approach in high-risk patients undergoing major vascular surgery: the DECREASE-V Pilot Study. J Am Coll Cardiol, 2007. 49(17):1763–9.

79. Parodi, J.C., J.C. Palmaz, and H.D. Barone, Transfemoral intraluminal graft implantation for abdominal aortic aneurysms. Ann Vasc Surg, 1991. 5(6):491–9.

80. Zarins, C.K., et al. AneuRx stent graft versus open surgical repair of abdominal aortic aneurysms: multicenter prospective clinical trial. J Vasc Surg, 1999. 29(2): 292–305; discussion 306–8.

81. EVAR Trial Participants. Endovascular aneurysm repair and outcome in patients unfit for open repair of abdominal aortic aneurysm (EVAR trial 2): randomised controlled trial. Lancet, 2005. 365(9478):2187–92.

82. Lifeline registry of EVAR Publications Committee. Endovascular aneurysm repair: long-term primary outcome measures. J Vasc Surg, 2005. 42(1):1–10.

83. Brewster, D.C., et al. Initial experience with endovascular aneurysm repair: comparison of early results with outcome of conventional open repair. J Vasc Surg, 1998. 27(6):992–1003; discussion 1004–5.

84. Conrad, M.F., et al. Long-term durability of open abdominal aortic aneurysm repair. J Vasc Surg, 2007. 46(4):669–75.

85. Dillavou, E.D., S.C. Muluk, and M.S. Makaroun, Improving aneurysm-related outcomes: nationwide benefits of endovascular repair. J Vasc Surg, 2006. 43(3): 446–51; discussion 451–2.

86. Cronenwett, J.L., Vascular surgery training: is there enough case material? Semin Vasc Surg, 2006. 19(4):187–90.

87. LaCroix, H., The optimal surgical approach for elective reconstruction of the infra- and juxtarenal abdominal aorta: a randomized prospective study. ACTA Biomed Lovaniensia, 1997. 157(1–131).

88. Sicard, G.A., et al. Transabdominal versus retroperitoneal incision for abdominal aortic surgery: report of a prospective randomized trial. J Vasc Surg, 1995. 21(2): 174–81; discussion 181–3.

89. Cambria, R.P., et al. Transperitoneal versus retroperitoneal approach for aortic reconstruction: a randomized prospective study. J Vasc Surg, 1990. 11(2):314–24; discussion 324–5.

90. Quinones-Baldrich, W.J., et al. Endovascular, transperitoneal, and retroperitoneal abdominal aortic aneurysm repair: results and costs. J Vasc Surg, 1999. 30(1): 59–67.

91. Sieunarine, K., M.M. Lawrence-Brown, and M.A. Goodman, *Comparison of transperitoneal and retroperitoneal approaches for infrarenal aortic surgery: early and late results.* Cardiovasc Surg, 1997. 5(1):71–6.

92. Ali, Z.A., et al. *Perioperative myocardial injury after elective open abdominal aortic aneurysm repair predicts outcome.* Eur J Vasc Endovasc Surg, 2008. 35(4):413–419.

93. Elkouri, S., et al. *Perioperative complications and early outcome after endovascular and open surgical repair of abdominal aortic aneurysms.* J Vasc Surg, 2004. 39(3):497–505.

94. Miller, D.C. and B.D. Myers, *Pathophysiology and prevention of acute renal failure associated with thoracoabdominal or abdominal aortic surgery.* J Vasc Surg, 1987. 5(3):518–23.

95. West, C.A., et al. *Factors affecting outcomes of open surgical repair of pararenal aortic aneurysms: a 10-year experience.* J Vasc Surg, 2006. 43(5):921–7; discussion 927–8.

96. Brandt, C.P., J.J. Piotrowski, and J.J. Alexander, *Flexible sigmoidoscopy. A reliable determinant of colonic ischemia following ruptured abdominal aortic aneurysm.* Surg Endosc, 1997. 11(2):113–5.

97. Boley, S.J., L.J. Brandt, and F.J. Veith, *Ischemic disorders of the intestines.* Curr Probl Surg, 1978. 15(4):1–85.

98. Boley, S.J., *1989 David H. Sun lecture. Colonic ischemia – 25 years later.* Am J Gastroenterol, 1990. 85(8):931–4.

99. Brewster, D.C., et al. *Intestinal ischemia complicating abdominal aortic surgery.* Surgery, 1991. 109(4):447–54.

100. Bjorck, M., D. Bergqvist, and T. Troeng, *Incidence and clinical presentation of bowel ischaemia after aortoiliac surgery – 2930 operations from a population-based registry in Sweden.* Eur J Vasc Endovasc Surg, 1996. 12(2):139–44.

101. Longo, W.E., et al. *Ischemic colitis complicating abdominal aortic aneurysm surgery in the U.S. veteran.* J Surg Res, 1996. 60(2):351–4.

102. Levison, J.A., et al. *Perioperative predictors of colonic ischemia after ruptured abdominal aortic aneurysm.* J Vasc Surg, 1999. 29(1):40–5; discussion 45–7.

103. Pittaluga, P., et al. *Revascularization of internal iliac arteries during aortoiliac surgery: a multicenter study.* Ann Vasc Surg, 1998. 12(6):537–43.

104. Van Damme, H., E. Creemers, and R. Limet, *Ischaemic colitis following aortoiliac surgery.* Acta Chir Belg, 2000. 100(1):21–7.

105. Bast, T.J., et al. *Ischaemic disease of the colon and rectum after surgery for abdominal aortic aneurysm: a prospective study of the incidence and risk factors.* Eur J Vasc Surg, 1990. 4(3):253–7.

106. Batt, M., J.B. Ricco, and P. Staccini, *Do internal iliac arteries contribute to vascularization of the descending colon during abdominal aortic aneurysm surgery? An intraoperative hemodynamic study.* Ann Vasc Surg, 2001. 15(2):171–4.

107. Kuttila, K., et al. *Tonometric assessment of sigmoid perfusion during aortobifemoral reconstruction for arteriosclerosis.* Eur J Surg, 1994. 160(9):491–5.

108. Schiedler, M.G., B.S. Cutler, and R.G. Fiddian-Green, *Sigmoid intramural pH for prediction of ischemic colitis during aortic surgery. A comparison with risk factors and inferior mesenteric artery stump pressures.* Arch Surg, 1987. 122(8):881–6.

109. Lederle, F.A., et al. *Quality of life, impotence, and activity level in a randomized trial of immediate repair versus surveillance of small abdominal aortic aneurysm.* J Vasc Surg, 2003. 38(4):745–52.

110. Flanigan, D.P., et al. *Elimination of iatrogenic impotence and improvement of sexual function after aortoiliac revascularization.* Arch Surg, 1982. 117(5):544–50.

111. Weinstein, M.H. and H.I. Machleder, *Sexual function after aorto-lliac surgery.* Ann Surg, 1975. 181(6):787–90.

112. Rosenthal, D., *Spinal cord ischemia after abdominal aortic operation: is it preventable?* J Vasc Surg, 1999. 30(3):391–7.

Chapter 6

Patient Selection Criteria for Endovascular Aortic Aneurysm Repair

Venkataramu N. Krishnamurthy and John E. Rectenwald

Abstract Endovascular aortic aneurysm repair (EVAR) is being increasingly applied as a less-invasive alternative to open surgical repair of abdominal aortic aneurysms (AAAs). It is an excellent treatment option for AAA when performed on appropriately selected patients and with adequate preoperative planning. Recent trials have reported lower short-term operative mortality rates for EVAR than open surgical repair, but the long-term results of endograft repair are unknown. Preoperative planning and patient selection are essential for good short-term and long-term results and crucial to the successful widespread adoption of EVAR. A thorough understanding of the basic anatomic criteria for EVAR is essential before contemplating the procedure or selecting the appropriate device. When assessing the arterial anatomy of a patient for potential EVAR, multiple factors need to be considered. These include the quality of ilio-femoral access, the proximal landing zone (infrarenal neck), the anatomy of the aneurysm itself, the anatomy of the distal aorta, and the distal landing zones (most commonly in the common iliac arteries but can be more distal, depending on the patient's pelvic anatomy). Anatomical assessment dictates the particular endograft most suitable, as each endograft design addresses different anatomical issues and may better accommodate an individual patient's aneurysm. A thorough understanding of these devices is also necessary before a sound clinical decision can be made about which device is the most appropriate fit for a particular patient's aneurysm. Poor patient or endograft selection will inevitably lead to poor results and significant long-term complications.

Keywords Abdominal aortic aneurysm, Endovascular aortic aneurysm repair, Patient selection

Introduction

Despite advancements in anesthesia and surgical techniques, abdominal aortic aneurysm (AAA) remains a significant cause of morbidity and mortality worldwide. AAAs are estimated to occur in as many as 5% of older men with

G. Upchurch and E. Criado (eds.) *Aortic Aneurysms, Contemporary Cardiology*
DOI: 10.1007/978-1-60327-204-9_6, © Humana Press, a part of
Springer Science+Business Media, LLC 2009

a history of smoking.[1] The most feared complication of AAA, rupture, is associated with a high mortality rate (as high as 80%) with an estimated 9000 deaths per year in the United States.[2,3] In fact, AAA is the 13th leading cause of death in the United States in persons 65–74 years old.[4] Given the abysmal survival rate for ruptured aneurysms, it is not surprising that approximately 40,000 elective AAA repairs are performed each year to prevent rupture with an estimated surgery-related mortality of 1500 (~4%) per year.[5]

Currently, two very different treatment options are available for the patient with an infrarenal AAA – the traditional standard open surgical repair and endovascular aortic aneurysm repair (EVAR). Traditional open surgical repair of AAAs has been the standard of care since its introduction in the 1950s and remains the gold standard to which all other treatment options are compared. EVAR was developed in the mid-1990s as a less invasive alternative to open surgical repair and its frequency of use is rapidly increasing due to its decreased mortality and morbidity compared with open AAA repair. Currently, nearly 45% of all elective AAAs are being repaired endovascularly and similarly an increasing number of ruptured AAAs are being treated with EVAR.[5,6] Because most AAAs never progress to rupture, deciding when to electively repair an AAA and by what technique can be challenging.[7] The goal of this chapter is to briefly describe the criteria for selecting patients for AAA repair, regardless of method, and then discuss patient selection for EVAR in detail. Since infrarenal AAA comprises approximately 80% of all AAAs, this chapter will emphasize the specific guidelines used in selecting patients for EVAR of infrarenal AAAs. A brief review of the selection criteria and endovascular techniques for repair of AAA extending into suprarenal aorta and emergent treatment of the symptomatic and ruptured AAA will also be included in this chapter.

Standard Criteria for AAA Repair

Without question, one single concept is paramount when considering EVAR for patients with an AAA and cannot be overemphasized. *Proper patient selection for EVAR is the key to a successful outcome.* To be considered for EVAR, certain special patient and aneurysmal characteristics must be present in addition to the standard criteria for surgical AAA repair. The objectives of the patient selection are deceptively simple and twofold: First, does the patient meet criteria for AAA repair in general and, if so, does the patient meet anatomical criteria for endovascular repair?

The first step in considering patients for EVAR is to determine if the patient with AAA meets the standard indications for open surgical treatment. The Society for Vascular Surgery and the International Society for Cardiovascular Surgery guidelines for the repair of AAA[8] include the following:

1. Any patient with a documented rupture or suspected rupture;
2. A symptomatic or rapidly expanding aneurysm, regardless of its size;
3. Aneurysms larger than 4.5 cm in diameter if low operative risk, otherwise 5.5 cm in diameter for average or higher operative risk[9];
4. Complicated aneurysms with embolism, thrombosis, or symptomatic occlusive disease; and
5. Atypical aneurysms (e.g., dissecting, mycotic, and saccular).

Table 1 Aneurysm diameter and estimated risk of rupture.

Aortic diameter (cm)	Rupture risk (% per year)
< 4	0
4–5	0.5–5
5–6	3–15
6–7	10–20
7–8	20–40
>8	30–50

Current best estimated of risk of rupture of abdominal aortic aneurysms for a given size. Modified from Schermerhorn and Cronenwett[135]

These guidelines must be considered in relation to each patient's comorbidities and existing clinical risk factors.

The driving force for elective repair of AAA remains the risk of aneurysm rupture and subsequent risk of death. The decision to operate on AAAs is largely related to the size of the aneurysm and its associated rupture risk (Table 1). Currently, scientific data to support the decision to treat AAAs greater than 5.5 cm is based primarily on two randomized controlled trials: The Aneurysm Detection and Management (ADAM) study conducted at US VA hospitals[10] and the UK Small Aneurysm Trial.[9,11] Both these trials compared early surgery to surveillance for AAAs with sizes between 4.0 to 5.4 cm. These two trials independently concluded that a surveillance strategy for aneurysm less than 5.5 cm in diameter is prudent and that survival is not improved by repair of aneurysms smaller than 5.5 cm despite low operative mortality rates for other than patients of the lowest operative risk.

The decision between open or endovascular repair versus observation for patients with AAA can depend on factors other than solely the diameter of the aneurysm. These factors include aneurysm growth rate, risk of rupture while being observed, operative morbidity and mortality rates, the patient's life expectancy, and the patient's personal preferences concerning repair.[12,13]

Aneurysmal Growth Rate

Aneurysmal growth (expansion) rate is important predictor of rupture risk and timing of elective AAA repair. The rate of aneurysmal expansion varies with the size of the aneurysm according to the law of Laplace, with larger aneurysms growing much faster than smaller ones.[14–18] Reported mean expansion rates are 0.33 cm/year for AAAs 3.0–3.9 cm, 0.41 cm/year for AAAs 4.0–5.0 cm, and 0.51 cm/year for AAAs greater than 5.0 cm diameter.[19] Although aneurysm expansion rates can be estimated for a large population, individual aneurysms expand in a more erratic, stepwise fashion. Thus, for an individual patient, median expansion rates may be more useful for predicting aneurysm growth.[20] Several studies have estimated a median expansion rate of approximately 10% per year for clinically relevant AAAs in the size range of 4–6 cm diameter.[16,18,19,21,22]

In addition to large initial AAA diameter, other independent risk factors for rapid expansion of the AAA are current smoking, hypertension, widened pulse pressure, advanced age, severe cardiac disease, stroke, large thrombus burden within the aneurysm, and larger areas of contact between the aneurysmal wall and the thrombus.[16,17,20,23–29]

Risk of AAA Rupture While Under Observation

Clinical studies from 1960s[30] and autopsy studies[7,31] have shown a very high risk of rupture in large aneurysms (>5 cm diameter). These studies have reported AAA rupture in approximately 40% or more of patients with aneurysms larger than 5 cm or more in diameter. In current practice, AAA larger than 6 cm size is nearly always repaired unless the predicted operative mortality is prohibitive or the patient's life expectancy is short. This makes it difficult to perform population-based or natural history studies to precisely correlate the risk of rupture to the size of the AAA.

Current estimates of the risk of AAA rupture are based on reports of the natural history of small AAAs presented in the recent literature.[32] These studies have suggested a transition point between 5 and 6 cm, above which the risk of rupture is highly significant. For smaller size aneurysms (diameter 4.0–5.5 cm), the risk of rupture is relatively low (Table 1). Randomized Controlled Trials such as the ADAM study and UK Small Aneurysm Trials have reported AAA rupture in 0.6% and 1% per year, respectively, for aneurysms 4–5.5 cm diameter under regular surveillance.[9,10] Recent publication from UK Small Aneurysm Trial reported rupture risk of 0.3% for AAAs less than 3.9 cm, 1.5% for AAAs 4–4.9 cm, and 6.5% for AAAs 5–5.9 cm.[33] Moreover, the gender distribution of rupture was significantly unequal with a 4.5 times higher risk of rupture among females compared to males.

The annual AAA rupture risk varies significantly in the literature. The annual AAA rupture risk in population-based studies is estimated to be 0% for AAAs less than 4 cm, 1% for AAAs 4–4.9 cm, and 11% for AAAs 5–5.9 cm.[34] These population-based studies likely underestimate rupture risk because elective repair is offered to the AAAs at greatest risk for rupture within any size category during the follow-up, which in turn lowers the apparent rupture risk. In studies reporting AAA rupture risk among patients who are referred for surgery (referral-based studies), the estimated annual AAA rupture risk rates are highly variable and ranged from 0% to 0.25% for AAAs less than 4 cm, 0.5% to 5.4% for AAAs 4–5 cm, and 4.3% to 16% for AAAs larger than 5 cm.[14,35] These referral-based studies tend to overestimate the AAA rupture risk for the population as a whole since only patients referred for surgical repair are included. To overcome this limitation, Scott et al. combined rupture rate and operation rate and calculated maximal potential rupture rate (MPRR) that reflects a more realistic estimate of the rupture risk.[36] They reported MPRR of 2.1% per year for AAAs 3–4.4 cm and 10.2% per year for AAAs 4.5–5.9 cm. These data are interesting but, for an individual patient, it is difficult to deduce an accurate prediction rule for AAA rupture from these studies.

Biomechanical modeling using CT scan has been attempted for AAAs to study the impact of wall stress on the risk of rupture.[37,38] These studies report wall stress as the greatest predictor of rupture (hazard ratio 25) followed by female gender (hazard ratio 3). Aneurysm diameter did not predict rupture in an individual aneurysm. Computer modeling also suggested that focal bulges of the dilated aortic wall in aneurysms (saccular aneurysms) had a greater risk of rupture than fusiform aneurysms.[38–40]

In addition to the size of the aneurysm, a variety of factors have been shown to be independent predictors of rupture.[31,33,41,42] These include female gender, history of smoking, diastolic hypertension, COPD (chronic obstructive pulmonary disease), bronchiectasis, and positive family history for AAA.[41]

Mortality Risk from Surgical Repair of AAA

Reported mortality rates for elective surgical repair vary widely in the literature.[19,43–58] In general, mortality rates for open surgical repair average 5–6% in most large studies. Independent risk factors for operative mortality for elective AAA repair are serum creatinine (>1.8), congestive heart failure, myocardial ischemia, COPD, advanced age, and female gender.

Patient Life Expectancy

A good assessment of the patient's life expectancy is important in determining if surgical management of AAA should be offered. Because most patients with AAAs are, or have been, smokers, coexisting cardiopulmonary diseases, coronary artery disease, cerebrovascular disease, hypertension, hyperlipidemia, and cancer affect the overall survival after surgery. Many of these factors also increase the operative morbidity and mortality.

Patient Selection for EVAR

EVAR has been advocated as a less invasive alternative to open surgical repair of AAAs and, in general, EVAR is associated with less operative mortality and overall morbidity, and rapid patient recovery leading to a significantly shorter hospital stay when compared to conventional open repair.[59–62] The unknown durability of EVAR and the frequent need for secondary interventions after EVAR may, in the long-term, outweigh the early gains from this less invasive treatment option.[63,64] Fortunately, with continued innovation and improvement in stent graft design and technology, these perceived disadvantages may well be overcome in the future.

A number of factors need to be carefully evaluated before considering a patient for EVAR. *The process of patient selection for EVAR is of paramount importance* and includes the following steps:

1. Preoperative assessment: Detailed patient history and physical examination including evaluation of factors predictive of rupture such as aneurysm size, expansion rate, and risk of surgical treatment based on demographic factors, patient history, comorbidities, and life expectancy.
2. Preoperative imaging with high-quality contrasted and noncontrasted thin slice CT scan of the entire abdominal aorta from above celiac artery origin to the common femoral artery bifurcations.
3. Angiographic imaging with anterior–posterior and lateral views with contrast and a calibrated catheter with radiopaque marker bands. This study is frequently preformed at the time of endograft placement.
4. Evaluation of the risks of EVAR based on anatomical criteria.

5. Evaluation of the patient's ability to comply with required follow-up.
6. Patient counseling and determination of the most appropriate treatment strategy for each patient based on the relative risks and benefits of the available treatment strategies.

Of these, the two most important criteria that warrant specific attention are the anatomical criteria for EVAR and the ability of the patient to comply with the required clinical and imaging follow-up at regular intervals.

Preoperative Assessment

A detailed preoperative assessment determines the patient's risk factors for surgery and the basis for evaluating various treatment options. It is also important for counseling the patient about the likelihood of potential complications during and after the planned surgery. This should include, but not be limited to, patient-specific evaluation of the AAAs risk of rupture relative to risks of repair, relative benefits of EVAR compared to the conventional treatment, detailed assessment of the patient's overall health and comorbid conditions.

As a general rule, the aneurysm size criteria for EVAR are identical to elective open surgical repair. Renal, cardiac, pulmonary, and hepatic functions should be evaluated with appropriate laboratory and radiographic tests. Evaluation of any comorbidities such as hypertension, COPD, renal insufficiency, history of diabetes, myocardial ischemia/infarction, cerebrovascular disease, coagulopathy, potential sources of systemic infection, and allergies (specifically to intravenous contrast) should be evaluated in detail as these factors give a ballpark assessment of the operative risks and also the life expectancy of the patient. Other factors such as previous abdominal surgeries, the presence of abdominal wounds or ostomies, enteric fistulas, and morbid obesity may make an endoluminal approach more attractive than open repair in selected patients. Regardless of the selected approach to AAA repair, it is also important to evaluate the patient for the presence of other associated aneurysms, such as femoral and popliteal artery aneurysms, which may need to be addressed. Duplex ultrasound is an excellent modality for detection and screening for associated peripheral arterial aneurysms.

Preoperative Imaging Evaluation

Imaging evaluation is essential to decide patient suitability and technical feasibility of EVAR. Imaging must provide a thorough analysis of the vascular anatomy and aneurysm characteristics. Imaging provides the necessary information about:

1. The technical feasibility of EVAR by aortic anatomic criteria.
2. The type of the endograft that will be required.
3. Planning the size, length, and the number of the endograft components required.
4. Suitability of the access arteries for introducing the grafts and whether an iliac conduit or an alternative approach will be needed.
5. The probable technical risks involved in the EVAR procedure, and the formulation of appropriate "fallback" plans should these difficulties actually be encountered during endograft placement.

High-quality noncontrasted CT and contrast-enhanced helical CT angiography (CTA), catheter angiography, and intravascular ultrasound (IVUS) are all acceptable imaging modalities that may be used in the preoperative assessment for EVAR.[65] Both CTA and catheter angiography have limitations with regards to the accuracy of measurements and are not mutually exclusive techniques and frequently are used in combination. Most often, a preoperative CTA for proper preoperative sizing and planning and catheter angiography at the time of the procedure for confirmation of the size and length of endograft components are used in EVAR.

CT Scan Protocol

CT scan should be performed preferentially using a current generation Spiral CT or high-performance multidetector CT. A noncontrasted CT of the abdomen and pelvis should be performed from diaphragm to proximal femur with a slice thickness less than 3 mm and reconstructed at less than 2.5 mm intervals on a soft tissue algorithm. This should be followed by a contrast-enhanced CT with matching table positions, slice thickness, and IV contrast injection at a rate greater than 2.5 cc/s. Multiplanar reformatting and 3D reconstruction performed from CTA images are used as a reference standard for planning and sizing of the endografts.[59,66–70]

Axial CT slices and subsequent 3D reconstructed images are evaluated for the following:

1. *The morphology of the aneurysm:* CT scan is the most accurate modality for evaluation of the proximal and distal extent of the aneurysm, which is one of the key features for preoperative planning.[71,72] Additionally, CT scan also shows the thrombus within the aneurysm which is not well seen on catheter angiography and can clearly delineate the calcium burden in the aortic and iliac arteries. This is especially important when evaluating the proximal and distal landing zones and affects the ability of the endograft to effectively seal off the aneurysm and prevent type I endoleaks.

2. *Evaluation of the ilio-femoral arteries:* CT scan clearly shows the disease in iliac and femoral arteries which results from either the direct extension of the AAA (in the case of common and internal iliac aneurysms) or isolated aneurysms themselves. When windowed correctly, CT also determines the burden of atherosclerotic disease, calcification of the arterial wall, diameter of the ilio-femoral arteries (which is important as access for endografts), tortuosity of these vessels, and origins of the internal iliac arteries.

3. *Status of the renal and mesenteric arteries:* CT scan with multiplanar reformat and 3D reconstruction is very useful in evaluating the involvement of these vessels directly by the aneurysm itself or by generalized atherosclerotic disease, presence of accessory renal arteries, patency of the inferior mesenteric/lumbar arteries which potentially could be treated prior to the planned procedure to prevent future endoleak. Some publications have reported benefits (prevention of type II endoleak and greater shrinkage of aneurysm sac diameter) of routine preoperative embolization of the inferior mesenteric artery (IMA)[73]; however, this observation has not been consistently reproduced in more recent studies.[74] CTA also shows the presence of renal artery stenosis which may influence the decision to proceed to open surgery or require treatment prior to or at the time of EVAR.

4. *Precise measurement, planning, and simulation of the deployed devices for endovascular repairs:* These are described under anatomical assessment below. With the exception of 3D center-line studies, catheter angiography with a calibrated marker catheter is a more accurate method than standard

CT for determining the optimal length of the endograft. An aortogram also gives an excellent assessment of the angulation of the infrarenal aortic neck, the tortuosity, and lengths of the iliac arteries. The limitations of angiography are its inability to identify intraluminal thrombus and atherosclerotic plaques as well as assessment of the true size of the aneurysm since only the luminal flow channel is visualized on angiograms.

IVUS is an invasive method that requires significant skill and experience in both performing procedure and interpretation of the findings. IVUS is a very useful technique when iodinated contrast cannot be used for either CTA or catheter angiogram in patients with severe allergy or renal insufficiency. It allows for accurate assessment of the various diameters and guidance for accurate placement of the grafts under direct visualization. Like CTA, intraluminal thrombus and true aneurysm diameters can be accurately determined with IVUS.

Anatomical Criteria

The anatomical assessment for proceeding with EVAR includes evaluations of the proximal neck and distal landing zones for the endograft, diameter and morphology of the ilio-femoral arteries, location and morphology of the internal iliac arteries, involvement of the major visceral vessels with the aneurysm, and identification of small branches which may need to be excluded from the aneurysm. If a patient has suitable anatomic criteria for endograft placement, then worksheets specific for the endograft being placed facilitate appropriate endograft selection (Fig. 1).

Evaluation of the Proximal Attachment Site (Infrarenal Neck, Proximal Landing Zone)

Aortic neck morphology is critically related to effective sealing and stability of the aortic endograft. The sealing stent at the proximal fixation site should ideally be placed parallel to the axis of the nondilated aorta. Unsuitable proximal neck morphology (too wide, too short, or too angulated, Fig. 2) is the most common reason (>50% of cases) for a patient to be ineligible for EVAR.[75–77]

The infrarenal neck is evaluated for the following parameters – length, diameter, angulation, and presence of thrombus or calcification.

- A. *Length of proximal neck*: All currently available aortic endografts require a minimal neck length of 15 mm around the entire circumference of the infrarenal neck to adequately seal to prevent proximal endoleak (type 1a). A long neck provides better sealing and greater endograft stability.[75,78] Short proximal neck (<15 mm length) makes device deployment more difficult with less margin for error in relation to endograft placement near the renal arteries and consequent increased chances of type 1 endoleak and/or graft migration. The incidence of proximal endoleak is highest (6.25%) with neck length less than 15 mm and the lowest (0.46%) for neck longer than >25 mm.
- B. *Diameter of the proximal neck*: It is desirable to have a proximal neck diameter less than 3 cm diameter to get adequate sealing. Wider necks (>3 cm) make adequate proximal fixation of the stent graft difficult leading

COOK MEDICAL

Zenith Flex®
AAA ENDOVASCULAR GRAFT

DEVICE PLANNING AND SIZING WORKSHEET

Select Side of Main Body Introduction and Fixation Sites

☐ Right iliac   ☐ Left iliac

External Iliac (EI) measurement _____ mm
(Minimum diameter, inner wall to inner wall, from introduction site to aorta.)

Anatomical Measurements

CT table position at:

_____ lowest renal artery
15 mm below lowest renal artery,
check for 10% increase

_____ aortic bifurcation
_____ origin cl internal iliac
_____ origin il internal iliac

- When using CT for length, approximate lateral deviation/tortuosity and add to difference in table position.

Diameters: D1 [   ]   D2 [   ]   D3 [   ]

Lengths: L1 [   ]   L2 [   ]   L3 [   ]

D1: Largest aortic neck diameter throughout 15 mm neck length
D2: Largest iliac diameter throughout contralateral distal fixation site
D3: Largest iliac diameter throughout ipsilateral distal fixation site

L1: Lowest renal artery to aortic bifurcation + lateral deviation/tortuosity
L2: Lowest renal artery to contralateral distal fixation site + lateral deviation/tortuosity
L3: Lowest renal artery to ipsilateral distal fixation site + lateral deviation/tortuosity

Main Body

- From D1, select graft diameter.
- From L1, select the graft lengths.
- If choice of graft diameter or graft length is affected by other considerations, adjust accordingly.
- Using graft diameter and cl length, complete the Main Body Order Number.

Main Body Graft Diameters

D1 mm	Graft Diameter mm
18-19	22
20-21	24
22	26
23-24	28
25-26	30
27-28	32
29-32	36

Diameter 22-32

L1	cl Length*	il Length**
88-103	82	112
104-118	96	126
119-133	111	141
134-148	125	155
149-163	140	170

Diameter 36

L1	cl Length*	il Length**
101-120	95	125
121-139	113	143
140-158	131	161
159-177	149	179

*main body length on contralateral side
**main body length on ipsilateral side

Main Body Order Number = TFFB - [   ] - [   ]
Graft Diameter   cl Length/ Graft Length

ALL information must be complete:

Date: _____ Patient ID: _____
Hospital: _____
Physician Name: _____
Physician Signature: _____
Physician Phone #: _____
Physician e-mail: _____

Contralateral Iliac Leg

- From D2, select graft diameter.
- Using L2 and cl length, complete the following equation.

[L2] minus [cl Length] = _____ Contralateral Working Length

- If choice of graft diameter or graft length is affected by other considerations, adjust accordingly.

Contralateral Leg (TFLE) Graft Diameters

D2 mm	Graft Diameter mm
<8	8
8-9	10
10-11	12
12-13	14
14-15	16
16-17	18
18	20
19	22
20	24

Contralateral Leg (TFLE) Graft Lengths (mm)

Contralateral Working Length mm	Graft Length mm	Recommended Overlap stents
25-41	37*	1-1.5
42-58	54	1-1.5
59-75	71	1-1.5
76-92	88	1-1.5
93-109	105**	1-1.5
110-122	122**	1-1.5

*Assure adequate distal fixation length.
**Graft lengths 105 and 122 mm are available in 8-12 mm diameters only.

Contralateral Leg Order Number = TFLE - [   ] - [   ]
Graft Diameter   Graft Length

Ipsilateral Iliac Leg

- From D3, select graft diameter.
- Using L3 and il length, complete the following equation.

[L3] minus [il Length] = _____ Ipsilateral Working Length

- If choice of graft diameter or graft length is affected by other considerations, adjust accordingly.

Ipsilateral Leg (TFLE) Graft Diameters

D3 mm	Graft Diameter mm
<8	8
8-9	10
10-11	12
12-13	14
14-15	16
16-17	18
18	20
19	22
20	24

Ipsilateral Leg (TFLE) Graft Lengths (mm)

Ipsilateral Working Length mm	Graft Length mm	Recommended Overlap stents
20-33 graft diameter 18-24	37	1-2
20-33 graft diameter 8-16	54	1-3
34-40	54	1-2
41-57	71	1-3
58-74	88	1-3
75-91	105*	1-3
92-122	122*	1-3

*Graft lengths 105 and 122 mm are available in 8-12 mm diameters only.

Ipsilateral Leg Order Number = TFLE - [   ] - [   ]
Graft Diameter   Graft Length

© COOK 2007   AI-BPH-FLEXPSW-EN-0708

Fig. 1 An example of an aortic endograft sizing sheet. (Used with permission, Cook Medical, Inc., Bloomington, IN.)

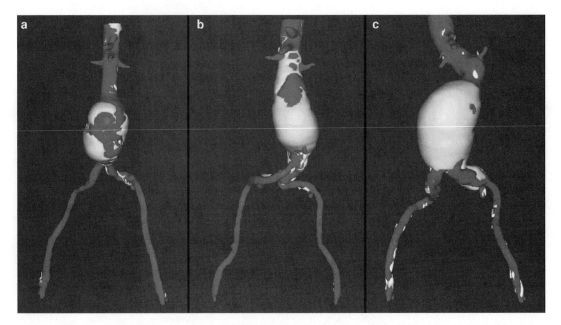

Fig. 2 Three-dimensional reconstructions demonstrating infrarenal aortic neck characteristics: Patients with the ideal infrarenal aortic neck (**a**), a nonideal conical infrarenal aortic neck (**b**), and the highly angulated infrarenal aortic neck (**c**) (*See Color Plates*)

to migration of the graft and endoleaks. However, Ingle et al. showed no statistically significant differences in the incidence of late proximal endoleak and the frequency of graft migration among patients treated with EVAR in smaller diameter (<3 cm) neck aneurysms compared with larger diameter (>3 cm) neck aneurysm.[79] Despite this finding, adherence to accepted Instruction for Use guidelines is recommended until such a time that long-term efficacy of EVAR is established with the exception of a few patients who have large aneurysms with very high operative risk.[75,80,81]

Currently, EVAR treatment of aneurysms with infrarenal neck diameters is limited to 32 mm in diameter. This is due to the fact that, with required endograft oversizing, endografts with diameters greater than 36 mm are not currently available (Table 2). Individuals with infrarenal neck diameters greater than 32 mm are currently being treated with either open surgery, aortic visceral artery "debranching" procedures with placement of thoracic aortic endografts or in selected institutions, fenestrated, or multibranched endografts.

- C. *Angulation of the proximal neck:* Two neck angles are evaluated in the preoperative assessment of EVAR. Suprarenal neck angulation refers to an angle measured between long axis of the immediate suprarenal and infrarenal aorta. A measurement less than 45° is favorable for EVAR. An angulation more than 45° predisposes to endoleak due to improper proximal seal by grafts. The second angle measured is aortic neck angulation. This is measured between long axis of the infrarenal neck to the long axis of the AAA. An angle less than 60° is considered favorable for EVAR as angulation greater than 60° predisposes to endoleaks and complicates device delivery.[82,83] Thus, in extremely tortuous aorta, EVAR should not be offered as the primary treatment option.

Multiple endografts have been or are currently in development to deal with AAAs with the highly angulated infrarenal neck. Examples include the Aorfix aortic endograft (Lombard Medical) and the Zenith Flex (Cook). These endografts have been designed with the highly angulated proximal aortic neck in mind and may provide an acceptable seal at the proximal endograft landing zone.

- D. *Shape of the proximal neck:* Abnormal shapes of the neck may result in graft malposition or migration. Nonparallel neck shapes, such as an hourglass configuration or an inverted funnel shape (aortic neck with >10% increase in diameter over 15 mm of proximal aortic neck length, Fig. 2b), result in difficult device delivery and increase the risk of device migration and subsequent type 1 proximal endoleaks. Endografts with fixation at the aortic bifurcation (Powerlink, Endologix Corporation) or suprarenal fixation (Cook Zenith) have been developed to address this issue and can be used judiciously in this situation.
- E. *Irregular calcification, plaque, or thrombus at the proximal neck*: These may interfere with proximal fixation and sealing of the endograft leading to migration of the endograft and/or endoleaks. However, the relevance of thrombus in the proximal neck is controversial since some small clinical studies have not found aortic thrombus at the proximal landing zone to increase the incidence of early or late proximal endoleaks.[84]

Evaluation of the Distal Attachment Site (Iliac Landing Zones)

The distal landing zones for endografts are most frequently the common iliac arteries unless they are involved by direct extension of the AAA or contain isolated iliac aneurysms. At least 10 mm of the nonaneurysmal vessel is needed for secure iliac limb endograft fixation, although 15 mm is recommended if at all possible. If the distal landing zone is short or nonexistent on one side, graft can be extended to land in external iliac arteries to obtain adequate seal.[85] This situation is commonly seen with aneurysmal involvement of the common iliac artery. In such cases, ipsilateral internal iliac artery is embolized either before or during the endograft placement to prevent type 2 endoleak from the internal iliac artery. Typically a single patent internal iliac artery with antegrade flow is sufficient to maintain adequate pelvic perfusion, although risk of clinically significant pelvic ischemia from bilateral iliac occlusions is very rare.[86] Care should be taken to embolize the most proximal portion of the ipsilateral internal iliac artery in order to preserve the anterior and posterior branches to maintain collateral blood flow to as much of the pelvis as possible. Bilateral internal iliac artery occlusion usually results in buttock claudication. In cases where both common iliac arteries do not provide adequate landing zone, such as when there are bilateral aneurysms, bilateral iliac limbs can be extended to external iliac arteries with surgical transposition or bypass grafting of one or both internal iliac arteries.[87] If there is only ectasia or minimal aneurysmal dilatation of the common iliac arteries, flared end (bell-bottomed) iliac limb grafts may be used to obtain adequate sealing without having to sacrifice internal iliac circulation.[88] At some institutions, iliac bifurcation or branched endografts are also available for use in these situations.

In summary, key aortic anatomical features that may exclude a patient form EVAR of the AAA are:

- short proximal aortic neck (<15 mm),
- severe proximal neck angulation (>60° between infrarenal neck and long axis of the AAA),
- severe suprarenal neck angulation (>45° between immediate suprarenal and infrarenal aorta),
- nonparallel, inverted funnel shape neck (>10% increase in diameter over 15 mm of proximal aortic neck length), and
- circumferential thrombus and/or calcification at the proximal and distal stent fixation sites.

Evaluation of the Diameter and Morphology of the Ilio-Femoral (Conduit/Access) Arteries

The endografts are generally introduced into the aorta via a femoral artery approach. A good preoperative assessment of the conduit arteries (common femoral, external, and common iliac arteries) guides the proper technique for delivery of the endografts and greatly reduces complications. Conduit arteries are evaluated for their inner diameter, burden of calcification, tortuosity, and angulation in addition to other morphological features in the distal landing zone. Proper evaluation of the femoral and iliac arteries will determine if an auxiliary procedure such as a retroperitoneal exposure of the iliac arteries with placement of iliac conduits is necessary.

- A. *Diameter of conduit vessels*: Inner diameter of the conduit arteries should be measured and documented prior to the procedure. The main body endograft introducer sheaths and the grafts themselves are of large diameter (up to 26 Fr), requiring these conduit vessels to be of sufficient diameter to prevent graft dislodgement during delivery or rupture of the vessel leading to catastrophic bleeding. Table 2 shows the maximum diameters of the aortic delivery devices for various commercially available endografts.

  Focal iliac stenoses may be pretreated with balloon angioplasty or by passage of a large diameter vascular dilator to allow delivery of the endograft. Adequate precautions should be taken not to excessively dilate a stenosis due

Table 2 Description of characteristics of commonly used endograft devices.

Device name/ Manufacturer	Maximum available size of aortic/ Main body component (mm)	Maximum recommended diameter of infrarenal aortic diameter that can be treated (mm)	Recommended oversizing at infrarenal neck level (%)	Size (outer diameter) of the aortic/ main body component (Fr)
Zenith/Cook	36	32	15–20	24
Powelink/ Endologix	28	25	15	20
Excluder/Gore	31	28	5–10	18
Ancure/Guidant	26	25	15–20	23.5
AneuRx/Medtronic	28	29	15–20	21.5
Talent/Medtronic	36	32	15–20	22–24

This table lists the currently available endografts with maximum available graft diameters, recommended maximum aneurysm neck diameters for endograft placement, and recommended graft oversizing at the proximal landing zone to the risk of rupture, particularly in highly calcified external iliac vessels. If external artery iliac stenosis persists despite balloon angioplasty, an iliac bypass conduit may be performed (a prosthetic graft attached to the common iliac artery via a retroperitoneal incision) to provide access for delivery of graft device.[89] This bypass conduit may be anastomosed to the ipsilateral common femoral artery to bypass external iliac stenosis at the end of the procedure. Alternatively, a focal recalcitrant iliac stenosis could be treated with a covered stent to allow passage of the endograft delivery catheters. Obviously, care must be taken to choose an appropriately sized covered stent in order to avoid stent migration or ensnarement upon passing the endograft delivery catheters. In cases of unilateral chronic long segment iliac occlusion or severely calcified long segment iliac stenosis, an aortouni-iliac endograft may be planned with an occluder cuff for the contralateral common iliac artery (if needed) and femoral–femoral bypass graft. Alternatively, the authors have successfully recannalized occluded common and external iliac arteries in order to place bifurcated endografts with and without iliac artery stent placement prior to endograft placement. This approach, when successful, avoids an aortouni-iliac endograft, preserves flow to the contralateral internal iliac artery, and avoids a femoral–femoral bypass graft.

- B. *Tortuosity and angulations*: Minor tortuosity and smaller angulation between common iliac artery and the AAA can often be corrected by the use of superstiff guide wires. Severe tortuosity and angulation of the iliac arteries must be accounted for when placing iliac limb grafts, especially into the external iliac arteries (Fig. 2c). These can cause difficulty in advancing the endografts and can cause kinks in the grafts after the graft deployment. The severe tortuosity of the native vessels can "reoccur" after removal of the stiff guide wires. The relatively stiffer stent grafts within the softer native artery can result in kinks within the native artery and a "T-bar" effect causing the last stent in the limb to circumferentially fully oppose the opposite wall of the iliac artery, resulting in an obstruction of the graft and thrombosis of the limb (Fig. 3).

Involvement of the Major Vessels in the Aneurysmal Sac

When the aneurysm is excluded by the endograft, vessels arising from the aneurysm sac, two potential problems can result: the potential for retrograde flow these vessels and resultant type II endoleak, and the potential for ischemia in the distribution of these branches, once direct aortic flow to these vessels is prevented by the aortic endograft.

Large lumbar arteries and widely patent IMAs need to evaluated and documented in the preprocedure work up as these could be potential source of type II endoleak and aneurysm sac progression in long term. Incidence of early endoleaks, mostly type II endoleaks, varies from 12% to 44%.[90] Most of these (~70%) type II endoleaks resolve spontaneously in 3–4 weeks postendograft placement and therefore not warrant aggressive treatment when identified on completion angiogram.[90,91] In those patients on anticoagulation with persistent type II endoleaks, careful reversal of anticoagulation should be considered as type II endoleak may potentially disappear after reversal.[91]

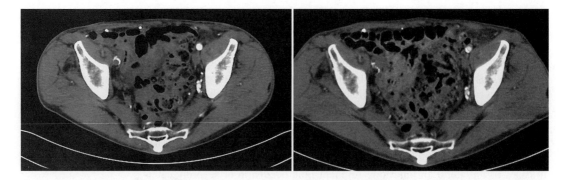

Fig. 3 Computed tomography angiogram (*CTA*) in a patient with right iliac graft limb occlusion from a graft-native artery "T-bar." The right iliac graft limb was extended into the right external iliac artery after coil emboliza-tion of the ipsilateral internal iliac artery for treatment of a right common iliac aneurysm. The distal stent of the right graft limb eventually opposed the posterior wall of the native external iliac artery (the "T-bar"), resulting in graft occlusion. The CTA image on the left is one slice (2.5 mm) above the image on the right. Note calcifications of the native posterior external iliac artery wall anterior to the anterior portion of the stent graft and position of the contralateral external iliac artery

Importantly, a large caliber IMA with very prominent marginal artery of Drummond's or arch of Riolan on preoperative imaging should raise a high index of suspicion for a significant superior mesenteric artery stenosis or occlusion. If this problem is not immediately recognized, risk of colonic ischemia after EVAR is high. Therefore, either the mesenteric stenosis should be addressed prior to EVAR by endovascular techniques or an open surgical repair with superior mesenteric revascularization should be performed.

Compliance with Follow-up Protocols

Because the long-term outcome and durability of EVAR is not fully estab-lished, the patient's ability to comply with the recommended clinical and imaging follow-up is essential when selecting patients for EVAR. Focused clinical examination and imaging with contrast-enhanced CT scan within 1 month of EVAR and then at 6, 12, 18 months, and annually thereafter are recommended.[92] The main features monitored are AAA sac size, structural integrity of the graft, device migration, and any evidence of clinically signifi-cant endoleak.

Special Circumstances in Patient Selection for EVAR

Unfortunately, many patients with AAA do not meet the anatomical criteria for EVAR. Graft designs and deployment techniques are being continuously improved to accommodate for these shortcomings, resulting in ever expanding indications for EVAR. Some of these have already been addressed earlier in this chapter.

Not-So-Ideal Neck/Proximal Attachment Site

The ideal neck for EVAR should be less than 30 mm in diameter, be at least 15 mm long from below the origin of the lowest renal artery, and be relatively straight and free of thrombus or irregular calcified plaques. This situation provides for proper fixation and sealing of the graft and decreases the likelihood of endoleak or graft migration. Unfortunately, such an aortic neck rarely exists and when the neck is not ideal, alterations in graft design and fixation systems have been developed to address this issue. These design enhancements include fixation hooks/barbs, suprarenal attachment stents, balloon expandable stent components, more precise deployment mechanisms, and fenestrated/scalloped graft designs.

Suprarenal attachment graft designs have a bare-stent segment above the level of the graft material and the proposed advantage is better fixation and prevention of early and late stent graft migration. Current generation endografts are being increasingly and safely used for shorter and wider necks with good results.[93] For individuals with a normal aortic segment at and above the level of renal arteries but with not so suitable infrarenal neck, fenestrated and multibranched endografts are being used in current clinical trials.[94-97]

Symptomatic and Ruptured AAA

EVAR is being increasingly used in many institutions to treat patients with symptomatic or ruptured AAA who are generally treated with open surgical techniques.[98-104] The numbers of patients with ruptured AAAs that are being treated with aortic endografts has steadily increased over the last several years, driven primarily by the improved survival rates reported in the literature.[6] Unfortunately, the proportion of patients with ruptured AAAs who are suitable for EVAR seems to be lower compared with asymptomatic AAAs because ruptured AAAs tend to have larger neck diameters and shorter neck length.[103] EVAR utility varies from 40% to 80% in patients with ruptured AAAs.[103-105]

The preoperative investigations used to assess patients before endovascular ruptured aneurysm repair (EVrAR) have varied among institutions. Whenever possible, thin slice contrast-enhanced CT using CT angiogram protocol on the way to operating room is useful in selecting patients for EVrAR. The old idea that patients with a suspected ruptured AAA should go straight to the operating room rather than the CT scanner is hardly applicable in today's world of helical CTA with scanning times in seconds and rarely is a patient transferred to the author's institution with a ruptured AAA without a CT scan. If the patient is too profoundly unstable to undergo CT scanning, an aortogram may be performed through brachial or femoral approach to decide the candidacy for EVrAR. In general, anatomical criteria to be considered for EVrAR of ruptured AAA are similar to that of asymptomatic AAA.

Although the basic techniques for endograft implantation in ruptured aneurysms are the same as for the elective situation, different strategies have been applied. Aortobi-iliac, aortouni-iliac, and aortouni-femoral grafts have all been used to a variable extent. Some centers have routinely used aortouni-iliac grafts for acute cases, whereas others have favored bifurcated devices, the choice of device depends upon the individual institution (device availability and experience). An aortouni-iliac device has the advantage of relatively rapid deployment of the primary graft, whereas it also requires implantation of a contralateral occlusion plug into the iliac artery and revascularization by a femorol–femoral crossover bypass. Rupture kits are being marketed by various manufacturers which enable most aneurysms to be repaired with a minimal amount of stock. Certain supplementary techniques such as placing occlusion balloon in the proximal abdominal aorta over a guide wire may also be required during EVrAR of ruptured AAAs to control hemorrhage.

Several single-center studies have reported significantly improved outcomes (morbidity, mortality, and length of hospital stay) in the short-term follow-up compared with open repair. Ohki et al. reported the use of an aortouni-iliac device in combination with an occlusion balloon placed via brachial artery approach for treating ruptured AAA with a survival of 61% over a mean follow-up of 15.6 months.[106] The mean survival duration in this study was significantly longer for EVrAR than survival in patients treated by open surgical repair (7.9 months).

Recently, Greco et al. reported a mortality rate of 39.3% for EVrAR compared with 47.7% for open repair.[107] There were significant reductions in pulmonary, renal, and bleeding complications. An analysis of the National US Medicare database (1999–2003) showed that this early survival benefit disappeared at 6 month follow-up and stayed nonsignificant on continued follow-up out to 2.5 years.[108]

In conclusion, development of a successful EVrAR program should include the treatment of ruptured or symptomatic AAA and requires the ready availability of an experienced endovascular team, a range of device sizes and ancillary equipment, the capability to perform rapid preoperative imaging (particularly CT), and excellent procedural imaging equipment in the operating room environment.

Aneurysms That Involve and Extend Above the Renal Artery: Juxtarenal/Suprarenal AAAs and Thoraco-Abdominal Aneurysms

The AAA that involves renal arteries, visceral branches, and/or extend into the thoracic aorta has complex anatomy making surgical repair challenging. The mortality rates associated with conventional surgical treatment are higher than the infrarenal AAA and range from 5% to 34%.[109–112] In addition, there is a significant incidence of major postoperative complications associated with these aneurysms such as paraplegia, cardiopulmonary issues, and renal failure resulting in a rate of hemodialysis that approaches 8% in some series.[113] The successful application of EVAR as a less invasive treatment option to this group of patients may provide improved outcomes compared to open surgery for these complex aneurysms than typical infrarenal AAA.

The intricacy of designing and implanting endografts for aneurysms that involve the visceral segment is more complex than infrarenal endografts. At present, three designs of endografts have been developed and are currently being evaluated for treating these complex aneurysms – fenestrated, reinforced fenestrated, and directional branch grafts.[114]

Fenestrated Endografts
These are the earliest endografts developed for juxtarenal aneurysms. These grafts are custom designed and have holes that are synchronized to visceral branches. A balloon expandable stent is then placed through the customized fenestration once the main body graft has been aligned with the target visceral ostia and deployed. The balloon is inflated to the size of the target vessel and further flared with a larger balloon to rivet the visceral stent against the graft and aortic wall. This is then repeated for the desired number of visceral

vessels. These are mainly applied in the endovascular treatment of juxtarenal aneurysms.[94,95,97,115,116]

Reinforced Fenestrated Endografts

This design is similar to the fenestrated endograft described above but with the addition of the nitinol ring to support the circumference of the customized fenestration, and the uncovered stent is substituted with a covered stent. The reinforced fenestrated endograft design can be used to treat aneurysms that involve the renal arteries or aneurysms involving all of the visceral vessels. This device implantation is more challenging than a simple fenestrated device as there exists a space between the fenestration and branch ostium which can complicate cannulation. The use of covered stents rather than bare stents for the visceral vessels requires longer and larger (less flexible delivery system) balloon-expandable stent grafts. This type of graft design makes the branch vessel origin relatively narrow and right-angled and this may make the renal and visceral perfusion less physiological.

Directional Branch Endografts

This type of endograft is designed to overcome many of the shortcomings seen in the reinforced fenestrated graft design. The directional branches are constructed in a manner to optimize the flow dynamics between the aorta and its branches. The branch allows more angulations between the aorta and the visceral branch to be accommodated, avoiding the steep angles seen in the reinforced fenestrated design. The length of the seal between the aortic component and the visceral branch graft in this device is longer than the joint within a reinforced fenestrated device (where the entire sealing region consists of a nitinol ring surrounding the fenestration). One limitation of this design is that these longer branches and sealing zones between the main body graft and the visceral branches take up space within the aneurysm as well as the delivery system making the device bulky (delivery device may be up to 24 F sheath compared with 18–20 F for fenestrated grafts). In addition, the more complicated visceral cannulations associated with branched endografts require extensive fluoroscopy exposure, contrast load, and significant proficiency with catheter and wire techniques.

Selection of patients for EVAR when the aneurysm involves and extends above the level of renal artery origin is a difficult and complex problem. It is heavily dependent on the availability of the various fenestrated grafts and experienced endovascular surgeons. Recent studies have demonstrated the mid-term safety and efficacy of fenestrated endografts.[116–118] In the largest series from the Cleveland Clinic, in which data on 119 patients was reported, the perioperative (30 day) mortality was under 2%, and survival at 12, 24, and 36 months was 92%, 83%, and 79%, respectively. Aneurysm sac shrinkage was noted in 79% at 12 months. Endoleaks were uncommon and noted in 9% of patients at 30 days (all type II), and 4%, 6%, and 3% at 12, 24, and 36 months, respectively. Results on the safety and efficacy of directional branched endografts are still evolving. Early reports show favorable outcomes.[119–121] Long-term durability is not known and therefore, as in infrarenal EVAR, long-term, indefinite imaging and clinical follow-up is essential. Thus, only those patients who can comply with the recommended follow-up protocol should be selected for EVAR of aneurysms that involve visceral segment and thoracoabdominal aneurysms.

Conclusions

EVAR is a landmark contribution in the management of AAAs providing acceptable outcomes with a significant decrease in perioperative morbidity and mortality rate compared to open surgical repair. There has been a significant increase in the number of patients being selected for EVAR of AAAs over the last decade. In recent years, the use of EVAR in the management of infrarenal AAAs has increased to approximately 45–80%.[76,80,122,123] This increased use of EVAR has been attributed to increased familiarity and improved clinical experience with endovascular techniques and significant technical advances in the graft design.

Early results show reduced operative mortality rates, but randomized clinical trials of EVAR versus open repair have not yet demonstrated differences in survival or quality of life over 4 years of follow-up.[124–126] More important, EVAR is associated with a unique set of complications, secondary interventions, and life-long imaging surveillance, leading to increased expense to society.[127–132]

Adverse anatomy of the infrarenal neck/proximal attachment site remains the most common reason for exclusion from EVAR repair, although recent developments, such as fenestrated endografts, are beginning to address this issue. Other common exclusion factors include severe bilateral iliac artery disease and female gender (generally due to smaller ilio-femoral/conduit arteries) but these issues will likely be addressed by decreasing the diameters of the delivery catheters and development of more flexible endografts.[133,134] One issue surrounding successful treatment of AAAs with EVAR that is unlikely to change is the fact that proper patient selection for EVAR will always remain the key to a successful outcome.

References

1. Fleming CC, Whitlock EP, Bell TL, Lederle FA. Screening for abdominal aortic aneurysm: A best-evidence systematic review for the US Preventive Services Task Force. Ann Intern Med 2005;142(3):203–11.
2. Adam DJ, Mohan IV, Stuart WP, Bain M, Bradbury AW. Community and hospital outcome from ruptured abdominal aortic aneurysm within the catchment area of a regional vascular surgical service. J Vasc Surg 1999;30(5):922–8.
3. Gillum RR. Epidemiology of aortic-aneurysm in the United States. J Clin Epidemiol 1995;48(11):1289–98.
4. Centers for Disease Control, National Center for Injury Prevention and Control. Retrieved February 19, 2008, from http://webappa.cdc.gov/sasweb/ncipc/leadcaus10.html
5. Nowygrod R, Egorova N, Greco G, et al. Trends, complications, and mortality in peripheral vascular surgery. J Vasc Surg 2006;43(2):205–16.
6. Cowan JA, Jr., Dimick JB, Henke PK, Rectenwald J, Stanley JC, Upchurch GR, Jr. Epidemiology of aortic aneurysm repair in the United States from 1993 to 2003. Ann NY Acad Sci 2006;1085(1):1–10.
7. Darling RR, Messina CR, Brewster DC, Ottinger LW. Autopsy study of unoperated abdominal aortic-aneurysms case for early resection. Circulation 1977;56(3):161–4.
8. Hollier LL, Taylor LM, Ochsner J. Recommended indications for operative treatment of abdominal aortic-aneurysms. Report of a subcommittee of the Joint Council of the Society for Vascular Surgery and the North American Chapter of the International Society for Cardiovascular Surgery. J Vasc Surg 1992;15(6):1046–56.

9. Powell JJ, Brady AR, Brown LC, et al. Mortality results for randomised controlled trial of early elective surgery or ultrasonographic surveillance for small abdominal aortic aneurysms. Lancet 1998;352(9141):1649–55.

10. Lederle FF, Wilson SE, Johnson GR, et al. Immediate repair compared with surveillance of small abdominal aortic aneurysms. N Engl J Med 2002;346(19):1437–44.

11. The United Kingdom Small Aneurysm Trial. Long-term outcomes of immediate repair compared with surveillance of small abdominal aortic aneurysms. N Engl J Med 2002;346(19):1445–52.

12. Katz DD, Littenberg B, Cronenwett JL. Management of small abdominal aortic aneurysms – early surgery vs watchful waiting. JAMA 1992;268(19):2678–86.

13. Brewster DD, Cronenwett JL, Hallett JW, Johnston KW, Krupski WC, Matsumura JS. Guidelines for the treatment of abdominal aortic aneurysms. Report of a sub-committee of the Joint Council of the American Association for Vascular Surgery and Society for Vascular Surgery. J Vasc Surg 2003;37(5):1106–17.

14. Limet RR, Sakalihassan N, Albert A. Determination of the expansion rate and incidence of rupture of abdominal aortic aneurysms. J Vasc Surg 1991;14(4):540–8.

15. Bengtsson HH, Nilsson P, Bergqvist D. Natural history of abdominal aortic aneurysm detected by screening. Br J Surg 1993;80(6):718–20.

16. Cronenwett JJ, Sargent SK, Wall MH, et al. Variables that affect the expansion rate and outcome of small abdominal aortic aneurysms. J Vasc Surg 1990; 11(2):260–9.

17. Grimshaw GG, Thompson JM. The abnormal aorta – a statistical definition and strategy for monitoring change. Eur J Vasc Endovasc Surg 1995;10(1):95–100.

18. Hirose YY, Hamada S, Takamiya M. Predicting the growth or aortic aneurysms – a comparison of linear vs. exponential models. Angiology 1995;46(5):413–9.

19. Hallin AA, Bergqvist D, Holmberg L. Literature review of surgical management of abdominal aortic aneurysm. Eur J Vasc Endovasc Surg 2001;22(3):197–204.

20. Santilli SS, Littooy FN, Cambria RA, et al. Expansion rates and outcomes for the 3.0-cm to the 3.9-cm infrarenal abdominal aortic aneurysm. J Vasc Surg 2002;35(4):666–71.

21. Bengtsson HH, Källerö SS, Bergqvist DD, Ekberg OO, Aspelin PP. Ultrasound screening of the abdominal aorta in patients with intermittent claudication. Eur J Vasc Surg 1989;3(6):497–502.

22. Englund RR, Hudson P, Hanel K, Stanton A. Expansion rates of small abdominal aortic aneurysms. Aust N Z J Surg 1998;68(1):21–4.

23. Schewe CC, Schweikart HP, Hammel G, Spengel FA, Zollner N, Zoller WG. Influence of selective management on the prognosis and the risks of rupture of abdominal aortic aneurysms. Clin Investig 1994;72(8):585–91.

24. Chang JJ, Stein TA, Liu JP, Dunn ME. Risk factors associated with rapid growth of small abdominal aortic aneurysms. Surgery 1997;121(2):117–22.

25. Macsweeney SS, Ellis M, Worrell PC, Greenhalgh RM, Powell JT. Smoking and growth-rate of small abdominal aortic aneurysms. Lancet 1994;344(8923):651–2.

26. Brady AA, Thompson SG, Greenhalgh RM, Powell JT. Cardiovascular risk factors and abdominal aortic aneurysm expansion: Only smoking counts. Br J Surg 2003;90(4):492–3.

27. Lindholt JJ, Heegaard NHH, Vammen S, Fasting H, Henneberg EW, Heickendorff L. Smoking, but not lipids, lipoprotein (a) and antibodies against oxidised LDL, is correlated to the expansion of abdominal aortic aneurysms. Eur J Vasc Endovasc Surg 2001;21(1):51–6.

28. Krupski WW, Bass A, Thurston DW, Dilley RB, Bernstein EF. Utility of computed tomography for surveillance of small abdominal aortic aneurysms – preliminary report. Arch Surg 1990;125(10):1345–50.

29. Wolf YY, Thomas WS, Brennan FJ, Goff WG, Sise MJ, Bernstein EF. Computed tomography scanning findings associated with rapid expansion of abdominal aortic aneurysms. J Vasc Surg 1994;20(4):529–38.

30. Szilagyi DD, Smith RF, Derusso FJ, Elliott JP, Sherrin FW. Contribution of abdominal aortic aneurysmectomy to prolong life. Ann Surg 1966;164(4):678.

31. Sterpetti AA, Cavallaro A, Cavallari N, et al. Factors influencing the rupture of abdominal aortic aneurysms. Surgery 1991;173(3):175–8.

32. Nevitt MM, Ballard DJ, Hallett JW. Prognosis of abdominal aortic aneurysms. A population based study. N Engl J Med 1989;321(15):1009–14.

33. Brown LL, Powell JT. Risk factors for aneurysm rupture in patients kept under ultrasound surveillance. Ann Surg 1999;230(3):289–96.

34. Reed WW, Hallett JW, Damiano MA, Ballard DJ. Learning from the last ultrasound. A population-based study of patients with abdominal aortic aneurysm. Arch Intern Med 1997;157(18):2064–8.

35. Guirguis EE, Barber GG. The natural history of abdominal aortic aneurysms. Am J Surg 1991;162(5):481–3.

36. Scott RR, Tisi PV, Ashton HA, Allen DR. Abdominal aortic aneurysm rupture rates: A 7-year follow-up of the entire abdominal aortic aneurysm population detected by screening. J Vasc Surg 1998;28(1):124–8.

37. Fillinger MM, Marra SP, Raghavan ML, Kennedy FE. Prediction of rupture risk in abdominal aortic aneurysm during observation: Wall stress versus diameter. J Vasc Surg 2003;37(4):724–32.

38. Fillinger MM, Raghavan ML, Marra SP, Cronenwett JL, Kennedy FE. In vivo analysis of mechanical wall stress and abdominal aortic aneurysm rupture risk. J Vasc Surg 2002;36(3):589–97.

39. Hunter GG, Smyth SH, Aguirre ML, et al. Incidence and histologic characteristics of blebs in patients with abdominal aortic aneurysms. J Vasc Surg 1996;24(1):93–101.

40. Vorp DD, Raghavan ML, Webster MW. Mechanical wall stress in abdominal aortic aneurysm: Influence of diameter and asymmetry. J Vasc Surg 1998;27(4):632–9.

41. Cronenwett JJ, Murphy TF, Zelenock GB, et al. Actuarial analysis of variable associated with rupture of small abdominal aortic aneurysms. Surgery 1985;98(3):472–83.

42. Darling RR, Brewster DC, Darling RC, et al. Are familial abdominal aortic aneurysms different? J Vasc Surg 1989;10(1):39–43.

43. Heller JJ, Weinberg A, Arons R, et-al. Two decades of abdominal aortic aneurysm repair: Have we made any progress? J Vasc Surg 2000;32(6):1091–8.

44. Semmens JJ, Norman PE, Lawrence-Brown MMD, Bass AJ, Holman CDJ. Population-based record linkage study of the incidence of abdominal aortic aneurysm in Western Australia in 1985–1994. Br J Surg 1998;85(5):648–52.

45. Pearce WW, Parker MA, Feinglass J, Ujiki M, Manheim LM. The importance of surgeon volume and training in outcomes for vascular surgical procedures. J Vasc Surg 1999;29(5):768–76.

46. Manheim LL, Sohn MW, Feinglass J, Ujiki M, Parker MA, Pearce WH. Hospital vascular surgery volume and procedure mortality rates in California, 1982–1994. J Vasc Surg 1998;28(1):45–58.

47. Kazmers AA, Perkins AJ, Jacobs LA. Outcomes after abdominal aortic aneurysm repair in those [3]80 years of age: Recent veterans affairs experience. Ann Vasc Surg 1998;12(2):106–12.

48. Huber TT, Wang JG, Derrow AE, et al. Experience in the United States with intact abdominal aortic aneurysm repair. J Vasc Surg 2001;33(2):304–10.

49. Galland RR. Mortality following elective infrarenal aortic reconstruction: A Joint Vascular Research Group study. Br J Surg 1998;85(5):633–6.

50. Bayly PP, Matthews JNS, Dobson PM, Price ML, Thomas DG. In-hospital mortality from abdominal aortic surgery in Great Britain and Ireland: Vascular Anaesthesia Society audit. Br J Surg 2001;88(5):687–92.

51. Becquemin JJ, Chemla E, Chatellier G, Allaire E, Melliere D, Desgranges P. Perioperative factors influencing the outcome of elective abdominal aorta aneurysm repair. Eur J Vasc Endovasc Surg 2000;20(1):84–9.

52. Collins TT, Johnson M, Daley J, Henderson WG, Khuri SF, Gordon HS. Preoperative risk factors for 30-day mortality after elective surgery for vascular

disease in Department of Veterans Affairs hospitals: Is race important? J Vasc Surg 2001;34(4):634–40.

53. Dardik AA, Lin JW, Gordon TA, Williams M, Perler BA. Results of elective abdominal aortic aneurysm repair in the 1990s: A population-based analysis of 2335 cases. J Vasc Surg 1999;30(6):985–92.

54. Dimick JJ, Stanley JC, Axelrod DA, et al. Variation in death rate after abdominal aortic aneurysmectomy in the United States – Impact of hospital volume, gender, and age. Ann Surg 2002;235(4):579–85.

55. Birkmeyer JJ, Siewers AE, Finlayson EVA, et al. Hospital volume and surgical mortality in the United States. N Engl J Med 2002;346(15):1128–37.

56. Blankensteijn JJ, Lindenburg FP, Van der Graaf Y, Eikelboom BC. Influence of study design on reported mortality and morbidity rates after abdominal aortic aneurysm repair. Br J Surg 1998;85(12):1624–30.

57. Brady AA, Fowkes FGR, Greenhalgh RM, Powell JT, Ruckley CV, Thompson SG. Risk factors for postoperative death following elective surgical repair of abdominal aortic aneurysm: Results from the UK Small Aneurysm Trial. Br J Surg 2000;87(6):742–9.

58. Bradbury AA, Adam DJ, Makhdoomi KR, et al. A 21-year experience of abdominal aortic aneurysm operations in Edinburgh. Br J Surg 1998;85(5):645–7.

59. May J, White GH, Yu W, et al. Endoluminal grafting of abdominal aortic aneurysms: Causes of failure and their prevention. J Endovasc Surg 1994;1(1):44–52.

60. Blum UU, Voshage G, Lammer J, et al. Endoluminal stent-grafts for infrarenal abdominal aortic aneurysms. N Engl J Med 1997;336(1):13–20.

61. Yusuf SS, Baker DM, Chuter TAM, Whitaker SC, Wenham PW, Hopkinson BR. Transfemoral endoluminal repair of abdominal aortic aneurysm with bifurcated graft. Lancet 1994;344(8923):650–1.

62. Moore WW, Vescera CL. Repair of abdominal aortic aneurysm by transfemoral endovascular graft placement. Ann Surg 1994;220(3):331–41.

63. Carpenter JJ, Baum RA, Barker CF, et al. Durability of benefits of endovascular versus conventional abdominal aortic aneurysm repair. J Vasc Surg 2002;35(2):222–8.

64. Laheij RJ, Buth J, Harris PL, Moll FL, Stelter WJ, Verhoeven EL. Need for secondary interventions after endovascular repair of abdominal aortic aneurysms. Intermediate-term follow-up results of a European collaborative registry (EUROSTAR). Br J Surg 2000;87(12):1666–73.

65. Beebe HH, Jackson T, Pigott JP. Aortic aneurysm morphology for planning endovascular aortic grafts – limits of conventional imaging methods. J Endovasc Surg 1995;2(2):139–48.

66. Trout HH, Tanner HM. A new vascular Endostaple: A technical description. J Vasc Surg 2001;34(3):565–8.

67. Malina MM, Nilsson M, Brunkwall J, Ivancev K, Resch T, Lindblad B. Quality of life before and after endovascular and open repair of asymptomatic AAAs: A prospective study. J Endovasc Ther 2000;7(5):372–9.

68. Arko FF, Hill BB, Reeves TR, et al. Early and late functional outcome assessments following endovascular and open aneurysm repair. J Endovasc Ther 2003;10(1):2–9.

69. Lawrence DD, Charnsangavej C, Wright KC, Gianturco C, Wallace S. Percutaneous endovascuar graft – experimental evaluation. Radiology 1987;163(2):357–60.

70. Kouchoukos NN, Dougenis D. Surgery of the thoracic aorta. N Engl J Med 1997;336(26):1876–88.

71. Balko A, Piasecki GJ, Shah DM, Carney WI, Hopkins RW, Jackson BT. Transfemoral placement of intraluminal polyurethane prosthesis for abdominal aortic aneurysm. J Surg Res 1986;40(4):305–9.

72. Finlayson SS, Birkmeyer JD, Fillinger MF, Cronenwett JL. Should endovascular surgery lower the threshold for repair of abdominal aortic aneurysms? J Vasc Surg 1999;29(6):973–84.

73. Axelrod DD, Lookstein RA, Guller J, et al. Inferior mesenteric artery embolization before endovascular aneurysm repair: Technique and initial results. J Vasc Interv Radiol 2004;15(11):1263–7.

74. Sheehan MM, Hagino RT, Canby E, et al. Type 2 endoleaks after abdominal aortic aneurysm stent grafting with systematic mesenteric and lumbar coil embolization. Ann Vas Surg 2006;20(4):458–63.

75. Stanley BB, Semmens JB, Mai Q, et al. Evaluation of patient selection guidelines for endoluminal AAA repair with the Zenith stent-graft: The Australasian experience. J Endovasc Ther 2001;8(5):457–64.

76. Zarins CC, Wolf YG, Lee WA, et al. Will endovascular repair replace open surgery for abdominal aortic aneurysm repair? Ann Surg 2000;232(4):501–5.

77. Wolf YY, Fogarty TJ, Olcott C, et al. Endovascular repair of abdominal aortic aneurysms: Eligibility rate and impact on the rate of open repair. J Vasc Surg 2000;32(3):519–23.

78. Greenberg RR. Abdominal aortic endografting: Fixation and sealing. J Am Coll Surg 2002;194(1):S79–S87.

79. Ingle HH, Fishwick G, Thompson MM, Bell PRF. Endovascular repair of wide neck AAA – Preliminary report on feasibility and complications. Eur J Vasc Endovasc Surg 2002;24(2):123–7.

80. Carpenter JJ, Baum RA, Barker CF, et al. Impact of exclusion criteria on patient selection for endovascular abdominal aortic aneurysm repair. J Vasc Surg 2001;34(6):1050–4.

81. Wolf YY, Hill BB, Lee A, Corcoran CM, Fogarty TJ, Zarins CK. Eccentric stent graft compression: An indicator of insecure proximal fixation of aortic stent graft. J Vasc Surg 2001;33(3):481–7.

82. Sternbergh WW, Carter G, York JW, Yoselevitz M, Money SR. Aortic neck angulation predicts adverse outcome with endovascular abdominal aortic aneurysm repair. J Vasc Surg 2002;35(3):482–6.

83. Cox DE, Jacobs DL, Motaganahalli RL, Wittgen CM, Peterson GJ. Outcomes of endovascular AAA repair in patients with hostile neck anatomy using adjunctive balloon-expandable stents. Vasc Endovascular Surg 2006;40(1):35–40.

84. Gitlitz DD, Ramaswami G, Kaplan D, Hollier LH, Marin ML. Endovascular stent grafting in the presence of aortic neck filling defects: Early clinical experience. J Vasc Surg 2001;33(2):340–4.

85. Parlani GG, Zannetti S, Verzini F, et al. Does the presence of an iliac aneurysm affect outcome of endoluminal AAA repair? An analysis of 336 cases. Eur J Vasc Endovasc Surg 2002;24(2):134–8.

86. Mehta MM, Veith FJ, Ohki T, et al. Unilateral and bilateral hypogastric artery interruption during aortoiliac aneurysm repair in 154 patients: A relatively innocuous procedure. J Vasc Surg 2001;33(2):S27–S32.

87. Parodi JJ, Ferreira M. Relocation of the iliac artery bifurcation to facilitate endoluminal treatment of abdominal aortic aneurysms. J Endovasc Surg 1999;6(4):342–7.

88. Kritpracha BB, Pigott JP, Russell TE, et al. Bell-bottom aortoiliac endografts: An alternative that preserves pelvic blood flow. Journal of vascular surgery 2002;35(5):874–80.

89. Abu-Ghaida AM, Clair DG, Greenberg RK, Srivastava S, O'hara PJ, Ouriel K. Broadening the applicability of endovascular aneurysm repair: The use of iliac conduits. J Vasc Surg 2002;36(1):111–7.

90. Buth JJ, Laheij RJF. Early complications and endoleaks after endovascular abdominal aortic aneurysm repair: Report of a multicenter study. J Vasc Surg 2000;31(1):134–45.

91. Resch TT, Ivancev K, Lindh M, et al. Persistent collateral perfusion of abdominal aortic aneurysm after endovascular repair does not lead to progressive change in aneurysm diameter. J Vasc Surg 1998;28(2):242–9.

92. Chaikof EL, Blankensteijn JD, Harris PL, et al. Reporting standards for endovascular aortic aneurysm repair. J Vasc Surg 2002;35(5):1048–60.

93. Greenberg RR, Fairman R, Srivastava S, Criado F, Green R. Endovascular grafting in patients with short proximal necks: An analysis of short-term results. Cardiovasc Surgery 2000;8(5):350–4.

94. Anderson JJ, Berce M, Hartley DE. Endoluminal aortic grafting with renal and superior mesenteric artery incorporation by graft fenestration. J Endovasc Ther 2001;8(1):3–15.

95. Stanley BB, Semmens JB, Lawrence-Brown MMD, Boodman MA, Hartley DE. Fenestration in endovascular grafts for aortic aneurysm repair: New horizons for preserving blood flow in branch vessels. J Endovasc Ther 2001;8(1):16–24.

96. Faruqi RR, Chuter TAM, Reilly LM, et al. Endovascular repair of abdominal aortic aneurysm using a pararenal fenestrated stent-graft. J Endovasc Surg 1999;6(4):354–8.

97. Greenberg RR, Hanlon S, Lyden SP, et al. Endovascular management of juxtarenal aneurysms with fenestrated endovascular grafting. J Vasc Surg 2004;39(2):279–86.

98. Yusuf SS, Whitaker SC, Chuter TAM, Wenham PW, Hopkinson BR. Emergency endovascular repair of leaking aortic aneurysm. Lancet 1994;344(8937): 1645–47.

99. Ohki TT, Veith FJ, Sanchez LA, et al. Endovascular graft repair of ruptured aortoiliac aneurysms. J Am Coll Surg 1999;189(1):102–12.

100. Verhoeven ELG, Prins TR, van den Dungen JJAM, Tielliu IFJ, Hulsebos RG, van Schilfgaarde R. Endovascular repair of acute AAAs under local anesthesia with bifurcated endografts: A feasibility study. J Endovasc Ther 2002;9(6):729–35.

101. Henretta JJ, Hodgson KJ, Mattos MA, et al. Feasibility of endovascular repair of abdominal aortic aneurysms with local anesthesia with intravenous sedation. J Vasc Surg 1999;29(5):793–8.

102. Veith FJ, Ohki T, Lipsitz EC, Suggs WD, Cynamon J. Endovascular grafts and other catheter-directed techniques in the management of ruptured abdominal aortic aneurysms. Sem Vasc Surg 2003;16(4):326–31.

103. Peppelenbosch NN, Yilmaz N, van Marrewijk C, et al. Emergency treatment of acute symptomatic or ruptured abdominal aortic aneurysm. Outcome of a prospective intent-to-treat by EVAR protocol. Eur J Vasc Endovasc Surg 2003;26(3):303–10.

104. Reichart MM, Geelkerken RH, Huisman AB, van Det RJ, de Smit P, Volker EP. Ruptured abdominal aortic aneurysm: Endovascular repair is feasible in 40% of patients. Eur J Vasc Endovasc Surg 2003;26(5):479–86.

105. Hinchliffe RR, Alric P, Rose D, et al. Comparison of morphologic features of intact and ruptured aneurysms of infrarenal abdominal aorta. J Vasc Surg 2003;38(1):88–92.

106. Ohki TT, Veith FJ. Endovascular grafts and other image-guided catheter-based adjuncts to improve the treatment of ruptured aortoiliac aneurysms. Ann Surg 2000;232(4):466–77.

107. Greco GG, Egorova N, Anderson PL, et al. Outcomes of endovascular treatment of ruptured abdominal aortic aneurysms. J Vasc Surg 2006;43(3):453–9.

108. McKinsey JF RA, Egorova NN. National outcomes for the treatment of ruptured abdominal aortic aneurysm: Comparison of open versus endovascular repairs. In: Society for Cardiovascular Surgery 2006 meeting abstracts; 2006.

109. Cambria RR, Clouse WD, Davison JK, Dunn PF, Corey M, Dorer D. Thoracoabdominal aneurysm repair: Results with 337 operations performed over a 15-year interval. Ann Surg 2002;236(4):471–9.

110. Coselli JJ. Thoracoabdominal aortic aneurysms – experience with 372 patients. J Card Surg 1994;9(6):638–47.

111. Hines GG, Busutil S. Thoraco-abdominal aneurysm resection. Determinants of survival in a community hospital. J Cardiovasc Surg 1994;35(6):243–6.

112. Cox GG, Ohara PJ, Hertzer NR, Piedmonte MR, Krajewski LP, Beven EG. Thoracoabdominal aneurysm repair – a representative experience. J Vasc Surg 1992;15(5):780–8.

113. Godet GG, Fleron MH, Vicaut E, et al. Risk factors for acute postoperative renal failure in thoracic or thoracoabdominal aortic surgery: A prospective study. Anesth Analg 1997;85(6):1227–32.

114. Greenberg RK. Aortic aneurysm, thoracoabdominal aneurysm, juxtarenal aneurysm, fenestrated dndografts, branched endografts, and endovascular aneurysm repair. Ann NY Acad Sci 2006;1085(1):187–96.

115. Browne TT, Hartley D, Purchas S, Rosenberg M, Van Schie G, Lawrence-Brown M. A fenestrated covered suprarenal aortic stent. Eur J Vasc Endovasc Surg 1999;18(5):445–9.

116. Greenberg RR, Haulon S, O'Neill S, Lyden S, Ouriel K. Primary endovascular repair of juxtarenal aneurysms with fenestrated endovascular grafting. Eur J Vasc Endovasc Surg 2004;27(5):484–91.

117. O'Neill SS, Greenberg RK, Haddad F, Resch T, Sereika J, Katz E. A prospective analysis of fenestrated endovascular grafting: Intermediate-term outcomes. Eur J Vasc Endovasc Surg 2006;32(2):115–23.

118. Verhoeven EE, Prins TR, Tielliu IFJ, et al. Treatment of short-necked infrarenal aortic aneurysms with fenestrated stent-grafts: Short-term results. Eur J Vasc Endovasc Surg 2004;27(5):477–83.

119. Chuter TAM, Gordon RL, Reilly LM, Pak LK, Messina LM. Multi-branched stent-graft for type III thoracoabdominal aortic aneurysm. J Vasc Interv Radiol 2001;12(3):391–2.

120. Anderson JJ, Adam DJ, Berce M, Hartley DE. Repair of thoracoabdominal aortic aneurysms with fenestrated and branched endovascular stent grafts. J Vasc Surg 2005;42(4):600–7.

121. Greenberg RR, West K, Pfaff K, et al. Beyond the aortic bifurcation: Branched endovascular grafts for thoracoabdominal and aortoiliac aneurysms. J Vasc Surg 2006;43(5):879–86.

122. Armon MM, Yusuf SW, Latief K, et al. Anatomical suitability of abdominal aortic aneurysms for endovascular repair. Br J Surg 1997;84(2):178–80.

123. Treiman GG, Lawrence PF, Edwards WH, Galt SW, Kraiss LW, Bhirangi K. An assessment of the current applicability of the EVT endovascular graft for treatment of patients with an infrarenal abdominal aortic aneurysm. J Vasc Surg 1999;30(1):68–74.

124. Greenhalgh RMRM, Powell JTJT, Thompson SGSG, Brown LCLC, Kwong GPGPS. Comparison of endovascular aneurysm repair with open repair in patients with abdominal aortic aneurysm (EVAR trial 1), 30-day operative mortality results: Randomised controlled trial. Lancet 2004;364(9437):843–8.

125. Endovascular aneurysm repair versus open repair in patients with abdominal aortic aneurysm (EVAR trial 1): randomised controlled trial. Lancet 2005;365(9478):2179–86.

126. Blankensteijn JJ, de Jong S, Prinssen M, et al. Two-year outcomes after conventional or endovascular repair of abdominal aortic aneurysms. N Engl J Med 2005;352(23):2398–405.

127. Veith FF, Baum RA, Ohki T, et al. Nature and significance of endoleaks and endotension: Summary of opinions expressed at an international conference. J Vasc Surg 2002;35(5):1029–35.

128. Sapirstein WW, Chandeysson P, Wentz C. The Food and Drug Administration approval of endovascular grafts for abdominal aortic aneurysm: An 18-month retrospective. J Vasc Surg 2001;34(1):180–3.

129. Lee WW, Carter JW, Upchurch G, Seeger JM, Huber TS. Perioperative outcomes after open and endovascular repair of intact abdominal aortic aneurysms in the United States during 2001. J Vasc Surg 2004;39(3):491–6.

130. Drury DD, Michaels JA, Jones L, Ayiku L. Systematic review of recent evidence for the safety and efficacy of elective endovascular repair in the management of infrarenal abdominal aortic aneurysm. Br J Surg 2005;92(8):937–46.

131. Hayter CC, Bradshaw SR, Allen RJ, Guduguntla M, Hardman DTA. Follow-up costs increase the cost disparity between endovascular and open abdominal aortic aneurysm repair. Journal of vascular surgery 2005;42(5):912–8.

132. Michaels JJ, Drury D, Thomas SM. Cost-effectiveness of endovascular abdominal aortic aneurysm repair. Br J Surg 2005;92(8):960–7.

133. Velazquez OO, Larson RA, Baum RA, et al. Gender-related differences in infrarenal aortic aneurysm morphologic features: Issues relevant to Ancure and Talent endografts. J Vasc Surg 2001;33(2):S77–S84.

134. Zannetti SS, De Rango P, Parlani G, Verzini F, Maselli A, Cao P. Endovascular abdominal aortic aneurysm repair in high-risk patients: A single centre experience. Eur J Vasc Endovasc Surg 2001;21(4):334–8.

135. Schermerhorn ML, Cronenwett JL. Abdominal aortic aneurysm, Chapter 21. *In* Cronenwett and Rutherford Eds., Decision Making in Vascular Surgery. Philadelphia, PA: W.B. Saunders Co., 2001.

Chapter 7

Endovascular Repair of Abdominal Aortic Aneurysms

Sheela T. Patel and Juan C. Parodi

Abstract Endovascular repair of abdominal aortic aneurysm has evolved dramatically during the last 15 years. From initially a promising experimental technique, applicable only to a minority of patients with aortic aneurysms, to currently a widespread technique that is used in more than one half of patients treated for aortic aneurysm. This chapter presents the current status of this treatment modality for abdominal aortic aneurysm.

Keywords EVAR, EVAR mortality/morbidity, Stent graft trials, AAA, Zenith endograft, Aneurx trial, DREAM trial, Stent graft durability

Introduction

Abdominal aortic aneurysm (AAA) is a common condition, occurring in approximately 1 in 20 older men who have ever smoked.[1] Population-based studies indicate that AAA is responsible for about 1.7% of deaths among adults aged 65–74 years. The natural history of AAA is characterized by progressive expansion and rupture with the rate of rupture and death for aneurysms > 6 cm in diameter exceeding 40% within 3 years of the initial diagnosis.[2] More than 15,000 deaths from aneurysm rupture occur annually in the US with an overall mortality rate for ruptured AAA approaching 90%. Rupture of these aneurysms has a mortality rate of 80%[3] and causes 9000 deaths per year in the US.[4] To prevent rupture, elective repair of an AAA is performed in nearly 40,000 patients each year in the US. Over the last 50 years, AAAs have been treated with prophylactic open surgical repair, a major surgical procedure consisting of laparotomy and cross-clamping of the aorta. The first resection and graft replacement of an AAA was performed in 1951 by Dubost et al.[5] The open repair is associated with a 30-day mortality of 4–12%[6] but the grafts are generally durable and last over 20 years. However, patients with aneurysms are generally elderly and often have significant comorbid medical conditions that increase the operative risks. More recently, endovascular repair was developed to provide a less-invasive alternative. In 1990, Juan C. Parodi

G. Upchurch and E. Criado (eds.) *Aortic Aneurysms, Contemporary Cardiology*
DOI: 10.1007/978-1-60327-204-9_7, © Humana Press, a part of
Springer Science+Business Media, LLC 2009

performed the first endovascular AAA repair in Buenos Aires, thus heralding a new era in the treatment. According to national hospital databases, there has been a 600% increase in the annual number of endovascular aortic aneurysm repair (EVAR) procedures performed in the US since 2000, comprising nearly half of all aneurysm repairs.[7] Continuing technological advances have made EVAR the first-line therapy for AAA in anatomically suitable patients. EVAR has become a mainstay in the arsenal of the vascular surgeon. This procedure has permitted physicians to treat a high-risk older group of patients that in the past would have been excluded from open aneurysm repair. In the last 5 years, there have been more than 30,000 endovascular graft devices implanted annually in patients to treat AAA size with favorable results.

Several studies have demonstrated decreased morbidity and mortality following endovascular repair of AAA. Other advantages include decreased blood loss, decreased transfusion requirements, decreased ileus, and quicker return to baseline functional status. This procedure can be performed in higher-risk patients for whom an open repair would not have been a viable option.

Patient Selection for Endovascular Repair

Currently EVAR is an FDA-approved alternative for open AAA repair. Patients with large (>5–5.5 cm) aneurysms or patients with smaller size (4–5 cm) aneurysms but rapidly enlarging should be considered for repair. Although many published series for endovascular AAA repair include patients with small AAA, findings of randomized clinical trials showed that, compared with surveillance by CT or ultrasonography, a strategy of immediate repair did not improve survival among patients who had AAA of 4–5.4 cm in diameter.[8,9]

In recent years, the number of patients treated with EVAR has steadily risen as a result of increased physician experience, availability of new and more versatile devices, and improvements in noninvasive imaging techniques. Some consider 25–30% of all treatable AAA to be eligible whereas others report that up to 80% can be treated.[10]

When considering EVAR, the patient's age, comorbid conditions, and life expectancy and anatomy should be considered. The primary factors that determine feasibility of endovascular repair are the diameter and length of the proximal neck of the aneurysm, the tortuosity of the aorta, and the anatomy of the iliac arteries. Unfavorable neck anatomy is the primary factor for exclusion from endovascular repair. If the angle between the neck of the aneurysm and the aorta is excessive, the graft may be displaced from its intended position with a subsequent leak at the attachment site. If the common iliac arteries are too large, the limb of the stent may not be well apposed to the wall of the artery, and a leak at the attachment site will result. Relative anatomic contraindications for EVAR include proximal neck < 15 mm, infrarenal aortic diameter > 26 mm, external iliac diameter < 7 mm or > 16 mm, and bilateral internal and external iliac aneurysms.

Patients considered for EVAR must undergo preoperative imaging to assess anatomy. CT with thin cuts of the abdomen and pelvis and subsequent reconstruction is used for operative planning including device selection and sizing. Anatomic and technical criteria must be fulfilled to enable EVAR to be performed successfully. Inadequate proximal neck anatomy is one of the most common reasons why patients are found unsuitable for EVAR. Ideally, an infrarenal neck length of at least 10–15 mm from the lowest renal artery is required for adequate proximal device fixation. Graft diameter usually is usually oversized by approximately 10–15% to ensure adequate radial forces to prevent migration and allow good apposition to the aortic wall. Current commercially available devices range up to 32 mm in diameter, therefore an aortic neck diameter ≤ 28 mm is necessary for adequate fixation. Treatment of aneurysms with larger infrarenal neck diameters may be possible with larger devices. An ideal neck should have minimal thrombus and calcification so that proximal fixation is easier and decrease the risk for migration or type I endoleaks. Aortic neck angulation greater than 60° can lead to imprecise proximal placement with kinking and poor fixation and is considered a relative contraindication to EVAR. Treatment of aneurysms with neck angle greater than 60° is determined by the conformability of the specific device.

Patients with a juxtarneal or suprarenal AAA are not amenable to EVAR with devices currently available in the US. With the development of branched and fenestrated grafts, full endoluminal aortic coverage can be achieved with preservation of visceral and pelvic perfusion. Branched graft technology is currently in use in some European countries and awaits FDA approval in the US, pending the completion of ongoing device-specific US clinical trials.

The guidelines of a subcommittee of the American Association for Vascular Surgery and the SVS concluded that EVAR should be limited to large aneurysms with suitable anatomy in patients unfit for open surgery.[11] A decision-model analysis of data from the European Collaborators on Stent Graft Techniques for Abdominal Aortic Aneurysm Repair (EUROSTAR) registry also suggested that EVAR is preferred for older patients with higher operative risk, whereas open repair is preferred for younger patients with low operative risk.[12] These positions reflect the lack of mortality benefit for EVAR and concerns over its durability.

Stent Graft Trials

After the initial success of homemade endovascular stent grafts, commercially manufactured devices were developed and are currently increasingly utilized as a minimally invasive alternative to open repair. Four have received approval from the US FDA: AneuRx (Medtronic, Inc., Minneapolis, MN), Excluder (W.L. Gore and Associates, Flagstaff, AZ), Zenith (Cook, Inc., Bloomington, IN), PowerLink (Endologix, Irvine, CA) and Talent (Medtronic). Other devices that have received approval for use in the European Union or Canada or are at the clinical trial stage in the US include Fortron (Cordis, Inc., Sommerville, NJ), and Anaconda (Sulzer Vascutek, Austin, TX). The majority of these devices are modular units and have available separate extension segments for each iliac segment, allowing for more customization to fit the patient's particular anatomy.

Zenith Trial Overview

The Zenith endograft (Cook, Inc., Bloomington, Indiana) approved by the FDA in 2003 is a supported, bifurcated, self-expandable stent graft with multiple stainless steel Z stents placed inside the graft. It attaches to the vessel wall with barbs. It has a proximal noncovered stent for suprarenal fixation to prevent migration and enhance graft-to-vessel attachment. FDA approval was based on a comparison between four groups of patients: a control group, a standard-risk group, a high-risk group, and roll-in group. A total of 352 patients were prospectively enrolled. Eighty concurrent surgical controls were enrolled with the intent of comparing them to the standard repair endovascular group. Significantly decreased cardiac, pulmonary, and renal morbidities were noted at 30 days in the endograft group. EVAR patients had fewer transfusion requirements, diminished blood loss, shorter hospital stay, decreased intensive care unit (ICU) stay, and quicker return to daily activities. Kaplan-Meier analysis demonstrated no difference in all-cause mortality and aneurysm-related death between the standard-risk EVAR group and the surgical control group. No acute conversions occurred. Three late conversions to open surgery were reported. Migration was not seen in any patients at 1 year. The majority of aneurysms were smaller in diameter at 1 and 2 years of follow-up. The Zenith endograft demonstrated a reduction in morbidity, mortality, and recovery time, as well as a high rate of aneurysm shrinkage.[13,14] Procedural morbidity was also significantly lower for patients treated with endovascular grafts. The endoleak rate was 4.9% at 12 months in the standard-risk group.

Excluder Trial Overview

The Excluder (W.L. Gore and Associates, Inc., Flagstaff, AZ) was approved by the FDA in 2002. It is a bifurcated endograft with an outer self-expanding nitinol support structure covered with ePTFE. The device is wrapped around the delivery system and tied with a PTFE thread. Two-year outcome data from the pivotal US multicenter, prospective Gore Excluder trial showed that patients treated with the Excluder endograft had less blood loss, required fewer transfusions, and had faster inpatient recovery compared to those treated with open repair.[15] Early major adverse events were reduced significantly in patients treated with the endograft (14% vs 57%, $p < .0001$) and this persisted at 2 years. There was no difference in overall survival rate. Endoleak occurred in 20%, persistent aneurysm growth in 14%. Overall, there was a 7% annual reintervention rate in the endograft group in the first 2 years. However, at 3-year follow-up, the investigators noted pressurization or increase in the aneurysm size in the absence of leaks in up to 20% of patients. The thin ePTFE material with high porosity used in the first-generation device was felt to be responsible for the endotension. Therefore, the device was modified and a low permeability design was introduced in 2004. The new material is engineered to reduce the potential for serous fluid movement through the graft wall.

AneuRx Trial Overview

The AneuRx (Medtronic, Inc., Minneapolis, MN) was the first modular device approved by the FDA in 1999. The modular system consists of a main bifurcated segment and a contralateral iliac leg. The initial multicenter study involved 250 patients with infrarenal aneurysms.[16] A total of 190 patients underwent endovascular repair using AneuRx and 60 underwent open surgical repair. During an 18-month period, there was no significant difference in mortality rates between the groups but patients who underwent EVAR had significant reduction in blood loss and days in the ICU. The major morbidity rate was reduced from 23% in the surgery group to 12% in the endovascular group ($p < .05$). Pooled data from the US Phase I, Phase II, and Phase III clinical trials of 1192 patients treated with AneuRx over 3 years of follow-up showed that the device has markedly reduced the risk of aneurysm rupture while eliminating the need for open surgery in 98%

of patients at 1 year and 93% of patients at 3 years. The overall patient survival rate was 93% at 1 year and 86% at 3 years.[17]

Endologix Trial Overview

The Endologix PowerLink system is a one-piece bifurcated graft composed of PTFE supported by nitinol. A prospective multicenter trial using this device was conducted at 15 sites. Between 2000 and 2003, 258 patients were enrolled. Patients treated with this device had significantly decreased perioperative mortality, blood loss, operative time, ICU, and hospital stay compared to the open surgery control group. There were no reported type I, III, or IV endoleaks at the 48-month follow-up, nor were there any ruptures, graft fabric defects, or stent wire fractures. The authors concluded that the PowerLink device is safe and protects treated patients from rupture, with longer follow-up needed to determine durability.

Registries

The two most important registries are the UK registry for Endovascular Treatment for Aneurysm (RETA) based in Sheffield, England, and the EUROSTAR registry based in Holland. These registries, although voluntary, have provided important information on EVAR, and data from the RETA registry was used in the design of the UK EVAR trials. Open audit in the form of voluntary registries is a useful tool for clinical evaluation of new technologies but do not replace randomized controlled trials in that they are incomplete and open to data entry bias.

The RETA registry was set up in 1996 to audit EVAR deployments within the UK. It contains retrospective and prospective data on 1823 procedures. However, it is voluntary and audited in an open fashion, possibly leading to selection bias. The midterm results from the RETA registry show that at 30 days, 5.8% of patients had died. Postprocedural complications within 30 days occurred in 27.8% of cases and 6.1% had persistent endoleaks. Mortality in the first year was 11%, and 10% per year thereafter up to 5 years. Complications related to the device and aneurysm occurred at a rate of approximately 15% per year (secondary endoleaks, graft migration, kinking, limb occlusion).

The EUROSTAR registry was launched in 1996 as a prospective audit of EVAR performance across 135 centers in 18 European countries. This registry is also voluntary but is the largest registry of devices in Europe. Over one thousand patients have been followed up for more than 5 years. Life table analysis shows a 5-year cumulative survival of 79.2%, a secondary intervention rate of 76.3%, and freedom from aneurysm rupture of 98.6%. This registry concluded that EVAR in high-risk patients may be justified if the patient's life expectancy is greater than 1 year, and that the medium-term outcome is significantly better in patients treated for small aneurysms.

The Lifeline Registry of Endovascular Aneurysm repair was established by the Society for vascular surgery in 1998 to evaluate the long-term outcome of EVAR using FDA-approved devices. This registry contains data on 2664 EVAR patients and 334 open surgical control patients collected under four multicenter IDE clinical trials (AnCure, AneuRx, Excluder, PowerLink). There was no difference in 30-day mortality between EVAR (1.7%) and open surgery (1.4%), and there was no difference in survival at 4 years between EVAR (74%) and surgery (71%). The EVAR group had significantly older and sicker patients than the open surgery group and included patients at high risk for open surgery. Kaplan-Meier analysis revealed a 1.3% cumulative risk of rupture at 5 years among 2664 EVAR patients. This is lower than the 1% per year rupture rate in patients with small aneurysms (<5.5 cm) followed in the UK Small Aneurysm Trial Participants.[8,9]

Randomized Trials of Open and Endovascular AAA Repair

EVAR Clinical Trial Overview

Since the early feasibility trials of EVAR, multiple trials have been performed comparing the results of EVAR with conventional open repair.[16,18–21] These trials were successful in confirming the perceived perioperative advantages of EVAR but were limited by their designs with regards to patient standardization and randomization. More recently, two large randomized trials that enrolled suitable candidates for either open repair or EVAR have been performed, including the Dutch Randomized Endovascular Aneurysm Management (DREAM) trial in the Netherlands and the Endovascular Aneurysm Repair Versus Open Repair (EVAR) trial in the UK. The European randomized trials have provided level-1 evidence to show that EVAR is more effective in preventing aneurysm-related death than conventional open surgery. The perioperative results of both DREAM trial and EVAR 1 trial confirmed the advantages of the less-invasive nature of EVAR.[22,23] In both trials, operative time, transfusion requirements, length of ICU stay, and overall length of stay were significantly less for patients undergoing EVAR. Furthermore, perioperative mortality was significantly lower after EVAR when compared with open repair in both trials. In addition to these results favoring EVAR, the perioperative EVAR 1 trial data, however, showed what has been perceived as one of the shortcomings of EVAR, a significantly higher rate of secondary interventions compared with open repair (9.8% vs 5.8%).

Although these randomized trials successfully showed the perioperative advantages of EVAR over open repair, there is still debate regarding the midterm and long-term advantages of EVAR. The midterm data from the DREAM trial obtained at the 2-year follow-up appear to suggest that the initial perioperative advantages of EVAR may not be maintained over time.[24] The overall survival rate 2 years after randomization was 89.7% for patients undergoing EVAR compared with 89.6% for those undergoing open repair. The midterm data from EVAR trial 1 drew similar conclusions.[25] All-cause mortality 4 years after randomization was similar between patients undergoing EVAR and patients undergoing open repair at approximately 28%. Additionally, both studies showed significantly higher rates of reintervention after EVAR compared with open repair (20% vs 6% in EVAR 1 and a nearly three times higher rate in the DREAM trial). Given the short-term and midterm data produced by these trials, a question remains with regard to the long-term advantages of EVAR over open surgery. In particular, the questions of whether survival will be different over the long term compared with patients undergoing open repair and if EVAR will prove to be cost-effective given the higher rates of reintervention. Longer-term data and cost analysis are necessary to help physicians determine which patients will most benefit from EVAR.

There are two additional ongoing trials of open repair versus EVAR that have not yet reported results: the Veteran Affairs Open versus Endovascular Repair (OVER) trial for abdominal aortic aneurysms and the French Aneurisme de l'aorte abdominale: Chirurgie versus Endoprosthese (ACE) trial.

A recent systematic review of four trials including over 1500 patients comparing open repair with endovascular repair[26] concluded that EVAR reduced 30-day mortality but not the 4-year mortality.

The DREAM Trial

The DREAM trial was a multicenter randomized trial of EVAR versus open surgery in which 351 patients were randomized with AAAs larger than 5.5 cm. Patients were enrolled if considered fit for open surgery and had suitable anatomy for EVAR. Initial results were reported in 2004[23] and revealed a 30-day mortality rate in favor of EVAR (1.2% EVAR, 4.6% OR). The combined rate of operative mortality and severe complications at 30 days was 9.8% for open and 4.7% for EVAR. At 2 years, the cumulative survival rates were 89.6% for open versus 89.7% for EVAR. The cumulative rates of aneurysm-related death were 5.7% and 2.1% for open and EVAR, respectively. Two-year follow-up results were reported in 2005[24] and demonstrated that all-cause mortality was not significantly different between the two groups (20.4% EVAR, 20.3% open). Although a trend toward reduced aneurysm-related death was noted for EVAR (2.1% EVAR, 5.7% open), this difference was not statistically different. Quality of life improved initially for EVAR, but after 6 months, it was equivalent for both groups. The authors concluded that the initial mortality advantage of EVAR over open was lost by 1 year because of nonaneurysm-related deaths.

The EVAR Trials

The UK EVAR trials were initiated in 1999.[27] EVAR 1 randomized suitable patients to either EVAR or open repair. Patients who were unfit to undergo open repair due to significant comorbidity were entered into the EVAR 2 trial. This randomized patients to either EVAR and best medical treatment or best medical treatment alone. Both EVAR trials were limited by long delays between randomization and treatment.

The EVAR 1 trial randomized 1082 patients over 60 years of age with an aneurysm of 5.5 cm or greater to either open repair or EVAR. A total of 512 patients in the EVAR group received their intended elective treatment compared with 496 in the open repair group. Thirty-day and in-hospital mortality were 2/3 lower in the EVAR group than in the open group (1.7% vs 4.7%, $p = .016$).[22] By 4 years, all-cause mortality had leveled off at about 28% for both groups.[28] However, there was a persistent difference in aneurysm-related mortality, 4% for the EVAR group and 7% for the open repair group. The overall rate of complications and reinterventions appeared to diverge between groups over time. Thirty-five percent of all patients receiving EVAR reported one or more postoperative complications, of whom 44% required a secondary intervention. In addition, there were 14 conversions to open repair following EVAR deployment. In contrast, complications and reinterventions were rare in open repair patients. The 30-day mortality for EVAR was 1.7% compared with 4.7% for open repair ($p = .007$). This mortality was lower than that reported by the RETA and EUROSTAR registries, perhaps because the patients randomized in EVAR 1 were those deemed fit to have an open repair compared to the registry data which included unfit patients. The EVAR 1 trial 30-day results reported that secondary procedures were necessary in 9.8% of EVAR patients compared with 5.8% in the open repair group. Endoleaks needed treatment in 3.4% of EVAR patients and ten patients required conversion to open repair intraoperatively. Reinterventions were required in three times as many patients who had EVAR, exceeding 20% at 4 years.

The EVAR 2 trial enrolled 338 patients aged more than 60 years who had aneurysm of at least 5.5 cm in diameter and who met high-surgical risk criteria for open repair due to cardiac, pulmonary, or renal comorbidities. Patients were randomized to EVAR or no intervention. The 30-day mortality for EVAR was 9%. AAA-related mortality at 4 years was 14% for EVAR and 19% for no intervention. Overall, 4-year survival was only 34% in EVAR and 38% in the no-intervention group. The authors concluded that EVAR "is not a safe procedure in such high-risk patients." High crossover and procedural mortality rates have led to controversy regarding the validity of this trial. It is uncertain whether these rates could be improved in another trial or whether they reflect the inherent difficulties of managing these sick patients. Twenty-seven percent of patients crossed over from nonoperative to EVAR and these patients had a lower procedure mortality from EVAR than those originally assigned to it (2% vs 9%). These 47 cases and the exclusion of 14 patients dying while waiting for EVAR appear to confer a survival advantage to those receiving EVAR over those receiving no treatment in a post hoc analysis, but the per protocol analysis did not show a significant difference in either all-cause or aneurysm-related mortality. Outcomes of the EVAR 2 trial have not settled the option for high surgical risk patients.

The trial used a "pragmatism rule" in which internists, cardiologists, radiologists, or surgeons were required to make a determination of whether the patient was unfit for surgery. The lack of objectivity inherent to this pragmatism is verified by the fact that a significant number of patients (47) form the surveillance arm crossed over to EVAR with a mortality of only 2%. The high-risk patient population likely lacks uniformity because no standard, objective criteria were used in making this determination.

Sicard et al.[29] identified high-risk patients (565 EVAR and 61 open) in five US multicenter controlled IDE clinical trials. Application of the EVAR 2 high-risk criteria to these trial data identified 565 patients who were certainly more ill than the 1651 normal-risk patients (4-year mortality: 44% high risk, 21% normal risk). High-risk was defined to match EVAR 2 and includes age 60 years or more with aneurysm size ≥ 5.5 cm and at least one cardiac, pulmonary, or renal comorbidity. The 30-day operative mortality was 2.9% in EVAR versus 5.1% in open ($p = .32$). Overall survival at 4 years after EVAR was 56% versus 66% in open ($p = .23$). The AAA-related death at 1 year was 3% for EVAR and 5.1% for open ($p = .37$). After treatment, EVAR successfully prevented rupture in 99.5% at 1 year and in 97.2% at 4 years.

Despite fitting the EVAR 2 definition of high risk, the US IDE trial mortality compares favorable with EVAR 2 in short-term (30-day mortality: 2.9% US IDE vs 9% in EVAR 2) and 4-year (44% US IDE vs 64% EVAR 2) results. They concluded that EVAR is safe and effective in most patients with advanced age, large aneurysms, and high-risk medical comorbidities. Sicard concluded that

EVAR provides excellent protection from aneurysm rupture and AAA-related death, with no significant difference from open surgical controls. High-risk patients found to have an extremely short-life expectancy from nonaneurysmal disorders may be appropriate candidates for watchful waiting.

Durability

Morphological and structural changes of the endograft leading to device failure have been reported. These changes include: suture breaks between the stent and the graft, fracture of the hooks used to anchor the proximal end of the endograft to the aortic wall, circular and longitudinal stent wire separation, separation of the connections between wire loops, graft fatigue, device migration, component separation, endograft, or vessel thrombosis. Most of these failures manifest with an endoleak.

Endoleak is defined as the incomplete exclusion of the aneurismal sac from the circulation with persistent perfusion of the aneurysm. Meta-analysis of 23 publications involving 1118 patients with successful EVAR yielded an endoleak rate of 24%.[30] Of these endoleaks, 66% were present immediately after stent graft placement and 37% were persistent over time. The clinical significance of endoleaks and their impact on the natural history of aneurysms is uncertain and poorly understood. Endoleaks are classified as:

- Type I: from the proximal or distal attachment sites of the graft. Treatment is usually graft extension.
- Type II: from side-branch vessels (lumbars or inferior mesenteric arteries) that continue to feed the excluded aneurysm sac; mainly treated with coil embolization, if necessary.
- Type III: due to fabric tear, modular or graft disconnection, or graft disintegration.
- Type IV: vascular flow caused by the high porosity of the graft, most likely created by the numerous suture holes holding the graft material to the stent.
- Type V (endotension): growth of the aneurysm sac but reperfusion of the sac could not be demonstrated.

Repair of Small Aneurysms

Traditional teaching dictates repair for AAAs when they reach a diameter of 5–6 cm. Two randomized prospective trials, the UK Small Aneurysm trial and the US Veterans Administration (ADAM) trial, compared early surgical repair with observation.[8,9] Both trials concluded that there is little benefit from early open surgical repair of aneurysms 4–5.5 cm. The perioperative complication rates associated with open surgery were not insignificant for the two trials (2–6%). The relatively high complication rates associated with open surgery raise the question of whether a trial of early EVAR versus serial surveillance might demonstrate benefits. The perioperative mortality rate was 1.8% (22/1193) in the AneuRx databases. EVAR of smaller aneurysms may be safer. The PIVOTAL trial was designed to assess the merits of early endovascular repair of infrarenal small AAAs. This multicenter prospective randomized study will compare EVAR with FDA-approved Medtronic stent grafts with surveillance every 6 months for management of 4–5 cm AAAs.

Evidence suggests that patients with larger aneurysms are less suitable for EVAR.[31] Larger aneurysms are often associated with arterial anatomy that is less favorable for EVAR.[32] It has been shown that patients with AAA > 6 cm and a proximal aortic neck > 26 mm have worse clinical outcome after EVAR.[33]

Cost-Effectiveness of EVAR

A recent cost analysis, modeled after the EVAR 1 and 2 trial scenarios, found that EVAR for a 70-year-old patient with a 5.5 cm AAA who was otherwise fit for surgery would provide an estimated benefit of only 0.10 quality-adjusted life years (QALYs) when compared with open surgery at an incremental cost close to $200,000 per QALY.[34] For an 80-year-old patient with a 6.5 cm AAA, who was unfit for open repair, EVAR would produce an estimated benefit of 1.64 QALYs compared with conservative management at an incremental cost of $15,000. Epstein et al.[35] used a decision-analytic model and found that EVAR costs 3800 pounds more per patient than open repair but produced fewer lifetime QALYs. Prinssen found that since there was almost no difference in all-cause mortality after 1 year in the DREAM trial, EVAR was not cost-effective given its higher cost. This approach assumed that mortality related to nonaneurysm caused during follow-up is greater in patients with EVAR and cancels out the early benefit in aneurysm-related mortality of EVAR.

Conclusions

Endovascular repair of AAA has improved the perioperative morbidity and mortality of patients undergoing AAA repair compared to open surgical repair, although further long-term follow-up is required to determine the durability of these repairs. The advent of branched and fenestrated graft technology will likely expand endovascular stent grafts to all aortic segments. Long-term success is best achieved if the devices are used in properly selected patients and are constructed of durable materials that can withstand the physiological milieu into which they are placed. Careful patient selection and meticulous surveillance postoperatively are essential for long-term success. With future advances in endograft technology, expanding operator experience, and improved surveillance techniques, the current trend of expanding indications for EVAR procedures is likely to continue.

References

1. Fleming C, Whitlock EP, Beil TL, Lederle FA. Screening for abdominal aortic aneurysm: a best-evidence systematic review for the U.S. Preventive Services Task Force. Ann Intern Med. 2005 Feb 1;142(3):203–11.
2. Szilagyi DE, Smith RF, DeRusso FJ, Elliott JP, Sherrin FW. Contribution of abdominal aortic aneurysmectomy to prolongation of life. Ann Surg. 1966 Oct;164(4):678–99.
3. Adam DJ, Mohan IV, Stuart WP, Bain M, Bradbury AW. Community and hospital outcome from ruptured abdominal aortic aneurysm within the catchment area of a regional vascular surgical service. J Vasc Surg. 1999 Nov;30(5):922–8.
4. Gillum RF. Epidemiology of aortic aneurysm in the United States. J Clin Epidemiol. 1995 Nov;48(11):1289–98.

5. Dubost C, Allary M, Oeconomos N. Resection of an aneurysm of the abdominal aorta: reestablishment of the continuity by a preserved human arterial graft, with result after five months. AMA Arch Surg. 1952 Mar;64(3):405–8.

6. Blankensteijn JD, Lindenburg FP, Van der Graaf Y, Eikelboom BC. Influence of study design on reported mortality and morbidity rates after abdominal aortic aneurysm repair. Br J Surg. 1998 Dec;85(12):1624–30.

7. Nowygrod R, Egorova N, Greco G, Anderson P, Gelijns A, Moskowitz A, McKinsey J, Morrissey N, Kent KC. Trends, complications, and mortality in peripheral vascular surgery. J Vasc Surg. 2006 Feb;43(2):205–16.

8. Mortality results for randomised controlled trial of early elective surgery or ultrasonographic surveillance for small abdominal aortic aneurysms. The UK Small Aneurysm Trial Participants. Lancet. 1998 Nov 21;352(9141):1649–55.

9. Lederle FA, et al. Immediate repair compared with surveillance of small abdominal aortic aneurysms. N Engl J Med. 2002 May 9;346(19):1437–44.

10. Becquemin JP. EVAR: new developments and extended applicability. Eur J Vasc Endovasc Surg. 2004 May;27(5):453–5.

11. Brewster DC, Cronenwett JL, et al. Guidelines for the treatment of abdominal aortic aneurysms. Report of a subcommittee of the Joint Council of the American Association for Vascular Surgery and Society for Vascular Surgery. J Vasc Surg. 2003 May;37(5):1106–17.

12. Schermerhorn ML, Finlayson SR, et al. Life expectancy after endovascular versus open abdominal aortic aneurysm repair: results of a decision analysis model on the basis of data from EUROSTAR. J Vasc Surg. 2002 Dec;36(6):1112–20.

13. Greenberg RK, Lawrence-Brown M, Bhandari G, Hartley D, Stelter W, Umscheid T, Chuter T, Ivancev K, Green R, Hopkinson B, Semmens J, Ouriel K. An update of the Zenith endovascular graft for abdominal aortic aneurysms: initial implantation and mid-term follow-up data. J Vasc Surg. 2001 Feb;33(2 Suppl):S157–64.

14. Greenberg R; Zenith Investigators. The Zenith AAA endovascular graft for abdominal aortic aneurysms: clinical update. Semin Vasc Surg. 2003 Jun;16(2):151–7.

15. Kibbe MR, Matsumura JS; Excluder Investigators. The Gore Excluder US multi-center trial: analysis of adverse events at 2 years. Semin Vasc Surg. 2003 Jun;16(2):144–50.

16. Zarins CK, White RA, Schwarten D, Kinney E, Diethrich EB, Hodgson KJ, Fogarty TJ. AneuRx stent graft versus open surgical repair of abdominal aortic aneurysms: multicenter prospective clinical trial. J Vasc Surg. 1999 Feb;29(2):292–305; discussion 306–8.

17. Zarins CK, White RA, Moll FL, Crabtree T, Bloch DA, Hodgson KJ, Fillinger MF, Fogarty TJ. The AneuRx stent graft: four-year results and worldwide experience 2000. J Vasc Surg. 2001 Feb;33(2 Suppl):S135–45.

18. Matsumura JS, Brewster DC, Makaroun MS, Naftel DC. A multicenter controlled clinical trial of open versus endovascular treatment of abdominal aortic aneurysm. J Vasc Surg. 2003 Feb;37(2):262–71.

19. Moore WS, Matsumura JS, Makaroun MS, Katzen BT, Deaton DH, Decker M, Walker G; EVT/Guidant Investigators. Five-year interim comparison of the Guidant bifurcated endograft with open repair of abdominal aortic aneurysm. J Vasc Surg. 2003 Jul;38(1):46–55.

20. Hua HT, Cambria RP, et al. Early outcomes of endovascular versus open abdominal aortic aneurysm repair in the National Surgical Quality Improvement Program-Private Sector (NSQIP-PS). J Vasc Surg. 2005 Mar;41(3):382–9.

21. Bush RL, Johnson ML, Collins TC, Henderson WG, Khuri SF, Yu HJ, Lin PH, Lumsden AB, Ashton CM. Open versus endovascular abdominal aortic aneurysm repair in VA hospitals. J Am Coll Surg. 2006 Apr;202(4):577–87.

22 Greenhalgh RM, Brown LC, Kwong GP, Powell JT, Thompson SG; EVAR trial participants. Comparison of endovascular aneurysm repair with open repair in patients with abdominal aortic aneurysm (EVAR trial 1), 30-day operative mortality results: randomised controlled trial. Lancet. 2004 Sep 4–10;364(9437):843–8.

23. Prinssen M, Verhoeven EL, Buth J, Cuypers PW, van Sambeek MR, Balm R, Aneurysm Management (DREAM)Trial Group. A randomized trial comparing conventional and endovascular repair of abdominal aortic aneurysms. N Engl J Med. 2004 Oct 14;351(16):1607–18.

24. Blankensteijn JD, de Jong SE, Prinssen M, van der Ham AC, Buth J, van Sterkenburg SM, Verhagen HJ, Buskens E, Grobbee DE; Dutch Randomized Endovascular Aneurysm Management (DREAM) Trial Group. Two-year outcomes after conventional or endovascular repair of abdominal aortic aneurysms. N Engl J Med. 2005 Jun 9;352(23):2398–405.

25. EVAR trial participants. Endovascular aneurysm repair versus open repair in patients with abdominal aortic aneurysm (EVAR trial 1): randomised controlled trial. Lancet. 2005 Jun 25–Jul 1;365(9478):2179–86.

26. Lederle FA, Kane RL, MacDonald R, Wilt TJ. Systematic review: repair of unruptured abdominal aortic aneurysm. Ann Intern Med. 2007 May 15;146(10):735–41.

27. Brown LC, Epstein D, Manca A, Beard JD, Powell JT, Greenhalgh RM. The UK Endovascular Aneurysm Repair (EVAR) trials: design, methodology and progress. Eur J Vasc Endovasc Surg. 2004 Apr;27(4):372–81.

28. EVAR trial investigators. Endovascular aneurysm repair versus open repair in patients with abdominal aortic aneurysm (EVAR trial 1): randomised controlled trial. Lancet. 2005 Jun 25-Jul 1;365(9478):2179–86.

29. Sicard GA, Zwolak RM, Sidawy AN, White RA, Siami FS; Society for Vascular Surgery Outcomes Committee. Endovascular abdominal aortic aneurysm repair: long-term outcome measures in patients at high-risk for open surgery. J Vasc Surg. 2006 Aug;44(2):229–36. Epub 2006 Apr 27.

30. Schurink GW, Aarts NJ, van Bockel JH. Endoleak after stent-graft treatment of abdominal aortic aneurysm: a meta-analysis of clinical studies. Br J Surg. 1999 May;86(5):581–7.

31. Thomas SM, Beard JD, Ireland M, Ayers S; Vascular Society of Great Britain and Ireland; British Society of Interventional Radiology. Results from the prospective registry of endovascular treatment of abdominal aortic aneurysms (RETA): mid term results to five years. Eur J Vasc Endovasc Surg. 2005 Jun;29(6):563–70. Epub 2005 Apr 14.

32. Peppelenbosch N, Buth J, Harris PL, van Marrewijk C, Fransen G; EUROSTAR Collaborators. Diameter of abdominal aortic aneurysm and outcome of endovascular aneurysm repair: does size matter? A report from EUROSTAR. J Vasc Surg. 2004 Feb;39(2):288–97.

33. Waasdorp EJ, de Vries JP, Hobo R, Leurs LJ, Buth J, Moll FL; EUROSTAR Collaborators. Aneurysm diameter and proximal aortic neck diameter influence clinical outcome of endovascular abdominal aortic repair: a 4-year EUROSTAR experience. Ann Vasc Surg. 2005 Nov;19(6):755–61.

34. Michaels JA, Drury D, Thomas SM. Cost-effectiveness of endovascular abdominal aortic aneurysm repair. Br J Surg. 2005 Aug;92(8):960–7.

35. Epstein DM, Sculpher MJ, Manca A, Michaels J, Thompson SG, Brown LC, Powell JT, Buxton MJ, Greenhalgh RM. Modelling the long-term cost-effectiveness of endovascular or open repair for abdominal aortic aneurysm. Br J Surg. 2008 Feb;95(2):183–90.

Chapter 8

Complications and Secondary Procedures after Elective Endovascular Aortic Aneurysm Repair

Matthew J. Sideman and Kevin E. Taubman

Abstract Endovascular aortic aneurysm repair has revolutionized the treatment of abdominal aortic aneurysms (AAAs). Since Juan Parodi first published his experience with custom-made stent grafts in 1991, there has been an explosion of interest in endovascular aortic aneurysm repair (EVAR). Manufactured devices have continued to improve leading to decreased operative time, blood loss, ICU stay, and overall hospital stays. As the technique improved, patients previously unfit for open repair were offered EVAR as treatment of their aneurysms that otherwise would have been left to grow and, approximately half of them, rupture. The decreased morbidity and mortality associated with EVAR and its broader application to patients that are not traditional surgical candidates gives some the false sense of safety when performing these procedures. Some think that EVAR is "complication free," but this is certainly not the case. EVAR cases are subject to many of the same complications as open AAA repairs and some that are unique to the procedure itself. It is imperative that physicians who plan on doing EVAR know the possible complications associated with this complex operation and be well versed on the secondary procedures utilized to manage them.

Keywords EVAR complication, endoleak, Limb ischemia, Endograft failure, Endograft infection, Post-implantation syndrome, Access-related complication

Endoleak

Endoleak refers to persistent filling of the aneurysm sac by arterial blood flow despite deployment of the stent graft. The term can cause confusion for other healthcare providers who are unfamiliar with EVAR. The word "leak" can be misinterpreted as extravascular bleeding leading to fear of anemia, hemorrhage, and hypotension. These are certainly not the case but the development of an endoleak is not without significance. It is the most common complication following EVAR. Presence of any type of endoleak at the completion of EVAR

G. Upchurch and E. Criado (eds.) *Aortic Aneurysms, Contemporary Cardiology*
DOI: 10.1007/978-1-60327-204-9_8, © Humana Press, a part of
Springer Science+Business Media, LLC 2009

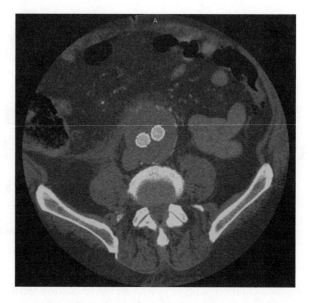

Fig. 1 Rupture of abdominal aortic aneurysm (*AAA*) due to endotension. Patient was hemodynamically stable but had severe back and flank pain.

has been reported in 12–44% of cases,[1–5] although these studies were on first-generation grafts. Initial endoleaks have been reported in anywhere from 15% to 22% in current generation grafts at 1 month.[6–9]

Endoleaks are divided into four (or five) types based on the anatomical source of the continued perfusion. They are as follows:

- Type I: Perfusion of the sac from either the proximal or distal endpoints of the stent graft, representing failure of adequate fixation.
- Type II: Retrograde perfusion of the sac via collateral flow from either lumbar branches or the inferior mesenteric artery.
- Type III: Antegrade perfusion of the sac from leaking between components of the graft.
- Type IV: Antegrade perfusion of the sac from needle holes in the graft material itself.
- Type V: Endotension: Serum transudation into sac through graft material.

The existence of the fifth type is debated but does exist.[10] Serum transudation due to the porosity of the graft can cause continued pressurization of the sac. Although the bloodstream is effectively diverted away from the aneurysm, it can continue to enlarge and even rupture (Fig. 1). Endotension occurred with early versions of polytetrafluoroethylene grafts due to large micron pores in the graft material. This is no longer felt to occur with current versions of these grafts which use a lower porosity material layer.[11]

Type IV endoleaks are also rarely seen today due to improvement in the manufacturing techniques of the grafts. If a type IV endoleak occurs, it likely represents flawed manufacturing of the device. It is also felt that most of these types of endoleaks will seal themselves once anticoagulation is reversed and the sac is allowed to thrombose.

Clinically Significant Endoleaks

Type I endoleaks are the most ominous. The presence of a type I endoleak at the end of an EVAR case essentially gives the patient no protection from rupture and mandates treatment. The first course of action should be to repeat balloon inflation at the seal zones with either longer inflation times or larger balloons. If the endoleak persists, it can usually be corrected by extending the proximal or distal endpoints with stent graft cuffs to improve the seal zone. The difficulty arises if there is no landing zone below the renal arteries to extend proximally or no landing zone before the internal iliac arteries distally. In these cases, the leaks can sometimes be overcome by placing an oversized Palmaz stent into the proximal neck. Distal type I endoleaks can be treated by stenting (balloon expandable or self-expanding) or by extending the stent graft to cover the hypogastric artery. If this is done, the hypogastric should first be embolized to prevent a type II endoleak with persistent filling of the aneurysm via retrograde flow through the hypogastric by pelvic collaterals. Careful consideration including the patient's baseline vascular status, presence of claudication, and patency of the contralateral hypogastic should be given before taking this approach. New onset of buttock claudication and/or pelvic ischemia is significant when the hypogastic is sacrificed.[12] Type I endoleaks that cannot be corrected require conversion to open repair for successful protection against aneurysm rupture.

Type III endoleaks can be present on initial implantation but more commonly occur later in the course of treatment due to partial component separation. Unibody grafts obviously do not carry the risk of type III endoleaks. When present, type III endoleaks mandate treatment to correct them.[13] The rupture and death rate for untreated type III endoleaks is prohibitively high. Most can be corrected with endovascular approaches by relining the component gap with extension cuffs.

Questionable Significant Endoleaks

There has been much debate over the significance of type II endoleaks.[10,13,14] They are the most common type of endoleaks to be present at the completion of an EVAR case. These leaks can be observed postoperatively since the majority of them will spontaneously seal given time (Table 1). It is widely believed that for a type II endoleak to persist, there must be at least two vessels feeding the sac. This allows continuous blood flow through the sac as one vessel becomes the "inflow" and the other becomes the "outflow." Even persistent type II endoleaks are of questionable importance. There are numerous reports of persistent

Table 1 Endoleak and migration rates of commercially available endografts.

Graft	Endoleak (%)		Migration (≥10 mm) (%)
	Initial	1 year	
AneuRx Medtronic	21	13.9	6.9
Excluder Gore	22	17	1.4
Zenith Cook	15	7.3	0
PowerLink Endologix	16	13.9	0.8

type II endoleaks being followed without enlargement of the aneurysm sac and without rupture. Intervention is warranted for a persistent type II endoleak, associated with growth of the aneurysm.[14] These leaks can be approached either operatively (open or laparoscopic[15]) with ligation of the feeding vessel(s) or endovascularly with embolization. A patent inferior mesenteric artery can be approached with a microcatheter via superior mesenteric artery collaterals. Lumbar vessels can be similarly approached with microcatheters through hypogastric collaterals. They can then either be embolized with coils or glue. If these maneuvers fail, the aneurysm can be punctured directly and glue is injected into the residual lumen.[16]

Late Occurring Endoleaks

Endoleaks can develop months to years after completion of an EVAR case even if there were previously none. Late onset endoleaks occur due to changing anatomy of the aneurysm and resultant changes in mechanical stress on the stent graft. Most late endoleaks are type I or type III and should be treated accordingly. The presence of late onset endoleaks underscores the necessity of long-term follow-up after EVAR. Clinical examination, abdominal radiographs, and CT scans at defined intervals are mandatory care for all EVAR patients. Willingness to comply with follow-up as well as radiation and contrast exposure should be considered when selecting patients for EVAR.

In summary, endoleaks are the most common complication after EVAR requiring a secondary procedure. Although most can be observed and resolve on their own, they mandate serial imaging of the patients to ensure aneurysm regression. All type I and III endoleaks require treatment, especially if they occur late. Persistent type II endoleaks with enlarging aneurysms also mandate treatment. Type IV endoleaks and endotension (type V) are rare occurrences but, like type II endoleaks, if they existent in the face of an enlarging aneurysm, they mandate treatment.

Migration

Migration is movement of the endograft after implantation. There is variability among the commercially available endografts in regards to the percentage of grafts that have been shown to migrate over time. Different companies have different definitions of migration leading to some confusion in the migration rates but there has been documented migration in all endografts to some degree. The generally accepted definition is movement of the graft greater than 10 mm. In general, endografts that rely solely on radial force for fixation have higher migration rates than grafts that have some type of active fixation.[17] It is also clear that the percentage of grafts that migrate increases over time.

The significance of migration is case specific. The spectrum ranges from no clinically significant effect to loss of proximal fixation with a new type I endoleak. Migration can also result in kinking of limbs leading to limb ischemia. Treatment of migration is directed by the clinical sequela, but is always aimed at maintaining freedom from aneurysm rupture. This likely indicates open or endovascular treatment of new endoleaks and/or reversal of limb ischemia.

There has been a wide range of migration rates reported in various studies. There is little uniformity between them upon which to draw conclusions about migration. For this reason, we reviewed the literature published by the manufacturing companies (both written and internet) in their IFUs, IDE trials,[6,7,9,18] and postmarket surveillance. The 1-year migration rates are listed in Table 1.

Limb Ischemia

Ischemic limb complications in the setting of EVAR are well described. Ischemia of the lower extremity may occur at the time of implantation or many months afterward. Earlier randomized data reported thrombosis rates as high as 7% within the first 30 days.[19] Another European study demonstrated rates of 2.5% within the first 30 days, 2.5% within 1 year, and 3.9% up to 39 months beyond initial graft deployment.[20] A more recent published review of the US Medicare database documented the annual incidence of limb ischemia at approximately 2% both in the initial perioperative period and over a subsequent 4-year follow-up period.[21]

Mechanisms of limb ischemia in the setting of EVAR are either anatomic and/or graft related. Examples of these mechanisms include kinking, stenosis, thrombosis, and progression of native arterial occlusive disease. It has been suggested that smaller graft limb diameter and extension to the external iliac system may promote graft limb occlusion.[22]

Kinking of the iliac limbs is a technical problem with the device that can occur at the time of implantation or as the result of graft migration. This resultant limb ischemia is created by either an acute graft limb thrombosis or a flow-limiting stenosis compromising inflow into the leg. Kinking identified at the time of implantation can generally be treated by stenting the iliac limb or extending the limb distally with an extension cuff.[23] If an extension cuff will cover the hypogastric artery, consideration should be given to embolizing the hypogastric first to prevent a type II endoleak. Early in the development of EVAR technology, kinking was a significant problem with grafts that had unsupported limbs, such as the Ancure graft (no longer available). Because of a recognized high rate of kinking, up to 28% of these graft had primary stenting done at the time of implantation to prevent this complication.[24] In part, this contributed to events leading the FDA to further investigate the device in postmarket analysis and ultimately resulted in its recall.

Limb ischemia can also occur from *thrombosis* of the iliac limbs. Acute thrombosis will result in limb threatening ischemia of the involved extremity. It mandates prompt diagnosis and treatment to prevent irreversible ischemia and limb loss. Options for therapy are dictated by several factors including institutional resources, patient condition including duration and degree of ischemia, and operator experience. If the patient's limb is not neurovascularly threatened, they may be anticoagulated and percutaneous treatment attempted. Endovascular techniques include thrombolysis (either pharmaceutical or mechanical) with treatment of any underlying anatomic lesion that led to the thrombosis. This may include angioplasty and stenting as indicated. Success is highly variable.[25]

If the extremity is profoundly ischemic with neuromotor or significant neurosensory compromise (Rutherford classification IIb), there is typically not sufficient time to attempt a minimally invasive (percutaneous) approach. In this circumstance or in the setting of a failed percutaneous therapy, an open surgical procedure (e.g., thrombectomy, endarterectomy, etc.) is necessary. This should include the option of extra-anatomic bypass reconstruction (e.g., femoral-to-femoral, axillary-femoral) as needed. Regardless of the employed method, if successful revascularization is achieved, a completion arteriogram is recommended to diagnose the presence of any underlying anatomic cause that may promote recurrence. If no etiology is identified, further consideration should be given to long-term therapeutic anticoagulation.

Finally, limb ischemia in the setting of EVAR may also be caused by *distal embolus* or *stenosis* of underlying peripheral arterial occlusive disease in the native vessels. In time, atherosclerotic lesions in the iliac and/or femoral vessels can lead to decreasing flow through the involved graft limb. If the flow decreases significantly, thrombosis will occur. Treatment of these complications seeks to preserve graft patency by improvement or restoration of the outflow of the involved extremity and maintain limb salvage. Specific interventions are dictated by the location and extent of the disease. Combined open and endovascular approaches may be required.[25]

Device Failure

There have been documented failures of endografts. These range from fractures of the stents, to fixation hook fractures, to perforation of graft materials. The significance of these failures can be variable.[26] There are numerous reports of device stent and hook fractures without untoward affects on the patient. There are also cases of graft material perforation by stents leading to reperfusion of the aneurysm sac, rupture, and death. The failure of the Vanguard (no longer available) device was due to six such ruptures from device failure.[27] Lessons learned from these early failures have lead to the improved technology of the newer generation grafts; however, they must stand the test of time to truly prove to be a durable repair.[28]

Graft Infection

Although rare (less than 0.05%), the occurrence of infected aortic endografts has been well described. When present, these circumstances result in catastrophic problems with the need for explantation and either extra-anatomic bypass or in situ reconstruction with autogenous or allograft tissue.[29–31] These necessary surgical interventions carry an exceedingly high morbidity and mortality rates. Limb loss, aortic stump blowout, and pelvic ischemia are among some of the devastating complications facing the surgeons involved with this scenario. Morbidity is further increased by extended operative durations. The literature supports conservatively estimated mortality rates of 10–15% at 30 days and up to 53% at 5 years.[29–31]

Staphylococcus and *Streptococcal* species remain the most common organisms involved. However, population-based studies of greater than 10,000 patients undergoing either EVAR or open abdominal aortic aneurysm (AAA) repair have suggested that the sources of contamination are multifactorial and are not solely related to intraoperative contamination. The same studies suggest that the presence of nosocomial infection, surgical site infections, and bloodstream septicemia during the perioperative period provides a significant contribution to the later manifestations of this pathological entity.[32]

Strict adherence to sterile technique and administration of appropriate preoperative antibiotics are mandatory to reduce the risk of this severe complication. Most graft infections are late-presenting findings occurring 6–36 months after implantation. Patients present with intermittent fevers, malaise, night sweats, and leukocytosis. Blood cultures may or may not be positive for the offending organism. Long-term antibiotic treatment is ineffective as the sole therapy for an aortic endograft infection.

Post-EVAR Implantation Syndrome

Post-EVAR implantation syndrome is a well-recognized complication of aortic endografting. Some cases series have documented up to a 45–56% occurrence.[33,34] Although the mechanisms are poorly understood, the syndrome is thought to be caused by activation of the inflammatory system. Various acute phase markers have been studied including C-reactive protein (CRP), IL-6, and a-1-antitrypsin, as well as markers for the coagulation cascade and fibrinolytic system.[35,36]

Post-EVAR implantation syndrome is classically described by the triad of fever, leukocytosis, and high CRP levels in the absence of sepsis or stent graft infection. However, the more fulminate clinical manifestations can progress to coagulopathy and severe inflammatory complications including renal failure and acute lung injury requiring hemodialysis and mechanical ventilation. There are no known factors to predict which patients are at risk or known adjuncts to prevent the syndrome from occurring. Treatment is supportive. The mild form usually runs its course over several days and antibiotics are not necessary.[34]

Access-Related Complications

Access-related complications include both vascular and wound problems. The occurrence of these complications varies widely between devices. Review of the IDE trials[6,7,9,18] shows that vascular complications range between 1.3% and 14.5% and that wound complications range from 3% to 11.2% (Table 2). The wide variability is due in part to differences in the size of access, rigidity of

Table 2 Vascular and wound complication rates of commercially available endografts.

Graft	Vascular (%)	Wound (%)
AneuRx Medtronic	4.8	7.9
Excluder Gore	1.3	3
Zenith Cook	14.5	3.7
PowerLink Endologix	5.6	11.2

grafts, and technique for deployment. This group of complications can include *dissection, rupture, embolus, thrombosis, lymphocele, pseudoaneurysm,* and *infection.*

Arterial Dissection

Arterial dissection may occur in the iliac vessel related to difficulty with the initial arterial access and placement of the introducer sheath. Several local factors will increase the risk of these events. This includes a disproportionately large sheath size requirement in relation to the native access vessels, concomitant occlusive disease of the access vessels, and tortuosity/angulation of the iliac vessels.

Preoperative imaging in the form of CT angiography and MR angiography is invaluable to avoid these pitfalls. In these circumstances, potential adjunctive maneuvers to prevent arterial dissection include predilation angioplasty of the iliac vessels prior to EVAR sheath placement, utilization of smaller access sheaths when possible, stiffer wires to aid in sheath placement, use of hydrophobic sheaths, and/or lubrication of the sheath with sterile mineral oil. Sheath placement should be done under fluoroscopic guidance and insertion halted for any significant resistance. Consideration should be given to using the contralateral side for the larger sheath access if amenable or conversion to an iliac conduit if unable to place the sheath in the native femoral or distal iliac artery.

If an arterial dissection does occur, it often remains undetected until completion of the EVAR graft deployment and upon removal of the access sheath. Also referred to as "iliac on a stick," large pieces of the dissected intima may be expelled after the sheath is removed. The dissected intima may also remain in the aorta or iliac arteries creating either an immediate or a delayed presentation of a flow-limiting stenosis or distal embolization. From our experience, we encountered the circumstance of an iliac dissection in the setting of a thoracic aortic EVAR that presented on the night of surgery with an acutely ischemic contralateral limb related to this mechanism. Upon exploration, the intima from the dissection of the right iliac system had embolized to the left popliteal artery (Fig. 2a and b).

Diagnosis and treatment of an iliac dissection requires a high index of suspicion. After closure of the access site, if the inflow into the limb is poor or the Doppler signals in the extremity are diminished in comparison to the preoperative examination, an arterial dissection should be considered. An arteriogram is indicated for any abnormal vascular examination findings to delineate the underlying anatomy. If a dissection is identified, the options for repair relate to the location and extent of the process. This may include endovascular procedures such as angioplasty and stenting. In the setting of failed endovascular therapy, an extra-anatomic bypass (e.g. femoral-femoral, axillary-femoral) is an alternative to reestablish arterial inflow. An arterial dissection that results in distal emboli should be treated with balloon thromboembolectomy or open embolectomy as the circumstances dictate.

Arterial Rupture

Rupture of the iliac artery occurs from persistent attempts to place large sheath access in iliacs that are too small, too diseased, and/or too tortuous. Iliac rupture

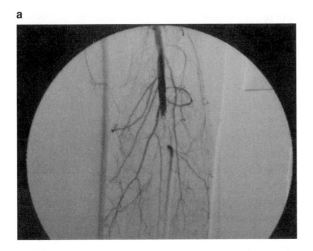

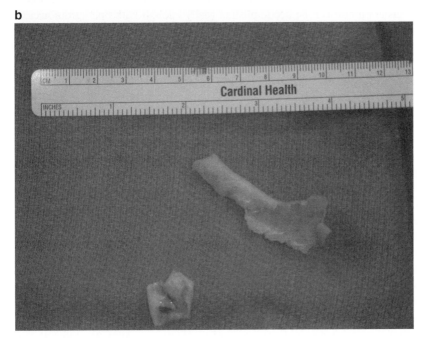

Fig. 2 (a) Arteriogram of left lower leg after distal embolization of iliac intima. (b) Iliac intima removed from the popliteal artery after exploration.

should be suspected when the patient experiences sudden pain or hemodynamic instability. Arteriogram will confirm retroperitoneal extravasation and hemorrhage. This should be controlled with inflation of balloons in the iliac to regain hemodynamic stability with appropriate resuscitation and transfusion of the patient by the anesthesiologist. Consideration should be given to open conversion at this time. If the rupture is small and the patient is hemodynamically stable, an endovascular solution can be attempted. This would involve placement of a covered stent across the perforation if wire access is maintained through the true lumen. If the hemorrhage is controlled with these maneuvers and the patient is stable, completion of the EVAR can be done. If the rupture is controlled, but the patient remains unstable, the EVAR should be aborted. If the rupture cannot be repair with covered stenting, open surgical conversion is necessary to prevent hemorrhagic death.

Embolus

Distal emboli can occur from the access site causing distal limb ischemia. These emboli can be intima from a dissection (as described above), athero-emboli from diseased iliac or common femoral arteries, or thrombotic from formation of clot on the sheath or in situ due to low flow distal to the large sheath access. It is imperative that the patient's distal vascular examination be documented prior to beginning the operation and reexamined after completion of the EVAR and closure of the access sites. Any significant change from preoperative baseline warrants further investigation with a runoff arteriogram. Treatment is then directed by the arteriogram findings but likely would require balloon thromboembolectomy and/or open thromboembolectomy. Treatment of distal emboli can be accomplished easily enough with open groin access. The problem becomes more challenging if percutaneous access is used for placement of the sheath(s).

Thrombosis

Access site thrombosis can occur acutely at the time of EVAR or subacutely presenting in the early postoperative period.[37] This is more likely to happen when accessing and then closing heavily diseased arteries. Whether using open arteriotomies or percutaneous access, if there is significant disease present at the access site, the lumen can be compromised with the repair. The artery should be examined if doing open access for disease after removal of the sheath. If it is extensive, consideration should be given to performing a local endarterectomy to prevent narrowing of the artery after closure. In extreme cases, replacement of the access artery with an interposition graft is necessary. For percutaneous access, closure devices can narrow the access vessel leading to thrombosis. Careful evaluation of the preoperative imaging should be undertaken before choosing to puncture an access artery percutaneously and use a closure device. Any heavily diseased or calcified arteries should be exposed surgically for sheath placement. If thrombosis occurs after percutaneous access and closure, the groin should be explored surgically and repaired as needed.

False Aneurysms

False aneurysms (FAs), or pseudoaneurysms, are defined by the absence of involvement of all three histological layers of the arterial wall. They may occur after EVAR regardless of whether the access is obtained via an open or percutaneous technique. However, the incidence is more common after percutaneous access and with newer generation devices of a size now capable of performing EVAR with percutaneous delivery, the occurrence may increase. Newer arterial closure systems may help to reduce this risk. A recent report of one device suggested a late complication rate of only 2% related to access closure.[38]

Risk factors for the development of these complications relate to access sheath size (≥7 FR), obesity, female gender, periprocedural anticoagulation, high/low femoral access entry sites, and perivascular infection. Diagnosis is made by either contrast-enhanced helical CT or MR angiography, Duplex sonography, or in some cases selective angiography.

Although there are a number of options for treating this complication including percutaneous thrombin and endovascular stenting, FAs detected after EVAR are likely best treated by open surgical exploration and repair. Typically, the defect in the artery is large related to either the percutaneous access sheath or the result of suture-line bleeding in open access circumstances. In the face of a wide-neck FA, thrombin injection may carry a prohibitive risk of native vessel thrombosis.[39]

Lymphocele

A lymphocele is a rare complication of open groin exposures. It is the result of a persistent lymphatic leak into the surgical site causing an accumulation of lymph. Often poor healing of the wound will result. There has been some debate as to whether the occurrence of this complication is higher in the setting of transverse/oblique versus vertical incisions.[40] Aggressive treatment of this complication in the setting of vascular procedures has been shown to reduce the subsequent wound infection rate.[41]

Local Wound (Surgical Site) Infections

Wound infections account for approximately 3% of the morbidity of EVAR, and when further examining for the occurrence of severe infection, this risk further diminishes to less than 1%.[19,20] Typical skin flora such as *Staphylococcus* and *Streptococcus* species are common offending organisms. Infection may range from mild cellulitis to wound dehiscence with purulent drainage. Treatment involves surgical debridement of devitalized tissue and culture-directed antibiotics. Rarely does the extent of infection require arterial reconstruction. However, if encountered to this level of severity, the same principles practiced in the setting of graft infections should be applied in terms of both in situ and extra-anatomic revascularization.

Strict adherence to sterile technique and judicious administration of appropriate perioperative antibiotics are necessary to decrease the incidence of surgical site infections. Tight control of blood glucose in the postoperative period has also been shown to substantially reduce the incidence of surgical site infections in cardiovascular surgery.[42]

Uncommon Complications

Spinal Cord, Colonic, and Pelvic Ischemia

The occurrence of pelvic, spinal, and colonic ischemia following EVAR of the infrarenal aorta is uncommon. Paraplegia following EVAR in the infrarenal aorta remains low with an estimated occurrence of 0.21%.[43,44] However, when present, this complication carries significant morbidity and mortality. This may occur in the setting of postgraft deployment or as a complication of secondary interventions to treat endoleak. Several papers have described an increased association between the appearances of this complication in the setting of perioperative embolization of the hypogastric arteries.

Preservation of one or both of the internal iliac arteries is typically recommended.

Similarly, the occurrence of colon and pelvic ischemia also remains acceptably low, but again when manifested may lead to a higher risk of death and disability. Based upon several trials, clinically significant colon ischemia only appears in 0.6–1.4% of cases.[19,20,44,45] Patients clinically presenting with aneurysm rupture and those requiring extended procedures appear to have elevated risk even in the setting of EVAR.[45] Mechanisms in colon ischemia appear to extend beyond interruption of formerly patent hypogastric vessels or the inferior mesenteric artery and may also relate to a complication of both macro- and microembolization to the capillary bed. Mortality in this setting was correlated with the amount of embolized material.[46]

Graft Enteric Fistula

An uncommon complication that was originally thought to only occur after open AAA repair is graft enteric fistula. This complication occurs approximately 1% of the time after open repair.[47] It is a catastrophic condition where the graft material erodes through an overlying segment of bowel. This results in bacterial contamination of the graft material and potentially massive GI bleeding. This has now been reported to occur after EVAR as well.[48,49] The presence of graft enteric fistula mandates explantation of the graft, repair of the enteric fistula, and either extra-anatomic bypass or reconstruction of the aorta with autogenous tissue. As described above, surgical treatment of this problem carries significantly high morbidity and mortality for the patient. Traditional therapy involves intestinal resection and explantation of the graft with either extra-anatomic or in-line reconstruction.

Conclusion

Although EVAR has expanded treatment of AAA to patients who were previously unfit for open repair with lower overall morbidity and mortality, these procedures are not without their complications. The responsible treating physician should be familiar with all possible complications, counsel their patients extensively on their causes, implications, and treatment, and be prepared to treat any complication that arises.

References

1. Blum U, Voshage G, Lammer J, et al. Endoluminal stent-grafts for infrarenal abdominal aortic aneurysms. N Engl J Med 1997;336:13–20.
2. Moore WS, Rutherford RB: Transfemoral endovascular repair of abdominal aortic aneurysms: Results of the North-American EVT phase 1 trial. J Vasc Surg 1996; 23:543–553.
3. Buth J, van Marrewijk CJ, Harris PL, et al. EUROSTAR Collaborators: Outcome of endovascular abdominal aortic aneurysm repair in patients with conditions considered unfit for an open procedure: A report on the EUROSTAR experience. J Vasc Surg 2002;35:211–221.
4. Mialhe C, Amicabile C, Becquemin JP: Endovascular treatment of infrarenal abdominal aneurysms by the Stentor system: Preliminary results of 79 cases. J Vasc Surg 1997;26:199–209.

5. Stelter W, Umscheid TH, Ziegler P: Three-year experience with modular stent-graft devices for endovascular AAA treatment. J Endovasc Surg 1997;4:362–369.

6. Zarins CK, White RA, Schwarten D, Kinney E, Diethrich EB, Hodgson KJ, Fogarty TJ: AneuRx stent graft versus open surgical repair of abdominal aortic aneurysms: Multicenter prospective clinical trial. J Vasc Surg 1999;29:292–305.

7. Matsumura JS, Brewster DC, Makaroun MS, Naftel DC: A multicenter controlled clinical trial of open versus endovascular treatment of abdominal aortic aneurysms. J Vasc Surg 2003;37:262–271.

8. Abraham CZ, Chuter TA, Reilly LM, Okuhn SP, Pethan LK, Kerian RB, Sawhney R, Buck DG, Gordon RL, Messina LM: Abdominal aortic aneurysm repair with the Zenith stent graft: Short to midterm results. J Vasc Surg 2002;36:217–224.

9. Carpenter JP: Endologix Investigators: Multicenter trial of the PowerLink bifurcated system for endovascular aortic aneurysm repair. J Vasc Surg 2002;36:1129–1137.

10. Veith FJ, et al. Nature and significance of endoleaks and endotension: Summary of opinions expressed at an international conference. J Vasc Surg 2002;35:1029–1035.

11. Haider SE, Najjar SF, Cho JS, Rhee RY, Eskandari MK, Matsumura JS, Makaroun MS, Morasch MD: Sac behavior after aneurysm treatment with the Gore Excluder low-permeability aortic endoprosthesis: 12-month comparison to the original Excluder device. J Vasc Surg 2006;44:694–700.

12. Lee WA, Nelson PR, Berceli SA, Seeger JM, Huber TS: Outcome after hypogastric artery bypass and embolization during endovascular aneurysm repair. J Vasc Surg 2006;44:1162–1168.

13. Buth J, Harris PL, van Marrewijk C, Fransen G: The significance and management of different types of endoleaks. Semin Vasc Surg 2003;16:95–102.

14. van Marrewijk CJ, Fransen G, Laheij RJ, Harris PL, Buth J: EUROSTAR Collaborators: Is a type II endoleak after EVAR a harbinger of risk? Causes and outcomes of open conversion and aneurysm rupture during follow-up. Eur J Vasc Endovasc Surg 2004;27:128–137.

15. Ho P, Law WL, Tung PH, Poon JT, Ting AC, Cheng SW: Laparoscopic transperitoneal clipping of the inferior mesenteric artery for the management of type II endoleak after endovascular repair of an aneurysm. Surg Endosc 2004;18:870.

16. Baum RA, Carpenter JP, Golden MA, Velazquez OC, Clark TW, Stavropoulos SW, Cope C, Fairman RM: Treatment of type 2 endoleaks after endovascular repair of abdominal aortic aneurysms: Comparison of transarterial and translumbar techniques. J Vasc Surg 2002;35:23–29.

17. Tonnessen BH, Sternbergh WC, Money SR: Mid- and long-term device migration after endovascular abdominal aortic aneurysm repair: A comparison of AneuRx and Zenith endografts. J Vasc Surg 2005;42:392–400.

18. Greenberg R, Zenith Investigators: The Zenith AAA endovascular graft for abdominal aortic aneurysms: Clinical update. Semin Vasc Surg. 2003;16:151–157.

19. Prinssen M, Verhoven E, Buth, Jaap, Cuypers, Philippe WM, van Sambeek: A randomized trial comparing conventional and endovascular repair of abdominal aortic aneurysms. NEJM 2004;351:1607–1618.

20. Drury D, Michaels JA, Jones L, Ayiku L: Systematic review of recent evidence for the safety and efficacy of elective endovascular repair in the management of infrarenal abdominal aortic aneurysm. Br J Surg 2005;92:937–946.

21. Schermerhorn ML, O'Malley AJ, Jhaveri A, Cotterill P, Pomposelli F, Landon BE: Endovascular vs. open repair of abdominal aortic aneurysms in the medicare population. NEJM 2008;358:464–474.

22. Carroccio A, Faries PL, Nicholas JM, Teodorescu V, Burks JA, Gravereaux EC, Hollier LH, Marin ML: Predicting iliac limb occlusions after bifurcated aortic stent grafting: Anatomic and device-related causes. J Vasc Surg 2002;36:679–684.

23. Sivamurthy N, Schneider DB, Reilly LM, Rapp JH, Skovobogatyy H, Chuter TA: Adjunctive primary stenting of Zenith endograft limbs during endovascular abdominal aortic aneurysm repair: Implications for limb patency. J Vasc Surg 2006;43:662–670.

24. Fairman RM, Baum RA, Carpenter JP, Deaton DH, Makaroun MS, Velazquez OC: Limb interventions in patients undergoing treatment with an unsupported bifurcated aortic endograft system: A review of the Phase II EVT Trial. J Vasc Surg 2002;36:118–126.

25. Becquemin JP, Kelley L, Zubilewicz T, Desgranges P, Lapeyre M, Kobeiter H: Outcomes of secondary interventions after abdominal aortic aneurysm endovascular repair. J Vasc Surg 2004;39:298–305.

26. Rutherford RB: Structural failures in abdominal aortic aneurysm stentgrafts: Threat to durability and challenge to technology. Semin Vasc Surg 2004;17:294–297.

27. Beebe HG: Lessons learned from aortic aneurysm stent graft failure; observations from several perspectives. Semin Vasc Surg 2003;16:129–138.

28. Leurs LJ, Buth J, Laheij RJ: Long-term results of endovascular abdominal aortic aneurysm treatment with the first generation of commercially available stent grafts. Arch Surg 2007;142:33–41.

29. Yeager RA, TaylorJr LM, Moneta GL, Edwards JM, Nicoloff AD, McConnell DB, Porter JM: Improved results with conventional management of infrarenal aortic infection. J Vasc Surg 1999;30:76–83.

30. Noel AA, Gloviczki P, Cherry KJ, Safi H, Goldstone J, Morasch MD, Johansen KH: Abdominal aortic reconstruction in infected fields: Early results of the United States Cryopreserved Aortic Allograft Registry. J Vasc Surg 2002;35:847–852.

31. Zhou W, Lin PH, Bush RL, Terramani TT, Matsumura JH, Cox M, Peden E, Guerrero M, Silberfein EJ, Dardik A, Rosenthal D, Lumsden AB: In situ reconstruction with cryopreserved arterial allografts for management of mycotic aneurysms or aortic prosthetic graft infections: a multi-institutional experience. Tex Heart Inst J 2006;33:14–18.

32. Vogel TR, Symons R, Flum DR: The incidence and factors associated with graft infection after aortic aneurysm repair. J Vasc Surg 2008;47:264–269.

33. Blum U, Voshage G, Lammer J, Beyersdorf F, Tollner D, Kretschmer G, Spillner G, Polterauer P, Nagel G, Holzenbein T, Thurnher S, Mathias L: Endoluminal stent-grafts for infrarenal abdominal aortic aneurysms. N Engl J Med 1997;336:13–20.

34. Görich J, Riliner N, Söldner J, Krämer S, Orend KH, Schütz A, Sokiranski R, Bartel M, Sunder-Plassmann L, Scharrer-Pamler R: Endovascular repair of aortic Aneurysms: treatment of complications. J Endovasc Surg 1999;6:136–146.

35. Storck M, Scharrer-Palmer R, Kapfer X, Gallmeier U, Görch J, Sunder-Plassman L, Brückner U, Mickley V: Does a postimplantation syndrome following endovascular treatment of aortic aneurysms exist? Vasc Surg 2001;35:23–29.

36. Shimazaki T, Ishimaru S, Kawaguchi S, Yoshihiko Y, Watanabe, Y: Blood coagulation and fibrinolytic response after endovascular stent grafting of thoracic aorta. J Vasc Surg 2003;37:1213–1218.

37. Aljabri B, Obrand DI, Mantreuil B, MacKenzie KS, Steinmetz OK: Early vascular complications after the endovascular repair of aortoiliac aneurysms. Ann Vasc Surg 2001;15:608–614.

38. Lee WA, Brown MP, Nelson PR, Huber TS, Seeger JM: Midterm outcomes of femoral arteries after percutaneous endovascular aortic repair using the Preclose technique. J Vasc Surg 2008 Mar 5 (Epub ahead of print)

39. Taubman, KE, Han, DC: False aneurysm and arteriovenous fistula. In: Cameron, JL editor: Current Surgical Therapy, 9th edition, Mosby, Philadelphia 2008.

40. Slappy AL, Hakaim AG, Oldenburg WA, Paz-Fumagalli, McKinney JM: Femoral incision morbidity following endovascular aortic aneurysm repair. Vasc Endovascular Surg 2003;37:105–109.

41. Schwartz MA, Schanzer H, Skladany M, et al. A comparison of conservative therapy and early selective ligation in the treatment of lymphatic complications following vascular procedures. Am J Surg 1995;170:206–208.

42. Lazar HL, Chipkin SR, Fitzgerald CA, Bao Y, Cabral H, Apstein CS: Tight glycemic control in diabetic coronary artery bypass graft patients improves perioperative outcomes and decreases recurrent ischemic events. Circulation 2004;109:1497–1502.

43. Berg P, Kaufmann D, van Marrewijk CJ, Buth J: Spinal cord ischaemia after stent-graft treatment for infra-renal abdominal aortic aneurysms. Analysis of the Eurostar database. Eur J Vasc Endovasc Surg 2001;22:342–347.

44. Maldonado TS, Rockman CB, Riles E, Douglas D, Adelman MA, Jacobowitz GR, Gagne PJ, Nalbandian MN, Cayne NS, Lamparello PJ, Salzberg SS, Riles TS: Ischemic complications after endovascular abdominal aortic aneurysm repair. J Vasc Surg 2004;40:703–709.

45. Becquemin JP, Majewski M, Fermani N, Marzelle J, Desgrandes P, Allaire E, Roudot-Thoraval F: Colon ischemia following abdominal aortic aneurysm repair in the era of endovascular abdominal aortic repair. J Vasc Surg 2008;47:258–263.

46. Dadian N, Ohki T, Veith FJ, Edelman M, Mehta M, Lipsitz EC, Suggs WD, Wain RA: Overt colon ischemia after endovascular aneurysm repair: The importance of microembolization as an etiology. J Vasc Surg 2001;34:986–996.

47. Schermerhorn ML, Cronenwett JL: Complications of abdominal aortic aneurysm repair. In: Rutherford, RB editor: *Vascular Surgery*, 6th edition, WB Saunders, Philadelphia 2005.

48. Ohki T, Veith FJ, Shaw P, Lipsitz E, Suggs WD, Wain RA, Bade M, Mehta M, Cayne N, Cynamon J, Valldares J, McKay J: Increasing incidence of midterm and long-term complications after endovascular graft repair of abdominal aortic aneurysms: a note of caution based on a 9-year experience. Ann Surg 2001;234:323–334.

49. Alankar S, Barth MH, Shin DD, Hong JR, Rosenberg WR: Aortoduodenal fistula and associated rupture of abdominal aortic aneurysm after endoluminal stent graft repair. J Vasc Surg 2003;37:465–468.

Chapter 9

Fenestrated Endovascular Stent-Grafts: Current Applications

E.L.G. Verhoeven, C.J. Zeebregts, I.F.J. Tielliu, T.R. Prins, W.T.G.J. Bos, A.O. Sondakh, and J.J.A.M. van den Dungen

Abstract Fenestrated stent-grafts are designed to treat short-neck abdominal aortic aneurysms. Thanks to customized fenestrations, patency of side branches such as the renal arteries and the superior mesenteric artery can be maintained, whilst positioning the graft across these aortic branches.

Stent-graft design improvement and technical refinements advanced the technique from experiment to a clinical application. In addition, further developments made it possible to treat juxtarenal, suprarenal, and some thoraco-abdominal aortic aneurysms (TAAA).

This chapter discusses the principles of the technique, the refinements in recent years, and the resulting applications. In addition, our results with this technique are here summarized.

Keywords Aortic aneurysm, Endovascular, Stent-graft, Fenestration, Branch

Introduction

During the last decade, endovascular aortic aneurysm repair (EVAR) has become an accepted alternative to open repair. Two prospective randomized trials have demonstrated short-term benefits compared to open surgery.[1,2] Although mid-term results of these two trials were disappointing due to a greater number of late complications and reinterventions in the endovascular group, the technique has continued to evolve with a clear trend towards increased durability and less reinterventions.[3,4] However, EVAR is still limited by certain aortic anatomical conditions: the technique is applicable only to infrarenal aneurysms with suitable proximal and distal landing zones to achieve a proper sealing. Sufficient calibre access vessels are mandatory to allow device insertion. Distally, adverse anatomy can usually be overcome with adjunct techniques, but a proximal neck is essential to achieve sealing and a long-lasting result. The Eurostar registry has demonstrated that EVAR in proximal necks shorter than 15 mm is associated with a higher risk of complications.[5] Consequently, an important number of aneurysms still have to

G. Upchurch and E. Criado (eds.) *Aortic Aneurysms, Contemporary Cardiology*
DOI: 10.1007/978-1-60327-204-9_9, © Humana Press, a part of
Springer Science+Business Media, LLC 2009

be classified as unsuitable for standard EVAR. On the other side, open repair of these short-necked and pararenal aneurysms is also associated with higher mortality and morbidity rates.[6,7]

The fenestrated stent-graft technique was developed in order to provide a solution to a neck unsuitable for standard EVAR. By using customized fenestrations to incorporate both renal and the superior mesenteric arteries, it is possible to treat these complex aneurysms by endovascular means.

This chapter discusses the basic principles of the fenestrated technique. Then, important changes in stent-graft design and technical refinements will be highlighted, and the current applications will be elaborated. To conclude, limitations of the technique will be addressed, followed by a summary of our results.

Principles and Technique

The fenestrated technique aims at achieving a durable seal in a short neck by positioning the first sealing stent proximal to the renal arteries or beyond the superior mesenteric artery, if necessary. Custom-made fenestrations are designed to maintain the patency of these vital side branches. The fenestrations allow positioning of the proximal sealing stent inside the suprarenal aorticneck, to provide a stable and durable anchoring of the graft. The different types of fenestrations have been described before.[8] A "standard" fenestrated graft usually involves two small fenestrations for the renal arteries and a scallop for the superior mesenteric artery, but other configurations are possible to conform to each patient's anatomy (Fig. 1).

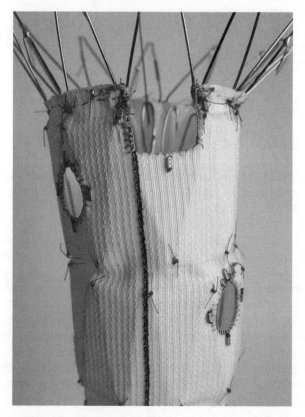

Fig. 1 A standard fenestrated stent-graft including two small fenestrations for the renal arteries and a scallop for the superior mesenteric artery

Fig. 2 Diameter Reducing Ties
Constraining The Deployed Graft

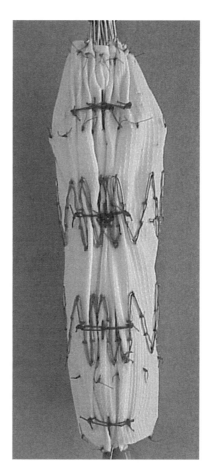

A complete comprehensive step-by-step technical approach has recently been published.[9] The increased complexity of fenestrated endograft deployment includes additional steps to the standard EVAR technique. The main body of the graft has to be partially deployed in the aorta, with a partially expanded diameter. For this purpose, diameter reducing ties constrain the graft to allow repositioning of the main body of the graft and catheterization of the fenestrations from the contralateral femoral artery (Fig. 2). Selective catheterization of the renal arteries is essential for correct deployment of the graft with the fenestrations aligned with the orifice of these vessels. It is important to realize that vessel catheterization can only be achieved by repositioning the graft until the fenestration faces the target vessel orifice. To facilitate correct position under fluoroscopy, fenestrated grafts have four radio-opaque markers around each fenestration, and three around scallops. The complete deployment of the graft requires releasing the diameter reducing ties and opening the top cap. The scallop for the superior mesenteric artery, if present, should automatically fall into position, without necessitating additional catheterization.

Evolution of the Technique

Over the years, a number of technical refinements related to the stent-graft configuration and various technical steps required for insertion of the graft have been introduced, to standardize the technique and increase the rate of technical success. Fenestrated bifurcated grafts have evolved towards composite grafts. Composite grafts include a tube graft containing the fenestrations which is deployed first, followed by a bifurcated graft, and completed with a contralateral limb. A tubular proximal body, including the fenestrations, is much easier to reposition during catheterization of the renal arteries. Deployment is easier and safer, without risk of torsion of the ipsilateral limb during repositioning (*see* "Results"). Another advantage of the composite system is the lower downwards migration force on the tubular part of the system containing the fenestrations.

An additional important improvement of the technique has been the application of routine stenting of renal artery fenestrations to optimize the appositioning. Even with meticulous pre-operative measurements and intra-operative positioning, renal artery appositioning with the graft fenestration may not be perfect since the procedural angiogram is unable to demonstrate the degree of appositioning accurately. The purpose of the renal stents is to optimize the apposition between fenestrations and ostia of the target vessels, and also to maintain this correct position over time. To provide better support to the stents, all fenestrations are now reinforced with a double nitinol ring. Finally, a better technique to guarantee the safe introduction and deployment of the stents has been developed. In the early stages, full deployment of the graft was executed with balloons inside the fenestrations and target vessels. Afterwards, the balloons were deflated and removed to allow insertion of the stents. This sequence carried a risk of loosing renal access, due to the stiffness of the stents. Currently, guiding catheters/sheaths are routinely introduced into the renal arteries. In this manner, the stents can be advanced through the guiding catheters before deploying the graft completely (Fig. 3). This guarantees safe deployment of the stents once the graft is fully open and the guiding

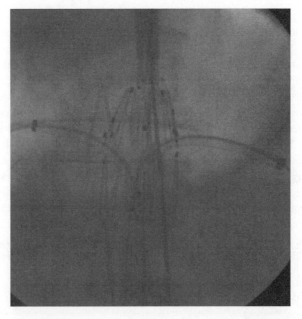

Fig. 3 Guiding catheters passing the fenestrations and positioned inside the renal arteries

sheath retracted. To prevent distal migration at the time of full deployment, it is advisable to push up the device slightly to counteract the aortic flow push. This manoeuver allows embedding of the hooks and minimizes downwards migration.[10]

Other improvements to this technique include ballooning of the proximal two stents of the main body graft before inserting stents into the renovisceral vessels. This improves apposition of the graft material against the aortic wall and results in a more secure position of the stents. It is important to allow sufficient overlap between the different graft components (i.e., at least three stents overlap between first tubular and second bifurcated graft, and 1.5 stents overlap between gate and contralateral limb).

Finally, it is essential to understand that meticulous pre-operative aortic measurements and planning are the key to technical success.

Current Applications of Fenestrated Endografts

From the anatomical point of view, fenestrated endografts are designed to treat infrarenal aortic aneurysms with a neck too short for standard EVAR. It is important to realize that appositioning of the graft against the wall is essential. Infrarenal aneurysms with a neck varying from 4 to 15 mm in length are most suitable for this technique. To treat juxtarenal, suprarenal, and TAAA, additional technical features are required. Turning a fenestrated graft into a branched graft by using covered stents instead of uncovered stents was an option, and developing truly branched grafts another. Both techniques are feasible and present with specific advantages and disadvantages.

For juxtarenal aneurysms, the fenestrated graft in conjunction with covered stents seems to be the logical option. The covered stent will not only provide apposition but also a seal with the fenestration. A safe seal with the aortic wall can be achieved if there is a sufficient neck available in the aortic portion between the celiac trunk and the renal arteries (Fig. 4a and b). By using multiple (up to four) small fenestrations and fitting each of them with covered stents, it becomes possible to treat suprarenal and TAAA, as demonstrated by Anderson et al.[11] (Fig. 5a and b). The Achilles' Heel of this technique is the questionable stability and durability of the seal between the nitinol ring of the fenestration and the covered stent, especially when there is a long gap to bridge from the fenestration to the ostium of the target vessel, such as in most TAAA. Exact positioning of the graft and the fenestrations is mandatory with this technique. Advantages of the technique are that the graft is not more bulky than a standard stent-graft and can be fitted in 22-Fr delivery systems, and that it is similar to the fenestrated technique used for short-necked aneurysms.

The second and probably better option for most TAAA is perhaps a fully branched endograft. This concept was initially developed by Chuter.[12] The theoretical advantage is that a branch provides a better seal and fixation for the bridging stent-graft. Another advantage is the less critical need to accurate positioning the graft branches relative to the target vessel orifices. Disadvantages include the required approach from the arm to catheterize the branches and target vessels, and the stiffness of the current range of available bridging stent-grafts. Because most side branches are directed straight downwards, the bridging stent-grafts have to accommodate an angle of up to 90° to enter the renal arteries, bearing in mind the physiological forces that promote kinking and

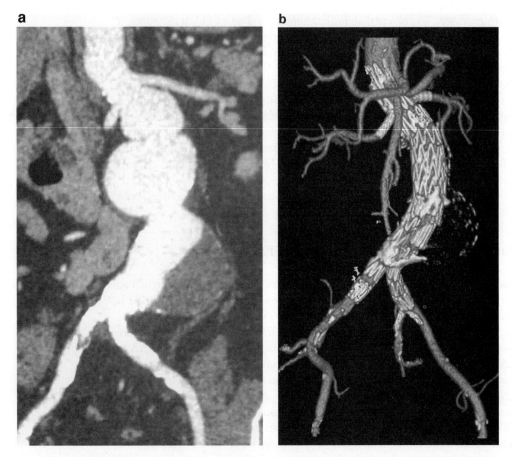

Fig. 4 (**a**) Pre-operative CT-scanning showing a juxtarenal aneurysm. (**b**) Post-operative CT-scanning reconstruction after fenestrated stent-grafting. Two covered stents were inserted in the renal artery fenestrations not only to optimize apposition but also to create a seal (*See Color Plates*)

occlusion of branched endografts (Fig. 6). To prevent this, a self-expandable stent can be additionally inserted inside the bridging stent-graft. The excess of fabric created by the side branches makes these branched grafts more bulky which often results in larger bore delivery systems.

Greater complexity sets apart this type of endovascular surgery from standard EVAR. Initially, we reserved the fenestrated technique for selected high-risk surgical patients only. This selection was either based on systemic co-morbidity (cardiac, renal, pulmonary) or because the patients presented with a hostile abdomen, precluding laparotomy or at least making laparotomy difficult and risky. With growing experience and confidence in the procedure, a more liberal use of the technique has included patients who are acceptable candidates for open surgery. However, an important number of patients are referred to us by other surgeons because of hostile abdominal conditions. These include patients with multiple laparotomies and those who require redo aortic surgery after previous open or endovascular aortic surgery.[13] Finally, patients are only accepted for fenestrated stent-grafting if their aneurysm was

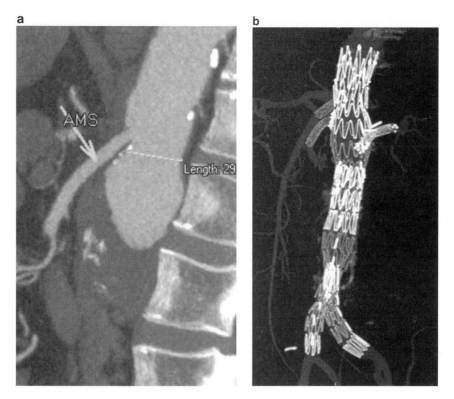

Fig. 5 (**a**) Pre-operative CT-scanning of a suprarenal aneurysm reaching to the level of the superior mesenteric artery (AMS, arrow). (**b**) Post-operative CT-scanning showing a graft with a short upwards facing branch for the left renal artery, two fenestrations for the right renal artery and the superior mesenteric artery, and a scallop for the celiac trunk (*See Color Plates*)

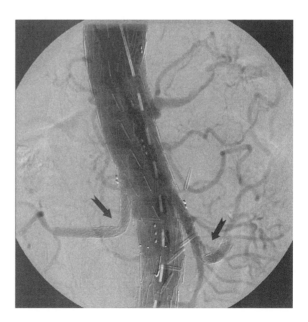

Fig. 6 Completion angiogram showing kinking in the two bridging stent-grafts to the renal arteries (arrows)

large enough to justify treatment with this complex technique; this was defined as aneurysm with a maximal diameter of at least 5.5.cm for men and 5.0 cm for women. In patients with smaller aneurysms, conservative treatment with routine aneurysm surveillance was advocated.

Limitations of the Technique

The limitations of the standard fenestrated technique become obvious considering the necessary steps for deployment. The graft needs to be repositioned to its final position during catheterization, and the insertion of the renal stents must be achieved correctly. Every anatomical feature rendering these two processes difficult to execute makes this already complex technique even more challenging. Severe angulation of the neck or iliac arteries, narrow iliac arteries, and previously inserted surgical grafts can all pose problems to reposition the graft. Insertion of stents into the renal arteries and renal artery patency are questionable in case of small or diseased renal arteries, short renal arteries with early bifurcations, and a sharp takeoff of the renal arteries. Other anatomical peculiarities can also increase the difficulty of this procedure: aortic side branches in proximity to each other render designing the graft more difficult, angulation of the neck makes difficult to determine the correct level of the small fenestrations for the renal arteries, thrombus inside the proximal neck poses a risk not only for endoleak but also for embolization during repositioning, and a small neck diameter can render the catheterization process more difficult because of the small space to manoeuver with shaped catheters.

Results

Our experience with different fenestrated and branched grafts includes 166 patients (Table 1). In Table 1, all fenestrated grafts fitted with covered stents, as well as hybrid grafts (combination of true branches and fenestrations), were classified as branched. With regard to procedure and follow-up, we dealt with three categories of patients: first, patients who have both the procedure and follow-up in our hospital; second, patients that were treated in our hospital but were followed by other centres; and third, patients that were treated in another hospital in conjunction with a Groningen team member. This situation is probably similar to other specialized centres and presents important consequences for follow-up reporting. Most reported results, albeit from a few specialized

Table 1 Fenestrated and branched stent-graft experience in Groningen, according to anatomical location and type of stent-graft.

Location	Fenestrated	Branched	Total
Abdominal	79	48	127
Thoracic (arch)	3	1	4
Thoraco-abdominal aortic aneurysm (TAAA)	6	9	15
Iliac branched		20	20

centres only, are good, with mortalities in the range of standard EVAR and a target vessel patency of around 95%.[14–16] Nevertheless, renal arteries need to be carefully monitored as imperfect technical results can lead to complications and eventually renal artery occlusion.[17]

Our own results are encouraging, including published mid-term outcome.[13,18] In the present study, we report on 76 patients (category I with procedure and follow-up in our hospital) who had a fenestrated/branched graft for complex aortic aneurysms (short-necked, juxta-, and suprarenal aneurysms, TAAA excluded). Technical success was 81/84 (96%) patients: in one case, we aborted the procedure in favour of a shorter quicker standard procedure with intentional sacrifice of two accessory renal arteries; in a second case, a heavily stenosed renal artery was treated surgically the day after the initial procedure; the third case (juxtarenal aneurysm after previous open surgery) had to be converted to open surgery. The reason for this conversion was that the bifurcated fenestrated graft became twisted and the top cap stuck. In this particular case, it was impossible to use a composite three-part graft due to length issues. Fortunately, the patient made an uneventful recovery. The overall mortality was 1.2%. One patient died 8 days after surgery from mesenteric ischaemia. Autopsy revealed a patent superior mesenteric artery. During follow-up, 10 (12%) patients died between 4 and 51 months after the procedure of unrelated causes. Occlusion occurred in 7 of 211 (3.3%) target vessels, all being renal arteries. As a result, seven (5%) kidneys were lost, but none of the patients required dialysis. If we exclude the 4 patients that had no technical success (3) or died (1), the risk of loosing a renal artery in a patient is 7/80 or 8.7%. Renal function overall remained stable during follow-up, but aneurysm size decreased significantly and no proximal type I endoleaks were seen. Reinterventions were required in 9/83 patients (10.8%); one patient excluded who received standard endovascular repair, but there were no late transabdominal reinterventions. These include three reinterventions within 30 days: one conversion, one surgery at day 1, and one laparotomy at day 7 in the patient who died from mesenteric ischaemia (all three mentioned above). There were six late reinterventions, three of which were angiographies with or without renal artery stenting. Two patients had angiographic reinterventions for type II endoleaks. Finally, the last patient developed a late groin infection that eventually needed surgical debridement.

Conclusion

Although the fenestrated endograft technique is still not widely available, there are several reasons to warrant its further development and careful widespread. First, the results with fenestrated grafts for short-necked and juxtarenal aneurysms are good in the expert hands. Second, the advantages of a less-invasive technique are probably greater in more complex aneurysms such as suprarenal and TAAA because of the high morbid–mortality of open surgery. Finally, we will always encounter patients who are at high surgical risk, due to co-morbid conditions, hostile abdomen, or with previous aortic surgery.

References

1. Greenhalgh RM, Brown LC, Kwong GP, Powell JT, Thompson SG. EVAR trial participants. Comparison of endovascular aneurysm repair with open repair in patients with abdominal aortic aneurysm (EVAR trial 1), 30-day operative mortality results: Randomised controlled trial. Lancet 2004;364: 843–8.
2. Prinssen M, Verhoeven EL, Buth J, et al. A randomized trial comparing conventional and endovascular repair of abdominal aortic aneurysms. N Engl J Med 2004;351: 1607–18.
3. EVAR trial participants. Endovascular aneurysm repair versus open repair in patients with abdominal aortic aneurysm (EVAR trial 1): Randomised controlled trial. Lancet 2005;365: 2179–86.
4. Blankensteijn JD, Jong de SE, Prinssen M, et al. Two-year outcomes after conventional or endovascular repair of abdominal aortic aneurysms. N Engl J Med 2005;352: 2398–405.
5. Leurs LJ, Stultiëns G, Kievit J, Buth J. Adverse events at the aneurismal neck identified at follow-up after endovascular abdominal aortic aneurysm repair: How do they correlate? Vascular 2005;13: 261–7.
6. Jean-Claude JM, Reilly LM, Stoney RJ, Messina LM. Pararenal aortic aneurysms: The future of open aneurysm repair. J Vasc Surg 1999;29: 902–912.
7. Zeebregts CJ, Geelkerken RH, Palen van der J, Huisman AB, Smit de P, Det van RJ. Outcome of abdominal aortic aneurysm repair in the era of endovascular treatment. Br J Surg 2004;91: 563–568.
8. Verhoeven EL, Prins TR, Tielliu IF, et al. Treatment of short-necked infrarenal aortic aneurysms with fenestrated stent-grafts: Short-term results. *Eur J Vasc Endovasc Surg* 2004;27: 477–83.
9. Moore R, Hinojosa CA, O'Neill S, Mastracci TM, Cina CS. Fenestrated endovascular grafts for juxtarenal aortic aneurysms: A step by step technical approach. *Catheter Cardiovasc Interv* 2007;69: 554–71.
10. Zhou SSN, How TV, Vallabhaneni SR, Gilling-Smith GL, Brennan JA, Harris PL, McWilliams R. Comparison of the fixation strength of standard and fenestrated stent-grafts for endovascular abdominal aortic aneurysm repair. *J Endovasc Ther* 2007;14: 168–75.
11. Anderson JL, Adam DJ, Berce M, Hartley D. Repair of TAAA with fenestrated and branched endovascular stent grafts. J Vasc Surg 2005;42: 600–7.
12. Chuter TA, Gordon RL, Reilly LM, Goodman JD, Messina LM. An endovascular system for thoracoabdominal aortic aneurysm repair. J Endovasc Ther 2001;8: 25–33.
13. Verhoeven EL, Muhs BE, Zeebregts CJ, Tielliu IF, Prins TR, Bos WT, et al. Fenestrated and branched stent-grafting after previous surgery provides a good alternative to open redo surgery. Eur J Vasc Endovasc Surg 2007;33: 84–90.
14. Anderson JL, Berce M, Hartley DE. Endoluminal aortic grafting with renal and superior mesenteric artery incorporation by graft fenestration. J Endovasc Ther 2001;8: 3–15.
15. Greenberg RK, Haulon S, Lyden SP, et al. Endovascular management of juxtarenal aneurysms with fenestrated endovascular grafting. J Vasc Surg 2004;39: 279–87.
16. Scurr JRH, Brennan JA, Gilling-Smith GL, Harris PL, Vallabhaneni SR, McWilliams RG. Fenestrated endovascular repair for juxtarenal aortic aneurysm Br J Surg 2007 (in press).
17. Haddad F, Greenberg RK, Walker E, et al. Fenestrated endovascular grafting: The renal side of the story. J Vasc Surg 2005;41: 181–90.
18. Muhs BE, Verhoeven EL, Zeebregts CJ, et al. Midterm results of branched and fenestrated endografts. *J Vasc Surg* 2006;44: 9–15.

Chapter 10

Open Surgical Treatment of Pararenal Abdominal Aortic Aneurysms

James C. Stanley

Abstract Pararenal abdominal aortic aneurysms (AAAs) are classified as to being juxtarenal or suprarenal. They account for 2–7% of all aortic aneurysms, with men affected twice as often as women. Precise anatomic imaging with computed tomographic arteriograms or conventional aortography is required for optimal surgical therapy. The morbidity of open surgical repair is most often related to renal insufficiency. The operative mortality averages 5% being slightly greater than that accompanying open infrarenal aortic aneurysmectomy.

Keywords Pararenal aneurysm, Juxtarenal aneurysm, Suprarenal aneurysm, Aortic aneurysm surgery

Introduction

Pararenal AAAs account for 2–7% of all aortic aneurysms. The open surgical treatment of pararenal AAAs is complex and requires a detailed knowledge of the anatomic disease, careful attention to thorough preoperative patient preparation, precise operative intervention, and contemporary intensive care in the early postoperative period.

Pararenal AAAs are classified as juxtarenal or suprarenal, depending on involvement of the renal artery (Fig. 1). Juxtarenal AAAs outnumber suprarenal AAAs, 4-to-1. Juxtarenal AAAs extend superiorly to just below the renal arteries such that no normal aorta exists between the aneurysm and the renal arteries. Suprarenal AAAs extend superiorly to include the orifices of the renal arteries to one or both kidneys. Pararenal AAAs, by definition, do not involve the superior mesenteric or celiac arteries, or extend above the diaphragm to involve the thoracic aorta. Coexistent renal artery arteriosclerosis is near universal with pararenal AAAs, but it is severe enough in only 10–25% of cases to cause renovascular hypertension or ischemic nephropathy.

G. Upchurch and E. Criado (eds.) *Aortic Aneurysms, Contemporary Cardiology*
DOI: 10.1007/978-1-60327-204-9_10, © Humana Press, a part of
Springer Science + Business Media, LLC 2009

a   b

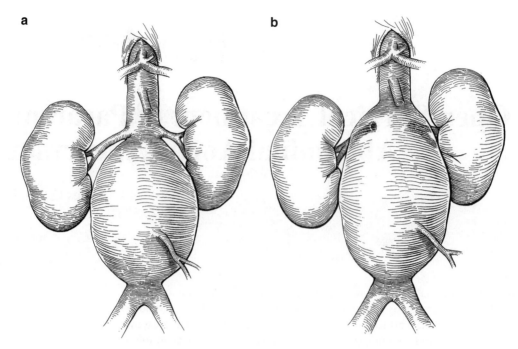

Fig. 1 Pararenal aortic aneurysms: Juxtarenal aneurysms (**a**) outnumber suprarenal aneurysms (**b**), 4-to-1. Reprinted with permission from Henke and Stanley.[26(p. 229)]

Clinical Presentation

Most pararenal AAAs are asymptomatic. In contemporary times, pararenal AAAs are usually discovered as incidental findings during imaging studies undertaken for other illnesses. The average age at the time of diagnosis is 67 years. Men are twice as likely as women to have pararenal AAAs.[1–4] This gender predilection is not as great as the 3.5- to 4-fold male predominance that exists with infrarenal AAAs. It is conceivable that the increased proportion of women having pararenal AAAs compared to infrarenal AAAs may be due to practice patterns with more common delays in treating women until their AAAs become larger. It is well known that larger AAAs carry a greater likelihood of aneurysmal changes in the more cephalic pararenal aorta. However, it is also possible that following menopause, the loss of reproductive hormones such as estrogen that enhance both elastin and collagen cross-linking may contribute to a more generalized form of aortic dilation, such that when infrarenal AAAs evolve in women, the juxtarenal aorta and suprarenal aorta are also likely to exhibit aneurysmal changes. Considerable anecdotal experience exists to support this contention.

Pararenal AAAs are usually larger than infrarenal AAAs. Nevertheless, their recognition on physical examination is uncommon. A definitive diagnosis of a pararenal AAA requires sophisticated imaging. In addition, the renal artery anatomy must be precisely delineated to plan optimal therapy of these aneurysms. Computed tomograms and 3-D tomographic arteriography are the studies used most often in contemporary practice (Figs. 2 and 3). Conventional arteriography is also frequently used (Fig. 4). Both the former studies require the use of iodinated contrast with its nephrotoxic risks. Magnetic resonance arteriography (MRA) is a frequent screening study, often obtained because of its noninvasive nature and avoidance of using nephrotoxic agents. However, in the case of

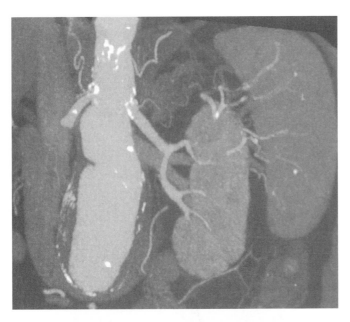

Fig. 2 Computed tomogram of a juxtarenal aortic aneurysm

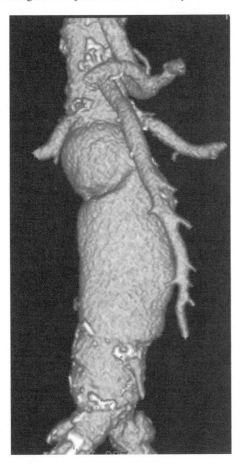

Fig. 3 Reformatted 3-D tomographic arteriogram of the juxtarenal aortic aneurysm in Figure 2 (*See Color Plates*)

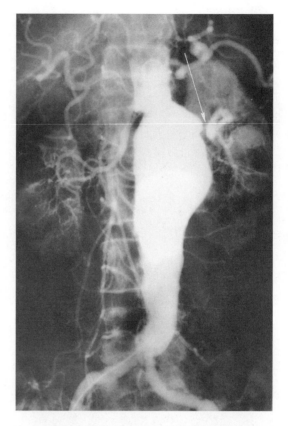

Fig. 4 Aortogram of a suprarenal aortic aneurysm with renal artery involvement (arrow). Reprinted with permission from Henke and Stanley.[26](p. 231)

pararenal AAAs, aortic branch disease may not be adequately defined by MRA studies because of turbulent flow and phase-dropout phenomenon.

Renal artery stenotic disease, severe enough to warrant endovascular or open operative therapy, complicates the treatment of patients with pararenal AAAs. In some series, renal artery interventions have been undertaken in more than 40% of cases.[5] Aortic spillover arteriosclerosis accounts for 80% of the renal stenoses, and critical narrowings exceeding 70–80% are bilateral in a third of the patients. The surgical therapy in many of these cases is controversial, in part due to the lack of clinical data to conclusively support renal artery reconstructive procedures in instances of ischemic nephropathy, as well as a paucity of clinical data that the renal artery is at high risk when clamping the perirenal aorta during the aneurysmectomy. Nevertheless, treatment of coexisting renal artery stenotic disease is justified when anatomic or functional studies support a diagnosis of renovascular hypertension. The technique of reconstructing the renal artery in these cases varies, with some favoring an aortorenal bypass[6] and others an aortorenal endarterectomy.[4,7–10]

Surgical risks attending operations for pararenal AAA are greater than for treatment of infrarenal AAAs. Three obvious factors contribute to these risks. First, a relatively extensive aortic dissection is required for repair of pararenal AAAs, which translates into increased surgical manipulation of the renal and superior mesenteric arteries as well as greater lengths of operative time.

Second, intraoperative renal ischemia due to having to clamp the aorta above the renal arteries is an inescapable part of these cases. Third, cardiac strain is greater due to the increased afterload necessitated by the more proximal aortic clamping in these cases.

Whereas most clinicians are selective with cardiac evaluations for infrarenal AAA repair, the magnitude of treating pararenal AAAs supports a more liberal screening of occult coronary artery disease. It is the author's advice that noninvasive pharmacological or exercise cardiac testing be undertaken in all patients with pararenal AAAs, and cardiac catheterization pursued if significant myocardial ischemia is suspected. Although by no means direct proof of the validity of such testing, preoperative cardiac studies have become common in most practices, resulting in an acceptable cardiac morbidity in those patients undergoing open surgical treatment of their pararenal AAAs.[2–5,9,11]

Operative Technique

Certain technical aspects of open surgical treatment of pararenal AAAs are well recognized by vascular surgeons, and are of importance to others who are advising these patients about their therapeutic options. Three basic means of exposing pararenal AAAs for optimal surgical therapy exist: (1) transabdominal, (2) retroperitoneal, and (3) thoracoabdominal. The patient's anatomic disease, prior abdominal surgery, body habitus, and the surgeon's personal preference are determining factors as to which approach is to be used. Each has distinct advantages and each carries different risks to the overall procedure.

A direct abdominal approach with a vertical midline or supraumbilical transverse incision is used in treating most pararenal AAAs.[4] Direct exposure of the pararenal aorta at the base of the mesentery and mesocolon is usually pursued, although indirect aorta exposure following medial visceral rotation may be undertaken as an alternative approach, especially in the case of unusually large pararenal AAAs. While medial visceral rotation yields excellent exposure of the aneurysm neck and renal vessels, pancreatitis is a potential complication.[4,12] In some patients, such as those with a very acute costophrenic angle, an abdominal approach alone limits the surgical exposure and increases the operative risks. In that setting, a thoracoabdominal incision allows greater visualization of the aorta and its branches.

A retroperitoneal approach through a flank or thoracic incision is preferred by some.[3,5,13,14] This approach is associated with less postoperative fluid requirements and a shorter hospital stay, but no difference in morbidity or mortality has been documented.[3] If a right renal artery or iliac artery reconstruction is required, it may be technically very difficult using this approach, and in such circumstances, a second abdominal incision may be required.

A major factor contributing to operative morbidity relates to the proximal aortic clamp placement at the suprarenal levels, be it between the renal and superior mesenteric arteries as well as above the superior mesenteric artery or celiac artery. The patient's anatomy and disease are often the primary determinants of where clamp placement is to occur.

Supraceliac aortic clamping is clearly easier in terms of dissection, and the aorta at that level is usually less atherosclerotic. This site provides positioning of the clamp away from the renal artery orifices and anastomotic area. Although some have reported no difference in patient morbidity and mortality between any of the potential clamp sites,[4] others have presented evidence that supraceliac control decreases mortality and postoperative renal failure.[1,2,15,16] The potentially severe coagulopathy accompanying supraceliac clamping in the experimental setting[17] has not been evident in recent clinical series.[1,2,15] Perhaps most important to choosing the level of aortic clamping is the significant mortality observed when clamping the proximal aorta between the renal and superior mesenteric arteries or between the superior mesenteric and celiac arteries.[1,2,15] Placement of a clamp below the superior mesenteric artery should only be done if a reasonable distance exists between the former vessel and the renal arteries.

If the segment of aorta being clamped is not free of extensive atherosclerosis or luminal thrombus, unclamping and repositioning the clamp to a more proximal site may be associated with atheroembolization, visceral infarction, and death.[2,3,9,11] In regard to the latter, once the pararenal aorta has been exposed, isolation and transient occlusion of the renal and mesenteric arteries with microvascular clamps before proximal aortic clamping is a very important means of preventing embolization of dislodged aortic debris that might cause irreversible injury to the kidneys and intestines.

The dominant cause of morbidity and a substantial cause of mortality following open pararenal AAA repair is renal failure.[9] Minimizing kidney ischemia during performance of the proximal aortic anastomosis to less than 30 min may decrease the incidence of postoperative renal insufficiency.[2,8,12] It has been noted that the duration of supravisceral clamp time is directly related to morbidity and mortality.[3,18,19] The proximal aortic anastomosis may often be completed in a more expeditious manner if the infrarenal aorta is transected and transposed to a position above the left renal vein where suturing can be completed in an unencumbered manner. Following completion of this anastomosis, the aorta and graft can be repositioned behind the left renal vein. Transecting the left renal vein to gain easier exposure of the pararenal aorta is not recommended and has been associated with greater postoperative renal insufficiency.[20] Replacing the clamp to the graft below the renal arteries and restoring flow to the kidneys after proximal aortic anastomosis completion will decrease renal ischemia, but caution must be taken to flush any aortic debris loosened by the proximal clamp, before restoring renal blood flow. If flushing is not done, loose material may embolize to the kidneys.

Another technique to minimize renal ischemic injury is with kidney hypothermia.[5] The author favors infusion of chilled (4°C) Ringer's lactate, to which is added 1000 U heparin, 12.5 g Mannitol, and 44.6 mEq of sodium bicarbonate/liter. Approximately 150 ml of this solution is infused through each renal artery orifice, with repeated administration if the occlusion time exceeds 30 min. This practice may be most efficacious for patients with preoperative renal insufficiency.[1–3,9] Ice-slurry packing of the kidneys may also lower the core kidney temperature, but such is more cumbersome and less often undertaken in most practices.

In most patients with *juxtarenal* aortic aneurysms, the proximal graft-to-aorta anastomosis occurs at the level of the renal artery orifices (Fig. 5). In some patients, the graft must be carried posteriorly above the renal arteries. In other instances, the anastomosis incorporates the proximal aorta and one renal artery with reimplantation of the other renal artery.

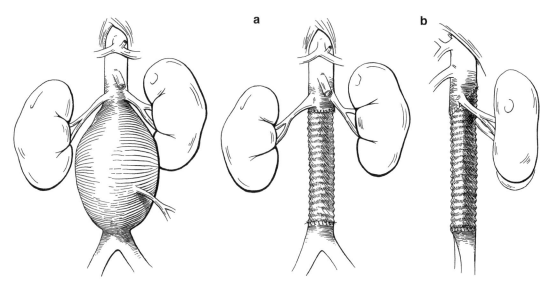

Fig. 5 Common open surgical reconstructive options used in treating juxtarenal aortic aneurysms: (**a**) juxtarenal graft placement, abutting the renal arteries and (**b**) tapered graft extending posteriorly above the renal arteries. Reprinted with permission from Henke and Stanley.[26(p. 231)]

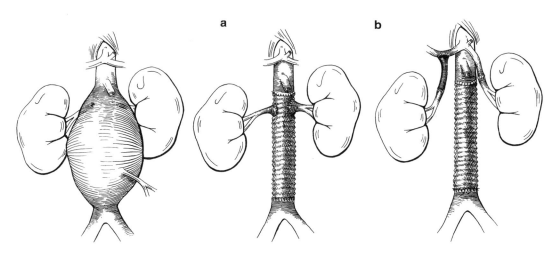

Fig. 6 Common open surgical reconstructive options used in treating suprarenal aortic aneurysms: (**a**) suprarenal graft placement with bilateral renal artery implantation and (**b**) suprarenal graft placement with right hepatorenal bypass and left splenorenal bypass. Reprinted with permission from Henke and Stanley.[26(p. 232)]

In most *suprarenal* aortic aneurysms, the graft anastomosis will be above the renal vessels with bilateral reimplantation of the renal arteries or some other means of maintaining normal renal blood flow. Nonanatomic renal revascularization with grafts to the kidney originating from the supraceliac aorta, or in some instances as hepatorenal or splenorenal bypasses, are of value in these circumstances (Fig. 6).

Surgical Outcomes

Open operative treatment of pararenal AAAs in contemporary series has been accompanied by modest morbidity and mortality rates (Table 1). Mortality figures from experienced institutions averages around 5%,[3,5,8,9,18-21] being slightly greater than that from contemporary series on infrarenal AAAs. Some have reported mortality rates nearly fourfold higher with suprarenal versus juxtarenal aneurysm repair.[18] Blood loss and fluid requirements are typically twice that of infrarenal AAA repairs but such is not an independent predictor of patient outcome.

Unfortunately, the morbidity associated with the open surgical treatment of pararenal AAAs remains high. The major complication of the operative treatment of pararenal AAAs and often times the cause of death, as previously mentioned, is renal failure. The incidence of postoperative renal failure ranges from 10% to 30%, and is highest among patients with preoperative renal insufficiency and in those requiring concomitant renal artery reconstruction.[2,4,5,8,18,20-22] However, the need for chronic hemodialysis in survivors is low. Intestinal ischemia and infarction is also a recognized cause of death in these patients.[9] Renal failure has accounted for more than half the mortality in several series.[1-3,5,8]

Treatment of coexisting renal artery disease causing renovascular hypertension results in improved blood pressure control in 50–70% of these patients, although only 20% are cured of their hypertension. Outcomes regarding reversal of ischemic nephropathy and prevention of renal artery disease progression are ill-defined in contemporary literature, with no evidence-based data supporting the routine reconstruction of the renal arteries in this subgroup of patients.

Overall survival at 5 years following the open surgical therapy of pararenal AAAs has been cited as low as 40% and as high as 75% with most late deaths due to cardiac causes,[8,19,23] not unlike that observed after infrarenal AAA repairs. It is relevant to any discussion of pararenal AAAs to recognize that serious comorbidities in certain patients may preclude safe endovascular or open operative repair of their aneurysms, and in these individuals, nonoperative therapy may be quite appropriate.[24,25] Nevertheless, given the lethal nature of aneurysmal expansion with rupture, operative treatment of pararenal AAAs is warranted in all patients who are otherwise acceptable surgical candidates.

Table 1 Operative outcomes of treating pararenal abdominal aortic aneurysm.[a]

Institution	Number of patients	Operative mortality (%)	New onset postoperative dialysis (%)
University of California, San Francisco, California[9]	257	5.8	7.0
Mayo Clinic, Rochester, Minnesota[20]	247	2.8	3.7
H San Raffaele Institute, Milan, Italy[21]	107	4.2	3.4
Methodist Hospital, Houston, Texas[8]	101	7.9	7.9
University of Michigan, Ann Arbor, Michigan[b]	84	3.5	2.4
Washington University, St. Louis, Missouri[5]	65	1.5	3.1
Henry Ford Hospital, Detroit, Michigan[3]	53	3.8	5.7

[a] Reported series composed of differing numbers of juxtarenal and suprarenal aneurysms, as well as differing numbers of patients subjected to concomitant renal revascularization procedures. This invalidates direct comparisons of one series to another

[b] Three year experience (1996–1999) originally presented in 2000

References

1. Green RM, Ricotta JJ, Ouriel K, and DeWeese JA. Results of supraceliac aortic clamping in the difficult elective resection of infrarenal abdominal aortic aneurysm. J Vasc Surg 1989;9:125–134.

2. Nypaver TJ, Shepard AD, Reddy DJ, Elliott JP, and Ernst CB. Supraceliac aortic cross clamping: Determinants of outcome in elective abdominal aortic reconstructions. J Vasc Surg 1993;17:868–876.

3. Nypaver TJ, Shepard AD, Reddy DJ, Elliott JP, Smith RF, and Ernst CB. Repair of pararenal abdominal aortic aneurysms. An analysis of operative management. Arch Surg 1993;128:803–813.

4. Qvarfordt PG, Stoney RJ, Reilly LM, Skioldebrand CG, Goldstone J, and Ehrenfeld WK. Management of pararenal aneurysms of the abdominal aorta. J Vasc Surg 1986;3:84–93.

5. Allen BT, Anderson CB, Rubin BG, Flye MW, Baumann DS, and Sicard GA. Preservation of renal function in juxtarenal and suprarenal abdominal aortic aneurysm repair. J Vasc Surg 1993;17:948–959.

6. Cambria RP, Brewster DC, L'Italien G, Koustas G, Atamian S, LaMuraglia GM, Gertler JP, and Abbott WM. Simultaneous aortic and renal artery reconstruction: Evolution of an eighteen-year experience. J Vasc Surg 1995;21:916–925.

7. Clair DG, Belkin M, Whittemore AD, Mannick JA, and Donaldson MC. Safety and efficacy of transaortic renal endarterectomy as an adjunct to aortic surgery. J Vasc Surg 1995;21:926–934.

8. Crawford ES, Beckett WC, and Greer MS. Juxtarenal infrarenal abdominal aortic aneurysm. Special diagnostic and therapeutic considerations. Ann Surg 1986;203:661–670.

9. Jean-Claude J, Reilly LM, Stoney RJ, and Messina LM. Pararenal aortic aneurysms: The future of open aortic aneurysm repair. J Vasc Surg 1999;29:902–912.

10. McNeil JW, String ST, and Pfeifer RB, Jr. Concomitant renal endarterectomy and aortic reconstruction. J Vasc Surg 1994;20:331–337.

11. Messina LM. Pararenal aortic aneurysms: The future of open repair. Cardiovasc Surg 2002;10:424–433.

12. Reilly LM, Ramos TK, Murray SP, Cheng SWK, and Stoney RJ. Optimal exposure of the proximal abdominal aorta: A critical appraisal of transabdominal medial visceral rotation. J Vasc Surg 1994;19:375–390.

13. Illig KA, and Green RM. Diagnosis and management of the "difficult" abdominal aortic aneurysm: Pararenal aneurysms, inflammatory aneurysms, and horseshoe kidney. Semin Vasc Surg 2001;14:312–317.

14. Pokrovsky AV, Karimov SI, Yermolyuk RS, Thursunov BZ, and Asamov RE. Thoracophrenolumbotomy as an approach of choice in reconstruction of the proximal abdominal aorta and visceral branches. J Vasc Surg 1991;13:892–896.

15. Hines GL, and Chorost M. Supraceliac aortic occlusion: A safe approach to pararenal aortic aneurysms. Ann Vasc Surg 1998;12:335–340.

16. Schneider JR, Gottner RJ, and Golan JF. Supraceliac versus infrarenal aortic cross-clamp for repair of non-ruptured infrarenal and juxtarenal abdominal aortic aneurysm. Cardiovasc Surg 1997;5:279–285.

17. Cohen JR, Angus L, Asher A, Chang JB, and Wise L. Disseminated intravascular coagulation as a result of supraceliac clamping: Implications for thoracoabdominal aneurysm repair. Ann Vasc Surg 1987;1:552–557.

18. Back MR, Bandyk M, Bradner M, Cuthbertson D, Johnson BL, Shames ML, and Bandyk DF. Critical analysis of outcome determinants affecting repair of intact aneurysms involving the visceral aorta. Ann Vasc Surg 2005;19:648–656.

19. Poulias GE, Doundoulakis N, Skoutas B, Prombonas E, Haddad H, Papaioannou K, Lymberiades D, and Savopoulkos G. Juxtarenal abdominal aneurysmectomy. J Cardiovasc Surg 1992;33:324–330.

20. West CA, Noel AA, Bower TC, Cherry KJ Jr, Gloviczki P, Sullivan TM, Kalra M, Hoskin TL, and Harrington JR. Factors affecting outcomes of open surgical repair of pararenal aortic aneurysms: A 10-year experience. J Vasc Surg 2006;43:921–928.
21. Chiesa R, Marone EM, Brioschi C, Frigerio S, Tshoma Y, and Melissano G. Open repair of pararenal aortic aneurysms: Operative management, early results, and risk factor analysis. Ann Vasc Surg 2006;20:739–746.
22. Breckwoldt WL, Mackey WC, Belkin M, and O'Donnell TF Jr. The effect of suprarenal cross-clamping on abdominal aortic aneurysm repair. Arch Surg 1992;127:520–524.
23. Faggioli G, Stella A, Freyrie A, Gargiulo M, Tarantini S, Rodio M, Pilato A, and D'Addato M. Early and long-term results in the surgical treatment of juxtarenal and pararenal aortic aneurysms. Eur J Vasc Endovasc Surg 1998;15:205–211.
24. Tanquilut EM, Veith FJ, Ohki T, Lipsitz EC, Shaw PM, Suggs WD, Wain RA, Mehta M, Cayne NS, and McKay J. Nonoperative management with selective delayed surgery for large abdominal aortic aneurysms in patients at high risk. J Vasc Surg 2002;36:41–46.
25. Veith FJ, Tanquilut EM, Ohki T, Lipsitz EC, Suggs WD, Wain RA, and Gargiulo NJ. Conservative observational management with selective delayed repair for large abdominal aortic aneurysms in high risk patients. J Cardiovasc Surg 2003;44:459–464.
26. Henke PK, and Stanley JC. Surgical treatment of pararenal aortic aneurysm. In Ernst CB, Stanley JC, eds. Current Therapy in Vascular Surgery, 4th edition, St. Louis, Mosby, 2001.

Chapter 11

Pelvic Ischemia During Endovascular Abdominal Aortic Aneurysm Repair

Juan Fontcuberta, Manuel Doblas, Antonio Orgaz, Angel Flores, Jose Gil, Ignacio Leal, and Enrique Criado

Abstract The advent of endovascular abdominal aortic aneurysm repair (EVAR) has led to a decrease in postoperative morbidity, shorter hospital stays, and quicker recovery time following abdominal aortic aneurysms repair. Nevertheless, EVAR continues to be burdened with similar ischemic complications as seen with open aortic surgery, and occurs in 3–10% of patients. Signs and symptoms of pelvic ischemia (PI) include buttock and thigh claudication (BC and TC), impotence, perineal necrosis, rectal necrosis, colonic necrosis, and distal spinal cord or lumbar plexus ischemic neuropathy. Some of the mechanisms that may contribute to PI include interruption of hypogastric arterial circulation and atheroembolization. Several case reports and small retrospective studies have found that preservation of direct internal iliac artery (IIA) perfusion is important in preventing PI complications. The incidence of colonic ischemia after EVAR is 1.5%, though multiple large series have reported no cases of ischemic colitis. Preserving direct blood flow to the IIAs is likely the key in preventing this complication, particularly in the presence of a patent inferior mesenteric artery.

Keywords Pelvic ischemia during EVAR, Collateral pelvic circulation, Pelvic ischemia, AAA repair, IIA occlusion during EVAR, Claudication and AAA repair, Bowel ischemia

Introduction

Signs and symptoms of pelvic ischemia (PI) include buttock and thigh claudication (BC and TC), impotence, perineal necrosis, rectal necrosis, colonic necrosis, and distal spinal cord or lumbar plexus ischemic neuropathy. Endovascular abdominal aortic aneurysm repair (EVAR) has proven to be safe and effective in preventing aneurysm expansion and rupture.[1–4] Successful endovascular treatment of abdominal aortic aneurysms (AAAs) requires undilated arterial segments, relatively free of disease proximal and distal to the aneurysm.[5]

G. Upchurch and E. Criado (eds.) *Aortic Aneurysms, Contemporary Cardiology*
DOI: 10.1007/978-1-60327-204-9_11, © Humana Press, a part of
Springer Science + Business Media, LLC 2009

These undiseased arterial sites are necessary for the fixation of the endovascular prosthesis to the arterial wall. Tight apposition and fixation is necessary to achieve exclusion of the aneurysm from the arterial circulation.[6,7]

Extension of the aneurysm to the bifurcation of the common iliac artery (CIA) necessitates deployment of the distal aspect of the endovascular graft in the external iliac artery (EIA). This in turn results in interruption of arterial flow to the ipsilateral internal iliac artery (IIA).[8] In addition, when the IIA exhibits significant aneurysmal dilatation, its perfusion must be interrupted to prevent rupture.[9,10] The effects of IIA occlusion vary greatly in their severity and are dependent on the circumstances under which occlusion occurs.[11] These effects range from asymptomatic occlusion to the development of significant pelvic and spinal cord ischemia.[12–15]

Complications resulting from unilateral IIA occlusion associated with EVAR have been observed in 12–45% of cases.[16–19] Unilateral IIA occlusion may be a relatively innocuous event; however, the occlusion of both IIAs appears to be associated with a greater likelihood of development of an ischemic complication.[16,18,19]

The advent of EVAR has led to a decrease postoperative morbidity, shorter hospital stay, and quicker recovery time following AAA repair. Nevertheless, EVAR continues to be burdened with similar ischemic complications as seen with open aortic surgery. Ischemic complications after EVAR occur in 3–10% of patients. The mechanisms that may contribute to PI include interruption of hypogastric arterial circulation and atheroembolization.

Pelvic Collateral Circulation

Collateral pathways connect the midgut, hindgut, and pelvis via the superior mesenteric artery (SMA), inferior mesenteric artery (IMA), IIA, and profunda femoris arteries. Midgut to hindgut collaterals include the meandering artery, or the arch of Riolan, and the marginal artery of Drummond, both of which originate from the left branch of the middle colic artery and connect to the left colic artery or IMA.[20]

The sigmoid colon can receive collateral perfusion from the IIA via hemorrhoidal arteries. In the event of chronic occlusive disease of the IMA, the left IIA may provide most of the blood supply to the sigmoid colon. The IIA can also provide collateral circulation to the distal spinal cord and the lumbosacral nerve roots via iliolumbar and lateral sacral arteries. These collaterals are especially important when the artery of Adamkiewicz is occluded or originates very proximally.

The femoral arteries also can play a significant role in buttock and perineal perfusion via medial and lateral circumflex femoral arteries. The medial circumflex femoral artery terminates in the obturator artery, a branch of the IIA. The lateral circumflex femoral artery directly supplies the gluteal muscles. The superior and inferior gluteal arteries supplying blood to the buttocks are the main branches of the IIA.

Iliopoulos et al.[11] conducted a study measuring intraluminal IIA pressures and its variations after intermittent clamping of the pelvic branches from ten patients. The findings from the study suggested that ascending branches from the ipsilateral external iliac-deep femoral system provide a more significant collateral pathway to the region of the occluded IIA than the contralateral patent IIA. The authors then directly concluded that it is important to preserve vessels in the EIA-deep femoral system ipsilateral to an occluded IIA to minimize the risks of PI.

Pelvic Ischemia After Aortic Reconstruction

In vascular patients, the critical collaterals between the midgut, hindgut, pelvis, and the upper thigh can be compromised by occlusive disease. Therefore, in this population, interruption of direct blood supply to these territories during aortic reconstruction can result in PI.

Several case reports and small retrospective studies have found that preservation of direct IIA perfusion is important in preventing PI complications. BC and necrosis as well as lumbar plexus injury have been reported to occur after unilateral IIA occlusion. When direct IIA perfusion is occluded, collateral flow from the ipsilateral profunda femoris artery is essential to prevent PI. However, this collateral pathway may be inadequate to maintain pelvic perfusion in patients with arterial occlusive disease, particularly in patients with extensive occlusive disease involving the common femoral artery (CFA) and profunda femoris arteries.

Retrograde perfusion of the IAA after bypass to the femoral artery from the aorta is less reliable for pelvic perfusion. This approach has been associated with colonic infarction and PI after acute thrombosis of the retrogradely perfused EIA, even when occlusive disease of this artery is not severe. O'Connor et al.[20] showed that 67% of distal aortic segments bypassed by the end-to-side technique occlude within 1 year, but no patients in that series developed symptoms of PI, likely because the pelvic collateral supply had time to adapt while the distal aortic and common iliac aortic segments progressed to complete occlusion.

When faced with an occluded or aneurysmal IIAs that must be excluded, the IMA should be reimplanted, if patent and care should be taken to ensure adequate ipsilateral profunda femoris artery revascularization. Alternatively, a separate bypass to the patent distal portion of an aneurysmal IIA may be done when none of the other approaches to prevent PI is possible.

The internal pudendal artery, which originates from the IIA, provides circulation to the genitalia through the penile and the scrotal arteries. Because of the rich collateral supply in the genitourinary organs, ischemic complications involving the genitourinary organs as a result of PI are extremely uncommon. Catheter-directed coil embolization of the IIA may lead to the formation of minute fragments of thrombus that may migrate into the capillary bed and prevent adequate collateral vessel formation. As a result, irreversible tissue loss such as scrotal skin sloughing may occasionally occur.[21]

A grading system for PI was described by Yano et al.[19] in 2001. These criteria are used to quantify the clinical severity of PI after IIA occlusion:

Class 0 – no symptoms
Class I – nonlimiting claudication with exercise
Class II – new onset impotence or moderate-to-severe buttock pain, leading to
    physical limitations with exercise
Class III – Buttock rest pain with or without skin necrosis and/or colonic
    ischemia

Gluteal Blood Supply and Perioperative Monitoring

During open repair of aortoiliac aneurysm, various studies such as measurement of stump pressure in the IIA, assessment of intestinal viability by Doppler, or intramural oxygen saturation in the colon have been proposed to aid the intra-operative decision about IIA reconstruction.[22–25]

During EVAR, the IIA is often occluded as a necessary part of the procedure. The frequency of IIA occlusion during EVAR is two to three times higher than that for open surgery.[17,26–29] Several studies have reported that 26–41% of patients complain of persistent BC after IIA interruption during EVAR.[12,17,27,30–32] The incidence of new onset of impotence after IIA interruption during EVAR ranges between 4% and 12%.[17,27,33]

Inuzuka et al.[34] assessed pelvic circulation during EVAR in 12 patients who underwent aortouniiliac stent-graft with crossover bypass for exclusion of AAA measuring penile brachial pressure index (PBI) by pulse-volume-plethysmography and bilateral gluteal tissue oxygen metabolism with near-infrared spectroscopy to provide a gluteal tissue oxygenation index (TOI). They found an immediate reduction in PBI and gluteal TOI during EVAR in all patients. After revascularization of the ipsilateral limb of the stent-graft, the recovery of PBI and TOI was significantly less in aortouni-EIA stent-graft than following aortouni-CIA stent-graft. In contrast, contralateral gluteal TOI remained low in both groups after revascularization of the ipsilateral limb of the stent-graft and only after completion of crossover bypass did the contralateral TOI recover to baseline level in both groups. This study suggests that patency of uni-lateral IIA is sufficient for maintaining penile blood flow, but insufficient to maintain contralateral gluteal blood flow, because the ipsilateral collateral blood flow from the limb (i.e., via deep femoral artery or common femoral artery) is not sufficient to maintain ipsilateral gluteal flow. The PBI, before and after exercise, could be used to detect impaired hypo-gastric circulation in men. Further penile pressure cannot differentiate right from left arterial lesions.

Exercise TcPO$_2$, although a surface (and not muscle) perfusion measurement is a sensitive and reliable index for the management of patients suspected of exercise-related proximal ischemia.[35–38]

Arteriography, MRI, or angioscanners do show lesions on the aortoiliac tree; however, they are invasive, costly, and cannot be used as primary investigation. Transparietal and transanal ultrasound imaging or Doppler may allow direct visualization of the IIA, but the transparietal scanning is limited to nonobese patients with no intestinal gas. Finally, neither of these two imaging techniques proves the casual relationship between symptoms or ischemia and the presence of arterial lesions.[24]

In the absence of angiographically visible collateral supply to the IMA territory, a patient's ability to tolerate IIA embolization may be tested by temporary balloon occlusion of the artery while monitoring the superior rectal artery signal using a transrectal Doppler probe. Disappearance of the signal that does not reappear within 15 min may signal poor collateral circulation and a high risk of colonic ischemia.[24] Similarly, measuring the penile brachial index before and after IIA balloon occlusion can assess the risk of postprocedure impotence. A penile brachial index of less than 0.7 may indicate vasculogenic impotence.

Recently, Jaquinandi et al.[39] showed an estimation of the functional role of the arterial pathways to buttock circulation during treadmill walking in patients with claudication. The study suggested that the ipsilateral lumbar pathway has a major role in the buttock blood supply, whereas the contralateral IIA, IMA, and medial sacral pathways do not compensate for chronic buttock, exercise induced regional blood flow impairment.

Effects of IIA Interruption During EVAR

The occurrence of ischemia in cases of acute IIA occlusion, such as with coil embolization during EVAR, depends on the collateral pathway to the IIA. There are four collateral pathways to the IIA: the mesenteric route (the IMA, superior rectal artery, vessels in the colon, middle colic artery, and the IIA), the lumbar route (lumbar artery, iliolumbar artery, and the IIA), the IIA route (contralateral IIA, lateral sacral artery, and ipsilateral IIA), and the EIA route (the EIA, deep circumflex iliac artery or medial circumflex femoral artery, inferior gluteal artery, and the IIA).

Sugano et al.[22] made an evaluation of BC after open AAA repair with IIA stump pressure measurement and near-infrared spectroscopy. In this study, the contralateral IIA and ipsilateral EIA routes were apparently more important sources of collateral blood supply to the IIA than the IMA and lumbar routes. Also the collateral pathway from the EIA did not supply the superior gluteal artery, and BC after AAA repair thus appeared to be related to superior gluteal artery insufficiency. The IIA collateral route could develop after AAA repair in cases in which unilateral IIA preservation is performed. Arteriography after AAA repair (with the left IIA ligated) showed a blood supply to the superior gluteal artery from the contralateral (right) IIA by means of bilateral lateral sacral arteries.

A significant number (39%) of patients who sustain IIA occlusions after endovascular aortoiliac aneurysm repair have symptoms. Although most of these patients demonstrate some improvement of their symptoms, none return to their baseline levels of physical activity. They require, on average, almost 4 months to achieve symptomatic improvement.[32]

Mehta et al.[16] reported the results of interruption of one IIA (134/154) or both (20/154) IIAs as part of their endovascular or open repair of 154 patients with AAA, iliac aneurysm, or aortoiliac aneurysms. BC developed in 36% of the unilateral and 40% of the bilateral IIA interruptions within the first month. These symptoms persisted in only 12% of the unilateral and 11% of the bilateral IIA interruptions at 1 year. New-onset impotence resulted in only 9% of the unilateral and only 13% of the bilateral IIA interruptions.

Buttock Claudication

BC and impotence after stent-graft repair of AAA appear to be relatively common when internal iliac occlusion occurs as part of the procedure. Criado et al.[31] described 31 patients who underwent preoperative coil embolization of IIAs (20 unilateral and 11 bilateral) in preparation for stent-graft repair of AAA. No perineal necrosis or paralysis was seen in these patients, but impotence developed in 2%, and BC occurred in 13% of patients after unilateral IIA embolization and in no patients after bilateral embolization.

Razavi et al.[17] reported embolization/occlusion of IIAs in 32 patients and noted a 12% incidence of impotence and a 28% incidence of BC. The BC resolved in 78% of patients after a mean of 14 months.[17] After endovascular bilateral IIA interruption, proximal claudication seems to improve over time.[40] Lee et al.[27] found that patients treated with unilateral aortoiliac prosthesis and femorofemoral bypass were at higher risk for BC, possibly caused by loss of antegrade pelvic perfusion. Cynamon et al.[12] reported a 41% incidence of BC in 34 patients who underwent preoperative IIA embolization before aortic endografting. Patients undergoing embolization of the anterior and posterior branches of the distal IIA had a BC rate of 55%, whereas patients with proximal IIA embolization developed BC only in 10% of the cases. The diagnosis of the vascular origin of BC may be difficult, mainly if distal pulses are palpable. Routine distal pressure investigation in these patients is of low sensitivity in detecting abnormal blood flow to the pelvis.[41] Erectile dysfunction is perhaps the most underreported ischemic complication after IIAs for EVAR, but may occur in up to 46% of patients.[42] Recently, Maldonado et al.[43] reported ischemic complications following EVAR in 12.5% of patients with sacrificed IIA versus 6.3% in patients with bilaterally preserved IIA, but suggested that simultaneous bilateral IIA occlusion does not appear to increase the risk of pelvic or lower-extremity ischemia.

Bowel Ischemia After EVAR

The incidence of colonic ischemia after EVAR is 1.5%, but multiple large series have reported no cases of ischemic colitis.[20] This low incidence of colonic ischemia associated with EVAR is surprising because the IMA is patent in up to 50% of patients undergoing the procedure. Preserving direct blood flow to the IIAs is likely the key in preventing this complication, particularly in the presence of a patent IMA.

Geraghty et al.[44] suggested that embolization of atheromatous debris to the IIA beds during endovascular manipulations, rather than proximal IIA occlusion, is the primary cause of clinically significant ischemic colitis after EVAR. Pathological findings confirmed the presence of atheroemboli in the colonic vasculature in all patients who underwent colonic resection. Three of four patients who developed ischemic colitis had bilateral patent IIAs.

Maldonado et al.[45] described seven patients with PI after EVAR. All seven patients had copious thrombus in the aneurysms sac, and the cause of PI would appear to be more consistent with atheroembolism despite preservation of IIA circulation. Small bowel ischemia probably occurs more commonly in patients undergoing EVAR than open surgery, and is associated with high mortality.[46] The cause of small bowel ischemia after EVAR is presumed to be from thrombus or atheroma dislodgement into the SMA during the procedure. Microembolism may also occur into the renal arteries, IMA, and distal vessels, leading to acute renal insufficiency, colonic ischemia, buttock ischemia, and blue toes.

IIA Occlusion During EVAR

The IIA may be occluded unintentionally during EVAR because of arterial injury, embolization, or unintended endograft coverage.[18] Iliac artery injury has been reported in 4–13% of EVAR.[1,47,48] When necessary, coil embolization of the ipsilateral IIA is performed to prevent retrograde flow into the CIA

Color Plates

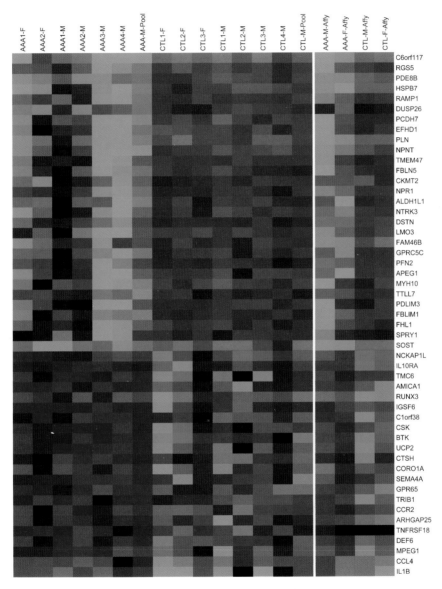

Chapter 1, Fig. 5 Whole-genome expression profile for AAA tissue. The 50 most significantly different genes between AAA and control tissue are shown as determined by the Illumina microarray platform in ascending order (the most differential genes are located on the top and bottom, with decreasing difference toward the center). To show consistency of the results between two platforms (Affymetrix and Illumina), data from both Illumina (15 left columns) and Affymetrix (4 right columns) platforms are presented. Sample IDs are on top of each column (AAA1-F = female aneurysm patient, CTL1-F = female control, etc.). The "Pool" samples were age, sex, and ethnicity-matched pools of RNA. All four samples run on Affymetrix arrays were pooled samples. Data were log2-transformed and gene-centered for each individual platform. Gene IDs shown on the right represent official IDs found at http://www.genenames.org/. For details, see study by Lenk et al.[104]

c

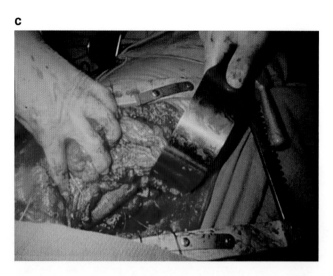

Chapter 5, Fig. 5 (**c**) Intraoperative picture demonstrating retroperitoneal exposure with completed aortic graft and reimplantation of left renal artery

d

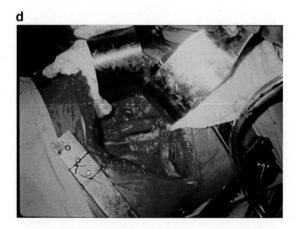

Chapter 5, Fig. 6 (**d**) Intraoperative view of infrarenal AAA repair with tube graft

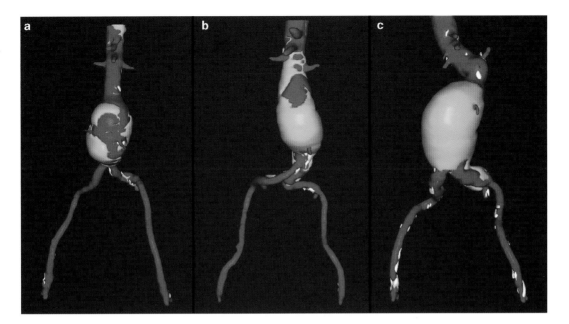

Chapter 6, Fig. 2 Three-dimensional reconstructions demonstrating infrarenal aortic neck characteristics: Patients with the ideal infrarenal aortic neck (**a**), a nonideal conical infrarenal aortic neck (**b**), and the highly angulated infrarenal aortic neck (**c**)

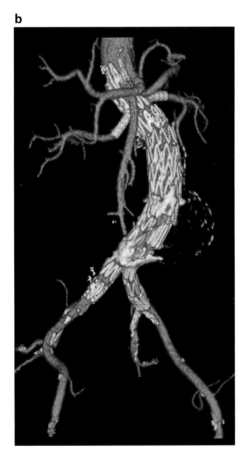

Chapter 9, Fig. 4 (**b**) Post-operative CT-scanning reconstruction after fenestrated stent-grafting. Two covered stents were inserted in the renal artery fenestrations not only to optimize apposition but also to create a seal

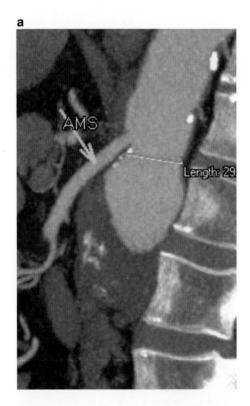

Chapter 9, Fig. 5 (**a**) Pre-operative CT-scanning of a suprarenal aneurysm reaching to the level of the superior mesenteric artery (AMS, arrow).

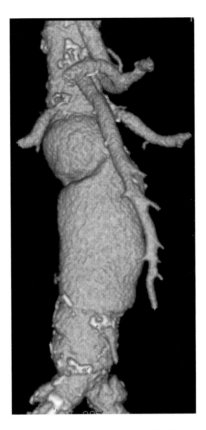

Chapter 10, Fig. 3 Reformatted 3-D tomographic arteriogram of the juxtarenal aortic aneurysm in Figure 2

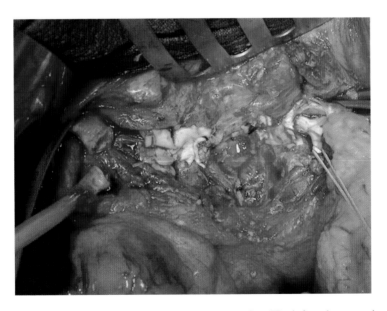

Chapter 15, Fig. 4 Retroperitoneum after mycotic aneurysm resection. The infected aorta and periaortic tissues from Fig. 3 have been debrided, leaving a large defect in the aorta and proximal iliac arteries

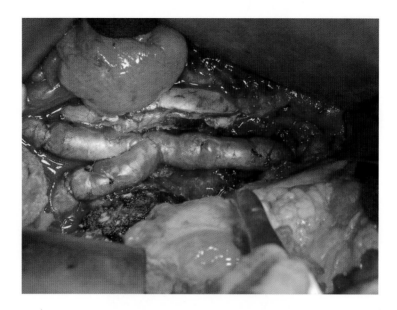

Chapter 15, Fig. 5 *In situ* aortic repair with superficial femoral vein (*SFV*). The SFV has been used to reconstruct the aorta and iliac segments after debridement of the mycotic aneurysm pictured in Figs. 3 and 4

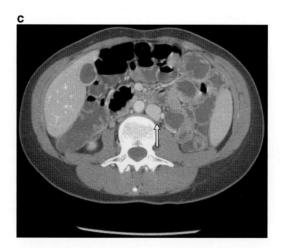

Chapter 20, Fig. 5 (**c**) Left-sided vena cava (*arrow*)

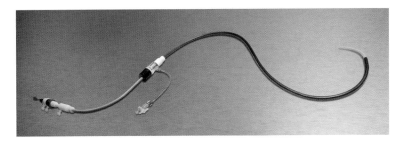

Chapter 25, Fig. 1 Photograph of the Superflex delivery system (TX2, Cook Medical, Inc., Bloomington, IN), showing its characteristic flexibility

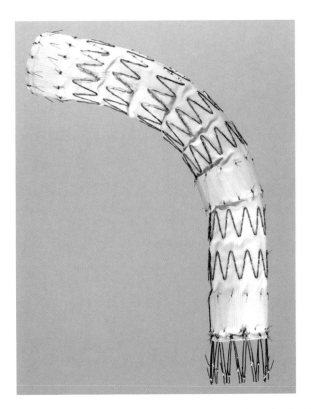

Chapter 25, Fig. 2 Photograph of the TX2 stent-graft, showing the barbed proximal and distal stents, and demonstrating narrowing of the gaps between stents on the inner curvature of a bend.

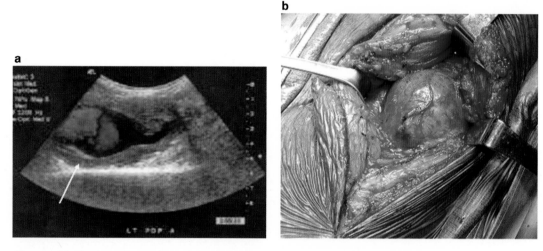

Chapter 28, Fig. 1 (**a**) Gray scale ultrasound image of a large left popliteal aneurysm (*white arrow*). (**b**) A large popliteal aneurysm after surgical exposure. Note this is a posterior approach, and proximal and distal arteries appear of reasonable size aneurysm and possibly into the native AAA sac, which may lead to aneurysm expansion and potential rupture.[18]

Coil embolization of the IIA has been shown to be technically feasible with a low procedural complication rate.[49–51] Coil embolization of the IIA can be performed before EVAR, or during endografting procedure itself, before graft deployment.[18] Access to the IIA is facilitated by an antegrade approach from the contralateral femoral or brachial artery. A generally large number of coils are required to achieve complete occlusion of this artery. In the case of an IIA aneurysm, the distal branches must also be occluded.[49]

Cynamon et al.[12] have published their experience with 13 patients who had BC after IIA coil embolization. They reported a substantial difference in the incidence of BC when coils were placed in the proximal IIA (10%) as opposed to its distal branches (55%). The IIA is embolized as close to the origin as possible, proximal to the bifurcation of the anterior and posterior divisions to maintain the collateral supply. Particular care has to be taken not to place coils distal to the gluteal bifurcation to avoid acute ischemic complications.[33]

Preoperative IIA embolization has the theoretical advantage of allowing collateral pelvic flow compensation before EVAR.[31]

The practice of bilateral IIA embolization is controversial and most surgeons view it as a highly risky if not contraindicated. Some reports appear to suggest that staged simultaneous bilateral IIA embolization is safe. It is generally accepted, however, that bilateral IIA occlusion should be avoided because of the high potential for ischemic complications. A number of clinical studies demonstrated that PI developed in 55–80% of patients with bilateral IIA occlusion, compared with 17–38% of patients with unilateral IIA occlusion.[17,19,52,53] Complete occlusion of the IIA at the time of EVAR may not be necessary to prevent type 2 endoleak.

Heye et al.[54] reported a total of 53 IIA embolization procedures performed in 45 patients. At the end of the embolization procedure, total occlusion of the postostial segment of the IIA was noted in 23 IIAs. In 30 cases, preservation of the antegrade flow through the coils was found. There was no significant difference in the incidence of type 2 endoleaks between patients with total occlusion of the IIA and those with residual flow in the IIA at the end of the embolization procedure.

The Amplatzer Vascular Plug (AGA Medical Corporation, Golden Valley, MN) is a nitinol wire self-expanding cylindrical device available in different diameters that allows precise occlusion at the origin of the IIA. It may reduce the risk of ischemic complications by preserving the distal branches and avoiding possible atheroembolization or occlusion of the major branch vessels by migrated coils.[55]

Gough and MacMahon[56] described a technique for ligation of the IIA that allows the entire procedure to be performed though the groin incision used for stent-graft insertion. In this technique, the inguinal ligament is partly divided to allow digital separation of the peritoneum from the EIA. The operative field is defined with two narrow bladed retractors, positioned anterior and medial to the EIA. Further dissection of the EIA, IIA, and distal CIA is achieved using a 10-mm laparoscope housed within a sheath and laparoscopic cholecystectomy forceps and diathermy scissors. Following identification of the IIA, it is occluded with either metal clips or a one linen ligature passed around the vessel close to its origin.

Wyers et al.[57] described a technique of intentional IIA coverage without concomitant coil embolization during EVAR in selected patients, based on the presence of adequate graft oversizing in the most distal 5 mm of the CIA and the most proximal 15 mm of the EIA. This approach is effective if the IIA orifice is small and close enough to the EIA orifice to be occluded by the side of a stent-graft. Mell et al.[58] reported good results with this approach. Twenty-one patients had unilateral IIA coverage without coil embolization. Immediate seal was achieved in all patients. No type 2 endoleaks were found from the origin of the IIA. This technique is simple, requires no additional equipment, minimizes intervention, and reduces cost. This technique, applied to properly selected patients, is effective in the prevention of IIA-associated endoleak.[57]

Preservation of IIA Perfusion During EVAR

The CIA anatomy plays a crucial role because it is the distal attachment zone for the stent-graft and must be completely sealed to assure exclusion of the aneurysm. One or both CIAs are dilated in 16–30% of endovascular stent-graft cases[16–19,27,31] making them unsuitable for adequate distal sealing with commercially available endovascular devices.

The so-called bell-bottom technique uses a flared cuff that anchors the device within the dilated CIA, thus preserving IIA patency.[59] A short aortic extension cuff is used in the distal CIA attachment zone to achieve a complete seal. The aortic extension cuff is oversized 10–20%.[60] A length of about 15 mm of distal contact between the extension cuff and the CIA is considered adequate for distal attachment and 20 mm length of the cuff proximally apposed within the endograft limb. The long-term durability of this technique remains unknown. Open surgery may still be a better treatment for complicated CIA aneurysms and IIA aneurysms associated with AAA.

As reported by Santilli et al.[61] small CIA aneurysms (<30 mm) rarely cause symptoms or rupture and expand very slowly. At least two devices (Talent, Medtronic AVE; Zenith, Cook, Inc.) provide iliac limbs large enough to achieve seal in CIAs 20–24 mm in diameter that may be deployed when the CIA is 20 mm in diameter or less.

External to internal artery bypass is usually performed with a 6- or 8-mm Dacron graft. The iliac bifurcation is mobilized though a small retroperitoneal incision. The IIA is clamped proximally and distally and divided between clamps. Proximally, the artery is oversewn for hemostasis. The distal artery is mobilized, and the graft is sutured end-to-end to the artery. The proximal end of the graft is anastomosed end-to-side to the EIA. The bifurcated endograft is then deployed.[62] Metal hemoclips are placed at the level of EIA anastomosis to aid in its identification during the endovascular procedure. This technique has a very low incidence of ipsilateral ischemic complications, and the associated patency rates are excellent. However, IIA bypass is technically challenging, increases the complexity of the EVAR, and may extend the hospital length of stay.

Lee et al.[63] reported a 27% incidence of BC immediately after EVAR and a primary patency rate for the IIA bypass of 91% at 36 months. However, concomitant IIA aneurysms, small diameter (<6 mm) IIA, severe calcification, a short common hypogastric trunk, severe obesity (deep pelvis), previous retroperitoneal surgery, or pelvic irradiation may preclude successful application of these techniques.[64]

Relocation of the iliac bifurcation with surgical implantation of the IIA onto the distal EIA to preserve pelvic blood flow as proposed by Parodi and Ferreira[65] is another option for the management of dilated CIA.

Bergamini et al.[66] described a novel approach to preserve pelvic perfusion during EVAR in patients with bilateral CIA aneurysms extending to the iliac bifurcation. He reported four cases treated with aortouniiliac endograft extended to the ipsilateral EIA, femorofemoral polytetrafluoroethylene bypass graft, and contralateral EIA-to-IIA endograft to preserve pelvic perfusion.

Another option to preserve at least one IIA is to place an aortouniiliac endograft with a femorofemoral bypass and contralateral CIA occlusion with a vascular plug. This technique may be the best option in some patients, but adds the risk of complications related to the presence of a prosthetic graft in the inguinal region. Perioperative morbidity associated with aortouniiliac endovascular aneurysm repair and femorofemoral crossover is similar to that reported with bifurcated endovascular stent grafts. In contrast to their use in iliac occlusive disease, the mode of graft failure appears to be related to problems of inflow rather than runoff. The durability of aortouniiliac endografting with a femorofemoral bypass has been deemed satisfactory with midterm and long-term follow-up. Hinchliffe et al.[67] showed 91% cumulative 3-year patency rate for the femorofemoral bypass graft and at the end of 5 years, 83% of grafts remained patent.

When the CIA diameter exceeds 24 mm, endograft landing proximal to the IIA is inadequate. Modular iliac bifurcated devices (IBDs) that perfuse both the external and internal iliac arteries are alternative to avoid IIA occlusion under investigation.[68] The technical success rates of the first-generation IBDs were disappointingly low (58%) related to the learning curve. The second-generation device success rates reached an 85% technical success rate.

Recommendations for the Prevention of PI During EVAR

It should always be considered that IIA occlusion is not a benign procedure. Neither inadvertent nor intentional hypogastric occlusion should be taken lightly during EVAR.

- Embolization and occlusion of the IIA should be avoided, if at all possible, and consideration should be given to adjunctive endovascular or surgical techniques to evascularize the IIA.
- IIA embolization and occlusion should be reserved for patients with aneurysm of the IIA.
- To avoid pelvic embolization, intra-arterial wire and catheter manipulations during the course of endoluminal aortoiliac aneurysms repair must be kept to a minimum.
- Staged preoperative unilateral IIA coil embolization and coil embolization performed concurrently with EVAR are not associated with increased risk for postoperative ischemic colitis.
- Collateral branches of the EIA and femoral arteries must be preserved.

- Bilateral IIA interruptions are safer if staged 1–2 weeks apart.
- Adequate heparinization of the patients and hemodinamic stability during these procedures are important factors to prevent PI.
- Open surgery may still be the optimal treatment for repair of large and complicated CIA aneurysms and IIA aneurysms associated with AAA.
- When possible, the IIAs are interrupted at their origin by oversewing, embolization, or stent-graft coverage. This preserves the extensive network of collateral connections between branches of the IIA, the EIA, and the femoral arteries.
- IMA exclusion or embolization in patients with SMA stenosis or previous partial colectomy, in which the collateral pathways between the IMA and SMA have been interrupted, pose a high risk of colonic/pelvic ischemic complications.

References

1. Zarins CK, White RA, Moll FL, Crabtree T, Bloch DA, Hodgson KJ, Fillinger MF, Fogarty TJ. The AneuRx stent graft: four-year results and worldwide experience 2000. *J Vasc Surg.* 2001;33(2 Suppl):S135–145.
2. Makaroun MS. The Ancure endografting system: an update. *J Vasc Surg.* 2001;33 (2 Suppl):S129–134.
3. Greenberg RK, Lawrence-Brown M, Bhandari G, Hartley D, Stelter W, Umscheid T, Chuter T, Ivancev K, Green R, Hopkinson B, Semmens J, Ouriel K. An update of the Zenith endovascular graft for abdominal aortic aneurysms: initial implantation and mid-term follow-up data. *J Vasc Surg.* 2001;33(2 Suppl):S157–164.
4. May J, White GH, Waugh R, Ly CN, Stephen MS, Jones MA, Harris JP. Improved survival after endoluminal repair with second-generation prostheses compared with open repair in the treatment of abdominal aortic aneurysms: a 5-year concurrent comparison using life table method. *J Vasc Surg.* 2001;33(2 Suppl):S21–26.
5. Woodburn KR, Chant H, Davies JN, Blanshard KS, Travis SJ. Suitability for endovascular aneurysm repair in an unselected population. *Br J Surg.* 2001;88(1):77–81.
6. Gitlitz DB, Ramaswami G, Kaplan D, Hollier LH, Marin ML. Endovascular stent grafting in the presence of aortic neck filling defects: early clinical experience. *J Vasc Surg.* 2001;33(2):340–344.
7. Zarins CK, White RA, Hodgson KJ, Schwarten D, Fogarty TJ. Endoleak as a predictor of outcome after endovascular aneurysm repair: AneuRx multicenter clinical trial. *J Vasc Surg.* 2000;32(1):90–107.
8. Faries PL, Morrissey N, Burks JA, Gravereaux E, Kerstein MD, Teodorescu VJ, Hollier LH, Marin ML. Internal iliac artery revascularization as an adjunct to endovascular repair of aortoiliac aneurysms. *J Vasc Surg.* 2001;34(5):892–899.
9. Deb B, Benjamin M, Comerota AJ. Delayed rupture of an internal iliac artery aneurysm following proximal ligation for abdominal aortic aneurysm repair. *Ann Vasc Surg.* 1992;6(6):537–540.
10. Perdue GD, Mittenthal MJ, Smith RB, 3rd, Salam AA. Aneurysms of the internal iliac artery. *Surgery.* 1983;93(2):243–246.
11. Iliopoulos JI, Hermreck AS, Thomas JH, Pierce GE. Hemodynamics of the hypogastric arterial circulation. *J Vasc Surg.* 1989;9(5):637–641; discussion 641–632.
12. Cynamon J, Lerer D, Veith FJ, Taragin BH, Wahl SI, Lautin JL, Ohki T, Sprayregen S. Hypogastric artery coil embolization prior to endoluminal repair of aneurysms and fistulas: buttock claudication, a recognized but possibly preventable complication. *J Vasc Interv Radiol.* 2000;11(5):573–577.
13. Connolly JE, Ingegno M, Wilson SE. Preservation of the pelvic circulation during infrarenal aortic surgery. *Cardiovasc Surg.* 1996;4(1):65–70.

14. Picone AL, Green RM, Ricotta JR, May AG, DeWeese JA. Spinal cord ischemia following operations on the abdominal aorta. *J Vasc Surg.* 1986;3(1):94–103.

15. Gloviczki P, Cross SA, Stanson AW, Carmichael SW, Bower TC, Pairolero PC, Hallett JW, Jr., Toomey BJ, Cherry KJ, Jr. Ischemic injury to the spinal cord or lumbosacral plexus after aorto-iliac reconstruction. *Am J Surg.* 1991;162(2):131–136.

16. Mehta M, Veith FJ, Ohki T, Cynamon J, Goldstein K, Suggs WD, Wain RA, Chang DW, Friedman SG, Scher LA, Lipsitz EC. Unilateral and bilateral hypogastric artery interruption during aortoiliac aneurysm repair in 154 patients: a relatively innocuous procedure. *J Vasc Surg.* 2001;33(2 Suppl):S27–32.

17 Razavi MK, DeGroot M, Olcott C, 3rd, Sze D, Kee S, Semba CP, Dake MD. Internal iliac artery embolization in the stent-graft treatment of aortoiliac aneurysms: analysis of outcomes and complications. *J Vasc Interv Radiol.* 2000;11(5):561–566.

18 Karch LA, Hodgson KJ, Mattos MA, Bohannon WT, Ramsey DE, McLafferty RB. Adverse consequences of internal iliac artery occlusion during endovascular repair of abdominal aortic aneurysms. *J Vasc Surg.* 2000;32(4):676–683.

19 Yano OJ, Morrissey N, Eisen L, Faries PL, Soundararajan K, Wan S, Teodorescu V, Kerstein M, Hollier LH, Marin ML. Intentional internal iliac artery occlusion to facilitate endovascular repair of aortoiliac aneurysms. *J Vasc Surg.* 2001;34(2):204–211.

20. O'Connor SE, Walsh DB, Zwolak RM, Schneider JR, Cronenwett JL. Pelvic blood flow following aortobifemoral bypass with proximal end-to-side anastomosis. *Ann Vasc Surg.* 1992;6(6):493–498.

21. Lin PH, Bush RL, Lumsden AB. Sloughing of the scrotal skin and impotence subsequent to bilateral hypogastric artery embolization for endovascular aortoiliac aneurysm repair. *J Vasc Surg.* 2001;34(4):748–750.

22. Sugano N, Inoue Y, Iwai T. Evaluation of buttock claudication with hypogastric artery stump pressure measurement and near infrared spectroscopy after abdominal aortic aneurysm repair. *Eur J Vasc Endovasc Surg.* 2003;26(1):45–51.

23. Krohg-Sorensen K, Kvernebo K. Laser Doppler flowmetry in evaluation of colonic blood flow during aortic reconstruction. *Eur J Vasc Surg.* 1989;3(1):37–41.

24. Iwai T, Sakurazawa K, Sato S, Muraoka Y, Inoue Y, Endo M. Intra-operative monitoring of the pelvic circulation using a transanal Doppler probe. *Eur J Vasc Surg.* 1991;5(1):71–74.

25. Vahl AC, Ozkaynak-Yilmaz EN, Nauta SH, Scheffer GJ, Felt-Bersma RJ, Brom HL, Rauwerda JA. Endoluminal pulse oximetry combined with tonometry to monitor the perfusion of the sigmoid during and after resection of abdominal aortic aneurysm. *Cardiovasc Surg.* 1997;5(1):65–70.

26. Lyden SP, Sternbach Y, Waldman DL, Green RM. Clinical implications of internal iliac artery embolization in endovascular repair of aortoiliac aneurysms. *Ann Vasc Surg.* 2001;15(5):539–543.

27. Lee CW, Kaufman JA, Fan CM, Geller SC, Brewster DC, Cambria RP, Lamuraglia GM, Gertler JP, Abbott WM, Waltman AC. Clinical outcome of internal iliac artery occlusions during endovascular treatment of aortoiliac aneurysmal diseases. *J Vasc Interv Radiol.* 2000;11(5):567–571.

28. Pittaluga P, Batt M, Hassen-Khodja R, Declemy S, Le Bas P. Revascularization of internal iliac arteries during aortoiliac surgery: a multicenter study. *Ann Vasc Surg.* 1998;12(6):537–543.

29. Johnston KW. Multicenter prospective study of nonruptured abdominal aortic aneurysm. Part II. Variables predicting morbidity and mortality. *J Vasc Surg.* 1989;9(3):437–447.

30. Sanchez LA, Patel AV, Ohki T, Suggs WD, Wain RA, Valladares J, Cynamon J, Rigg J, Veith FJ. Midterm experience with the endovascular treatment of isolated iliac aneurysms. *J Vasc Surg.* 1999;30(5):907–913.

31. Criado FJ, Wilson EP, Velazquez OC, Carpenter JP, Barker C, Wellons E, Abul-Khoudoud O, Fairman RM. Safety of coil embolization of the internal

iliac artery in endovascular grafting of abdominal aortic aneurysms. *J Vasc Surg.* 2000;32(4):684–688.

32. Lee WA, O'Dorisio J, Wolf YG, Hill BB, Fogarty TJ, Zarins CK. Outcome after unilateral hypogastric artery occlusion during endovascular aneurysm repair. *J Vasc Surg.* 2001;33(5):921–926.

33. Engelke C, Elford J, Morgan RA, Belli AM. Internal iliac artery embolization with bilateral occlusion before endovascular aortoiliac aneurysm repair-clinical outcome of simultaneous and sequential intervention. *J Vasc Interv Radiol.* 2002;13(7): 667–676.

34. Inuzuka K, Unno N, Mitsuoka H, Yamamoto N, Ishimaru K, Sagara D, Suzuki M, Konno H. Intraoperative monitoring of penile and buttock blood flow during endovascular abdominal aortic aneurysm repair. *Eur J Vasc Endovasc Surg.* 2006;31(4):359–365.

35. Cosson E, Paycha F, Tellier P, Sachs RN, Ramadan A, Paries J, Attali JR, Valensi P. Lower-limb vascularization in diabetic patients. Assessment by thallium-201 scanning coupled with exercise myocardial scintigraphy. *Diabetes Care.* 2001;24(5):870–874.

36. Larsen JF, Christensen KS, Egeblad K. Assessment of intermittent claudication by means of the transcutaneous oxygen tension exercise profile. *Eur J Vasc Surg.* 1990;4(4):409–412.

37. Schmidt JA, Bracht C, Leyhe A, von Wichert P. Transcutaneous measurement of oxygen and carbon dioxide tension (TcPO2 and TcPCO2) during treadmill exercise in patients with arterial occlusive disease (AOD) – stages I and II. *Angiology.* 1990;41(7):547–552.

38. Abraham P, Picquet J, Vielle B, Sigaudo-Roussel D, Paisant-Thouveny F, Enon B, Saumet JL. Transcutaneous oxygen pressure measurements on the buttocks during exercise to detect proximal arterial ischemia: comparison with arteriography. *Circulation.* 2003;107(14):1896–1900.

39. Jaquinandi V, Abraham P, Picquet J, Paisant-Thouveny F, Leftheriotis G, Saumet JL. Estimation of the functional role of arterial pathways to the buttock circulation during treadmill walking in patients with claudication. *J Appl Physiol.* 2007;102(3):1105–1112.

40. Mehta M, Veith FJ, Darling RC, Roddy SP, Ohki T, Lipsitz EC, Paty PS, Kreienberg PB, Ozsvath KJ, Chang BB, Shah DM. Effects of bilateral hypogastric artery interruption during endovascular and open aortoiliac aneurysm repair. *J Vasc Surg.* 2004;40(4):698–702.

41. Jaquinandi V, Picquet J, Bouye P, Saumet JL, Leftheriotis G, Abraham P. High prevalence of proximal claudication among patients with patent aortobifemoral bypasses. *J Vasc Surg.* 2007;45(2):312–318.

42. Lin PH, Bush RL, Chaikof EL, Chen C, Conklin B, Terramani TT, Brinkman WT, Lumsden AB. A prospective evaluation of hypogastric artery embolization in endovascular aortoiliac aneurysm repair. *J Vasc Surg.* 2002;36(3):500–506.

43. Maldonado TS, Ranson ME, Rockman CB, Pua B, Cayne NS, Jacobowitz GR, Adelman MA. Decreased ischemic complications after endovascular aortic aneurysm repair with newer devices. *Vasc Endovascular Surg.* 2007;41(3):192–199.

44. Geraghty PJ, Sanchez LA, Rubin BG, Choi ET, Flye MW, Curci JA, Thompson RW, Sicard GA. Overt ischemic colitis after endovascular repair of aortoiliac aneurysms. *J Vasc Surg.* 2004;40(3):413–418.

45. Maldonado TS, Rockman CB, Riles E, Douglas D, Adelman MA, Jacobowitz GR, Gagne PJ, Nalbandian MN, Cayne NS, Lamparello PJ, Salzberg SS, Riles TS. Ischemic complications after endovascular abdominal aortic aneurysm repair. *J Vasc Surg.* 2004;40(4):703–709; discussion 709–710.

46. Zhang WW, Kulaylat MN, Anain PM, Dosluoglu HH, Harris LM, Cherr GS, Dayton MT, Dryjski ML. Embolization as cause of bowel ischemia after endovascular abdominal aortic aneurysm repair. *J Vasc Surg.* 2004;40(5):867–872.

47. Henretta JP, Karch LA, Hodgson KJ, Mattos MA, Ramsey DE, McLafferty R, Sumner DS. Special iliac artery considerations during aneurysm endografting. *Am J Surg.* 1999;178(3):212–218.

48. Moore WS, Rutherford RB. Transfemoral endovascular repair of abdominal aortic aneurysm: results of the North American EVT phase 1 trial. EVT Investigators. *J Vasc Surg.* 1996;23(4):543–553.

49. Mori M, Sakamoto I, Morikawa M, Kohzaki S, Makino K, Matsunaga N, Amamoto Y, Hayashi K. Transcatheter embolization of internal iliac artery aneurysms. *J Vasc Interv Radiol.* 1999;10(5):591–597.

50. Henry M, Amor M, Henry I, Tzvetanov K, Buniet JM, Amicabile C. Endovascular treatment of internal iliac artery aneurysms. *J Endovasc Surg.* 1998;5(4):345–348.

51. Hollis HW, Jr., Luethke JM, Yakes WF, Beitler AL. Percutaneous embolization of an internal iliac artery aneurysm: technical considerations and literature review. *J Vasc Interv Radiol.* 1994;5(3):449–451.

52. Wolpert LM, Dittrich KP, Hallisey MJ, Allmendinger PP, Gallagher JJ, Heydt K, Lowe R, Windels M, Drezner AD. Hypogastric artery embolization in endovascular abdominal aortic aneurysm repair. *J Vasc Surg.* 2001;33(6):1193–1198.

53. Schoder M, Zaunbauer L, Holzenbein T, Fleischmann D, Cejna M, Kretschmer G, Thurnher S, Lammer J. Internal iliac artery embolization before endovascular repair of abdominal aortic aneurysms: frequency, efficacy, and clinical results. *AJR Am J Roentgenol.* 2001;177(3):599–605.

54. Heye S, Nevelsteen A, Maleux G. Internal iliac artery coil embolization in the prevention of potential type 2 endoleak after endovascular repair of abdominal aortoiliac and iliac artery aneurysms: effect of total occlusion versus residual flow. *J Vasc Interv Radiol.* 2005;16(2 Pt 1):235–239.

55. Ha CD, Calcagno D. Amplatzer Vascular Plug to occlude the internal iliac arteries in patients undergoing aortoiliac aneurysm repair. *J Vasc Surg.* 2005;42(6):1058–1062.

56. Gough MJ, MacMahon MJ. A minimally invasive technique allowing ligation of the internal iliac artery during endovascular repair of aortic aneurysms with an aorto-uni-iliac device. *Eur J Vasc Endovasc Surg.* 1998;16(6):535–536.

57. Wyers MC, Schermerhorn ML, Fillinger MF, Powell RJ, Rzucidlo EM, Walsh DB, Zwolak RM, Cronenwett JL. Internal iliac occlusion without coil embolization during endovascular abdominal aortic aneurysm repair. *J Vasc Surg.* 2002;36(6):1138–1145.

58. Mell M, Tefera G, Schwarze M, Carr S, Acher C, Hoch J, Turnipseed W. Absence of buttock claudication following stent-graft coverage of the hypogastric artery without coil embolization in endovascular aneurysm repair. *J Endovasc Ther.* 2006;13(3):415–419.

59. Karch LA, Hodgson KJ, Mattos MA, Bohannon WT, Ramsey DE, McLafferty RB. Management of ectatic, nonaneurysmal iliac arteries during endoluminal aortic aneurysm repair. *J Vasc Surg.* 2001;33(2 Suppl):S33–38.

60. Kritpracha B, Pigott JP, Russell TE, Corbey MJ, Whalen RC, DiSalle RS, Price CI, Sproat IA, Beebe HG. Bell-bottom aortoiliac endografts: an alternative that preserves pelvic blood flow. *J Vasc Surg.* 2002;35(5):874–881.

61. Santilli SM, Wernsing SE, Lee ES. Expansion rates and outcomes for iliac artery aneurysms. *J Vasc Surg.* 2000;31(1 Pt 1):114–121.

62. Arko FR, Lee WA, Hill BB, Fogarty TJ, Zarins CK. Hypogastric artery bypass to preserve pelvic circulation: improved outcome after endovascular abdominal aortic aneurysm repair. *J Vasc Surg.* 2004;39(2):404–408.

63. Lee WA, Nelson PR, Berceli SA, Seeger JM, Huber TS. Outcome after hypogastric artery bypass and embolization during endovascular aneurysm repair. *J Vasc Surg.* 2006;44(6):1162–1168; discussion 1168–1169.

64. Lee WA, Berceli SA, Huber TS, Seeger JM. A technique for combined hypogastric artery bypass and endovascular repair of complex aortoiliac aneurysms. *J Vasc Surg.* 2002;35(6):1289–1291.

65. Parodi JC, Ferreira M. Relocation of the iliac artery bifurcation to facilitate endoluminal treatment of abdominal aortic aneurysms. *J Endovasc Surg.* 1999;6(4):342–347.

66. Bergamini TM, Rachel ES, Kinney EV, Jung MT, Kaebnick HW, Mitchell RA. External iliac artery-to-internal iliac artery endograft: a novel approach to preserve pelvic inflow in aortoiliac stent grafting. *J Vasc Surg.* 2002;35(1):120–124.

67. Hinchliffe RJ, Alric P, Wenham PW, Hopkinson BR. Durability of femorofemoral bypass grafting after aortouniiliac endovascular aneurysm repair. *J Vasc Surg.* 2003;38(3):498–503.

68. Ziegler P, Avgerinos ED, Umscheid T, Perdikides T, Erz K, Stelter WJ. Branched iliac bifurcation: 6 years experience with endovascular preservation of internal iliac artery flow. *J Vasc Surg.* 2007;46(2):204–210.

Chapter 12

Open Operative Therapy for Ruptured Abdominal Aortic Aneurysm

Loay S. Kabbani and Gilbert R. Upchurch, Jr.

Abstract Abdominal aortic aneurysms (AAAs) usually remain asymptomatic for many years and, if left untreated, may rupture and cause death in as many as one-third of patients. When all patients experiencing a ruptured AAA (RAAA) are taken into account, including both those who arrive at the hospital alive and those who do not, overall mortality is between 77% and 88%, with over 50% of patients expiring before reaching the hospital. Those patients who reach the hospital usually have a contained rupture, most commonly into the left retroperitoneum. This may help to confine the bleed for a period of time. Despite making it to the hospital, RAAA patients still have a high mortality rate of 41% (though values as low as 19% and as high as 90% have been noted). There is evidence that repair of RAAA by high-volume surgeons with subspecialty training sustains significant survival, arguing in favor of regionalization. Endovascular repair has emerged as a less morbid therapy for RAAA, however, the need for suitable anatomy, availability of appropriate graft sizes, and technical experience in graft deployment are needed and usually available only in specialty centers.

Keywords Operative therapy, symptoms, Open AAA repair, Endo-leaks, Misdiagnosis of AAA, CT, Hardman index, Glasgow Aneurysm Score, Risk scoring

Clinical Presentation

The classic presentation for ruptured abdominal aortic aneurysm (RAAA) is a triad of severe abdominal or back pain, hypotension, and a pulsatile mass.[1,2] Unfortunately, this traditional presentation occurs in less than half of the patients. In a study of 116 patients with RAAAs preformed at the University of Michigan, 45% were hypotensive, 72% had back and abdominal pain, and 83% had a pulsatile abdominal mass.[3] Other common symptoms include syncope (30%), emesis (22%), flank ecchymosis (6%). Some less common presentations include trauma (motor vehicle accident)[2], hiccups,[4] gross

G. Upchurch and E. Criado (eds.) *Aortic Aneurysms, Contemporary Cardiology*
DOI: 10.1007/978-1-60327-204-9_12, © Humana Press, a part of
Springer Science+Business Media, LLC 2009

hematuria,[5,6] renal colic,[7] gastrointestinal bleeding,[8] crural neuropathy,[9,10] urethral obstruction,[11] obstruction of the left colon,[12] hip pain,[13] right testicular pain,[14,15] and even groin hernias and incarcerations.[16,17]

Patients who rupture into their vena cava, iliac vein or renal vein may present in congestive heart failure with distended neck veins, an abdominal bruit, microscopic or macroscopic hematuria, or an acute left varicocele. Aortocaval fistulas occur in as many as 2–4% of patients with RAAA.[18,19]

Accordingly, an episode of abdominal pain with hypotension in an elderly patient regardless of its duration or associated symptoms should lead to a serious consideration of a RAAA. It is essential not to have a false sense of security when evaluating a hemodynamically stable patient, especially when most patients are not aware that they harbor this potentially lethal lesion.

RAAA should not be excluded in patients who have undergone previous repair of their aneurysm. Anastomotic pseudoaneurysms may occur following open AAA repair, while endoleaks following endovascular repair may lead to RAAA. Synchronous aneurysms may also occur at sites remote from the previous repair (e.g., iliac artery aneurysms or pararenal aorta).[20–22]

Symptomatic or ruptured aortic aneurysms can mimic many other acute medical conditions and therefore are part of multiple differential diagnoses. The following conditions all may be confused with RAAAs[23]: (1) perforated viscous, (2) mesenteric ischemia, (3) strangulated hernia, (4) ruptured visceral artery aneurysm, (5) acute cholecystitis, (6) acute pancreatitis, (7) ruptured appendix, (8) ruptured necrotic hepatobiliary cancer, (9) lymphoma, (10) diverticular abscess, (11) acute myocardial infarction, and (12) renal colic. In one study, nearly one in five patients with symptomatic AAAs in an emergency department was originally diagnosed as having nephroureterolithiasis.[24] Fortunately, misdiagnosis of a RAAA is rare. Most patients who do undergo an operation for abdominal pain that was thought to be a RAAA either benefit from or at least are not harmed by the operation.[25]

Differentiation between symptomatic and ruptured aneurysms is important as they have different mortality rates. Patients with symptomatic aneurysms may have symptoms of variable severity (ranging from mild tenderness to pain indistinguishable from rupture); however, no blood is identified outside the aortic wall at laparotomy. The etiology of the pain is thought to be related to acute expansion of the aortic wall, intramural hemorrhage, and bleeding into the thrombus. These patients do not have hypotension, and their prognosis is much better than the prognosis of patients with rupture, but worse than with elective repair with an operative mortality five times that of elective AAA repair.[26]

Diagnostic Studies

Plain Films

Plain films of the lumbar region, routinely obtained in patients with back pain, may show a calcified shell of the aorta. In one review of 31 patients with surgically proven RAAAs, 65% had calcification of the aneurysm that was visible on a plain abdominal radiograph.[27] Ninety percent of the films had signs of rupture, when interpreted by a skilled radiologist.

Abdominal Ultrasound

Ultrasonography is typically not be used to diagnose RAAA. For despite having nearly 100% sensitivity in detecting AAAs,[28] ultrasound is very poor at detecting rupture. In one study, ultrasonography demonstrated extraluminal blood in only 4% of RAAAs in the emergency department.[29]

Computed tomography

Computed tomography (CT) is the best imaging technique to diagnose a RAAA. Retroperitoneal blood when used to diagnose RAAA on CT scan was found to be 77% sensitive and 100% specific. The positive predictive value was 100%, and the negative predictive value was 89%.[30]

Some of the signs used to help diagnose RAAA by CT are[31]:

1. A retroperitoneal hematoma adjacent to an AAA (Fig. 1a and b).
2. The draped aorta sign. This sign is present when the posterior wall of the aorta either is not identifiable as distinct from adjacent structures or closely follows the contour of adjacent vertebral bodies.
3. A focal discontinuity in the calcifications of the circumferential wall around the aorta.
4. A well-defined peripheral crescent of increased attenuation within the thrombus of a large AAA (Fig. 2).

With the development of multidetector CT scanners and the widespread use of endografts, the initial radiographic evaluation of patients with RAAA has changed. Some vascular surgeons think that it is prudent today to consider a CT scan on patients suspected of having a RAAA especially if they are stable or even quasi stable to see if they are an endograft candidates.[32] This view is being supported by the lower morbidity and mortality reported in patients undergoing endograft therapy for RAAA.[33] However, for the unstable patient, the operating room is the safest place for the patient.

MRI/MRA

Magnetic resonance (MR) imaging requires a much longer acquisition time, and MR imaging is less available and less convenient, therefore rarely used to diagnose RAAA.

Resuscitation and Transfer

First and foremost, if there are no personnel who are qualified in the institution, urgent transfer to a center with trained individuals is required. Centralization of emergency vascular services to include RAAA repair may benefit survival.[34]

Two large-bore intravenous accesses should be established with labs sent, a minimum of six units of packed red blood cells should be cross-matched. Transfusion devices that warm and rapidly transfuse blood products are extremely useful. A Foley catheter should be placed to help determine end organ perfusion. If the patient is hemodynamically stable, a baseline electrocardiogram and chest x-ray are rapidly acquired. An arterial line can be placed if it dose not delay transfer to the operative room. With the advent of endostenting and rapid multidetector CT scanners, some advocate trying to assess the ability to place an endograft prior to heading to the operative room.

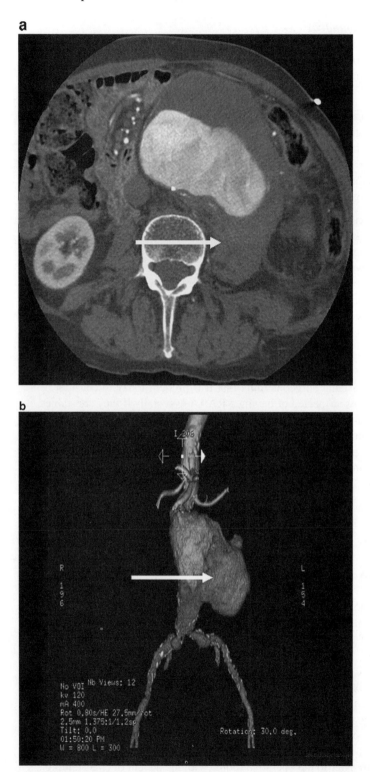

Fig. 1 (**a**) A computed tomography (*CT*) scan demonstrating a large retroperitoneal hematoma adjacent to an expanding abdominal aortic aneurysms (*AAA*). (**b**) Reformatted CT of an AAA with retroperitoneal rupture

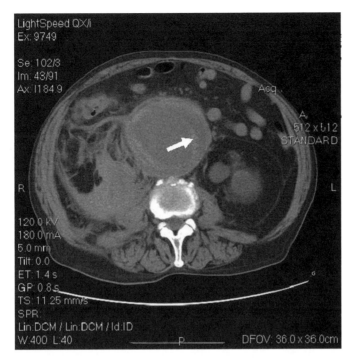

Fig. 2 Computed tomography (*CT*) image depicts a large abdominal aortic aneurysm with a hyperattenuated crescent sign, which may represent an acute hematoma or bleed within the aneurysm sac

   The optimal degree of preoperative resuscitation before operative intervention is controversial.[35,36] Crawford was the first to suggest minimal fluid resuscitation to maintain the systolic blood pressure at 50–70 mmHg.[37] Since then it has generally been accepted that attempts at complete resuscitation of the hemodynamically unstable patient before surgery are usually futile and may be detrimental. This is because normalization or even elevation of the blood pressure may lead to rupture of the temporary aortic seal. Although there are no randomized studies looking at minimal resuscitation in RAAA, the trauma literature supports this. Among patients with penetrating trauma and hypotension (systolic blood pressure < 90 mmHg), improved survival was observed in patients who received minimal fluid resuscitation therapy until they arrived in the operating room.[36] The mortality difference was small (30% with the delayed resuscitation group compared with 38% with immediate resuscitation). One must be sure that this may not apply to RAAA patients who are older and have significant cardiovascular comorbidities.

Risk Scoring

The cost of treating ruptured aneurysms is at least four times higher than elective cases and much higher for RAAA patients who have a complicated postoperative course.[38] This, along with the high morbidity and mortality, has driven physicians to attempt to devise a scoring system to identify those patients who will not benefit from attempted repair.[39] Prediction of immediate postoperative death allows for consoling the families, especially the elderly patient who may decide to forgo surgery. The last 20 years has seen more than 60 publications considering variables predictive of outcome after AAA rupture.[40]

Six predictive scoring systems are reported:

1. Hardman Index[41]

This is probably the simplest and most well-known scoring system. It was described in 1996 based on a retrospective series of 154 patients operated on for RAAA at a single institution in Australia. They looked at 67 perioperative variables and their association with 30 day mortality. Five independent variables were identified on multivariate analysis: (1) age > 76 years, (2) serum creatinine concentration of >0.19 mmol/liter (2.2 mg/dl), (3) loss of consciousness after arrival, (4) hemoglobin concentration of <9 g/dl, and (5) electrocardiographic signs of myocardial ischemia. Six studies showed a good correlation with outcome, initially reporting a mortality rate of 100% in patients with a score ≥3.[42,43] Subsequent studies did not confirm the totalitarian conclusions of this,[44–46] with a more recent study showing no correlation with outcome.[47]

2. Glasgow Aneurysm Score (GAS)[48]

This was based on a retrospective multicenter review of both ruptured and nonruptured aneurysm in 500 patients between 1980 and 1990. Multivariate analysis was preformed. The GAS was calculated after rounding the regression coefficients and accordingly a simple risk score was formulated.

Risk score = (age in years) + (17 points for shock) + (7 points for myocardial disease) + (10 points for cerebrovascular disease) + (14 points for renal disease)

The authors then evaluated this scoring system on a prospectively randomized study with similar results. Mortality was found to correlate well with GAS and a score >95 was related to a mortality of >80%, but not 100%. A more recent study found contradictory results with a mortality rate <50% for those patients with a score >110.[46]

3. Physiological and Operative Severity Score for Enumeration of Mortality and Morbidity (POSSUM)[49]

The POSSUM was primarily developed for auditing results, but has since been used to examine mortality rates. It uses 12 physiological variables and 6 operative variables to give a calculated risk of morbidity and mortality.[50] The validated modification of the POSSUM scoring system (V-POSSUM)[51] and the RAAA POSSUM (RAAA-POSSUM)[52] were developed by the Vascular Surgical Society of Great Britain and Ireland specifically for vascular patients and RAAA. The POSSUM and V-POSSUM have not shown good correlation with RAAA outcome,[53,44] and the RAAA-POSSUM has not been validated in any prospective studies.

4. Vancouver Scoring System (VSS)[54]

The VSS (also known as the Chen index) identified age, reduced conscious level, and preoperative cardiac arrest as significant predictors of death using multivariate analysis of a retrospective group of 147 RAAA. A predictive model was then created.

$$\text{mortality risk} = \frac{e^x}{1+e^x}$$

Where e is the base of the natural logarithm (≈ 2.71828) and $x =$ constant + sum of coefficients for all significant variables.

$X =$ [constant $= (-3.44)$] + [conscious (-1.14), or unconsciousness (1.14)] + [age $\times 0.062$] + [cardiac arrest (0.60) or no cardiac arrest (-0.60)].

It was then validated in a prospective series of 134 patients.[55] Like the other scoring systems, it was unable to predict a mortality of 100%.

5. Canadian Society for Vascular Surgery Aneurysm Study Group[56]

This study identified individual variables that were predictors of early survival, including preinduction blood pressure, creatinine, intraoperative urine output, site of cross-clamp (infrarenal vs. suprarenal), duration of cross-clamp, and postoperative occurrence of a myocardial infarction, respiratory failure, kidney damage, and coagulopathy. Since it takes into account preoperative, intraoperative, and postoperative variables, only at the conclusion of the case can one give a reasonable prognostic estimate.

6. Multiple Organ Dysfunction Score (MODS)[57]

Six key organ systems (respiratory, renal, hepatic, hematologic, neurologic, and cardiac) were looked at over time to determine the relationship between progressive organ dysfunction and mortality. The renal and hepatic components of the MODS were responsible for the progressive increase in MODS and were significantly higher in patients who died after 48 h compared with survivors. Renal dysfunction became significantly different between survivors and nonsurvivors on postoperative day 3, whereas it took until postoperative day 10 for the hepatic dysfunction scores to become significantly different. The conclusion of this study was that development of renal dysfunction followed by hepatic dysfunction indicates patients who are at the highest mortality risk.

In conclusion, no scoring system has been shown to have consistent or absolute validity,[40] in essence invalidating all scoring systems. In addition, surgical repair of RAAA appears to be cost-effective in comparison with no intervention.[58] Therefore, we maintain that only in the direst of situations (e.g., severe Alzheimer's, widely metastatic cancer, patient desires, etc.) should operative repair be denied.

Operative Strategy

The crucial element in the repair of a RAAA is safe, rapid, and effective proximal aortic control, as surgical repair is still the standard treatment for RAAA. However, as noted above, endovascular repair is being increasingly reported, and small studies suggest a lower morbidity and mortality rate.[59] The lack of experienced personnel, equipment, and a stock of endografts available to attempt RAAA repair do not allow this to be an option at smaller centers.

In the operating room while the patient is being prepped, broad-spectrum antibiotics are administered, the arterial line is placed along with a central venous catheter. The use of the cell saver is controversial,[60] and is surgeon-dependent. However, these procedures should not delay the operation as it is imperative that the bleeding is stopped. The patient is prepped and draped before anesthesia is induced with agents designed to have minimal effect on blood pressure. This practice allows the operation to be started immediately after induction. Hypotension after induction should be anticipated due to loss of sympathetic drive. One should be ready to gain rapid control of the aorta if this should happen. Some have suggested that in moribund patients experiencing severe shock, the surgeon should start even before the induction of anesthesia.

Proximal Control

The first goal of this operation is cessation of hemorrhage. Most surgeons prefer a transperitoneal, midline incision because it affords wide exposure to the abdominal aorta and allows rapid supraceliac control if necessary. This is accomplished initially by manual compression. The supraceliac aorta is exposed at the diaphragm by retracting the left lobe of the liver to the right, opening the gastrohepatic omentum and retracting the esophagus and stomach which are identified by the nasogastric tube to the left. The aorta is identified between the crura of the diaphragm which are divided with electrocautery. After isolating the aorta, the clamp is guided over the surgeon's index and middle fingers and placed on either side of the aorta.

Supraceliac aortic control is beneficial in cases of severe hypotension or uncontrolled bleeding. It also helps avoid renal and gonadal vein injury often associated with blind dissection in a hematoma to identify the infrarenal aortic neck. Supraceliac aortic clamping, however, incurs ischemia time to the viscera and along with it complications, notably postoperative bleeding and multisystem organ failure. Therefore, supraceliac aortic clamping is usually temporary, until the periduodenal aorta is dissected out to see if there is adequate room for infrarenal aortic clamping.

Other options for rapid proximal aortic control include[61]:

1. Aortic compression over the supraceliac aorta against the lumbar spine if rapid control is required before exposure can be obtained.
2. Direct placement of an aortic balloon (or Foley catheter) through the aneurysm sac. If this approach is used, try to thread the graft through the balloon before deployment. This maneuver facilitates the proximal aortic anastomosis.
3. Brachial or femoral artery puncture or cut down to insert an occlusion balloon into the visceral aorta using fluoroscopic guidance.
4. Thoracotomy with descending aortic clamping. There is some data to support worse outcomes for this approach when compared to transhiatal control.[62]

Caution needs to be used with these methods, as the aortic thrombus can be disrupted leading to embolization. Aortic balloons are associated with malpositioning or movement as the aneurysm sac is opened.[63] Recognize that aortic compression and balloon techniques are blind and may not provide complete control.

In the more stable patient, dissecting out the infrarenal aorta may reward you with a suitable neck where you can avoid a supraceliac aortic clamp. This is our first choice, however, if the patient becomes unstable, if there is a large hematoma around the renal arteries, or if we encounter significant bleeding, the supraceliac aorta is promptly clamped. Here, care must be taken to avoid injury to the left renal vein, the lumbar veins, and the IVC. The left renal vein can be ligated and divided, granted you need to preserve the venous collaterals to the left kidney, which include the left adrenal vein, the left gonadal vein, and the lumbar vein.

If a suprarenal AAA is approached anteriorly, medial visceral rotation is required to expose the suprarenal aorta. In this technique, the left colon is mobilized by incising the lateral peritoneal attachments. The colon, pancreas, spleen, and kidney are elevated, allowing access to the diaphragmatic crura, which cover the aorta at this level. Division of the crura allows access to the entire intra-abdominal aorta as well as the visceral and renal vessels.

Some surgeons prefer a retroperitoneal approach interring through the tenth intercoastal space. In one retrospective analysis,[64] the retroperitoneal approach was associated with less intraoperative hypotension and a lower mortality than the transperitoneal approach, although some patients with unusual features were excluded. This approach may be preferred if preformed routinely, in the stable patients with suprarenal aneurysms or in the hostile abdomen. This is not the ideal approach if you are concerned about other intra-abdominal pathology.[65]

After obtaining proximal aortic control, allow the anesthesiolologiol to fully resuscitate the patient and transfuse to an adequate blood pressure. This is important because after opening up the aorta, there is additional blood loss form the lumbar arteries.

Many surgeons avoid systemic heparinization because of bleeding complications, although heparinized saline can be given directly into the iliac arteries to try to reduce distal thrombosis. Some authors maintain that heparinization may be beneficial in decreasing the incidence of DIC and maintaining microcirculatory perfusion in patients with RAAA.[66]

Distal Control

This can be achieved with clamps on the iliac arteries or occasionally the distal aorta. Occlusion balloons can also be placed in the iliac arteries in a retrogude fashion after opening the aneurysm sac if there is a large hematoma and dissection is hazardous. Some surgeons open the aneurysm and get distal control by packing the iliac artery orifices under retractors.[67] Iliac aneurysms are left alone if they are not too large (<3–4 cm), as this ensures a rapid operation.

Operation

After eviscerating the small bowel and carefully mobilizing the duodenum from the aorta, the aneurysm is opened. The lumbar arteries and inferior mesenteric artery are suture ligated from inside the aneurysm. A Dacron or PTFE graft (usually 16–22 mm in diameter) is used and anastomosed proximally with a 3–0 permanent monofilament suture. A strip of telfa may be incorporated into the anastomosis in degenerative aortas on the aortic side as a continuous pledget.

Blood volume should have been restored by this time, and adequate fresh frozen plasma and platelets should be available. The anastomosis is tested with retrograde heparin flush prior to removing the clamp. Reperfusing the visceral and renal vessels may result in significant hypotension and requires careful coordination with anesthesia to ensure that the proper fluids are administered and that a presser agent and bicarbonate are prepared for use if required. If there are no significant leaks, the clamp is placed on the infrarenal aorta (or graft), packed, and attention turned to the distal anastomosis. A tube graft will suffice in 80–90% of the patients. If the repair involves the iliac arteries, an aortobi-iliac graft is used to maintain flow to at least one hypogastric artery to insure perfusion to the pelvis. Rarely is an aortobifemoral bypass required for RAAA.

If discovered intraoperatively, treatment of an aortocaval fistula is done after opening the aorta and placing pressure via sponge sticks on the cava distally and proximally. The vena cava is repaired by suturing the fistula from within the aneurysm. Care is taken to avoid air, thrombus, or other debris from entering the vena cava while repairing it.

The aneurysm sac is closed over the prosthesis, isolating it from the bowel. No attempt is made to decompress the retroperitoneal hematoma. The abdomen is closed with a heavy monofilament.

Hypothermia is associated with an increased incidence of surgical bleeding, wound infection, and an increased incidence of morbid cardiac events.[68] Prevention of hypothermia can reduce cardiac events in elective noncardiac surgery. Although this has not been specifically studied in RAAA, we advocate the prevention of hypothermia by the use of warmed anesthetic gases, warming of all intravenous fluids, and use of forced air warming devices.

Abdominal Closure After RAAA

In 25–30% of patients, the abdomen cannot be closed without significant tension secondary to swollen bowel or massive retroperitoneal hematoma or both and abdominal compartment syndrome (ACS) results if attempted.[69] This can be directly measured by obtaining a bladder pressure when the bladder volume is 50–100 ml. A bladder pressure of >25 is diagnostic of ACS. VAC closure for 3–5 days until the bowel edema and retroperitoneal blood decreases is prudent. A silastic bag closure or even closure with Mesh has been described. Secondary closer may take up to 28 days after aortic reconstruction.[70]

Postoperative Management

These patients need aggressive resuscitation and may have a very tumultuous postoperative course. There is at least a twofold increase in complications and a tenfold increase in mortality after RAAA. The overall cost of treating RAAA is 1.5–4 times that of elective AAA repair.[71] The early survival of patients after RAAA repair often has been quoted at 50%, with a range of 19–70%.[3,72]

Late Survival

In the Canadian aneurysm study, the 5-year survival for patients alive at 30 days was 53% compared with 71% of patients who had undergone elective repair.[56] In the VA system, the 5-year survival was 54% for RAAA patients compared with 69% for the elective group.[73] Importantly, there was a very good quality of life and good functional outcome of the survivors of RAAA, especially the younger patients.[74,75]

Conclusion

Operative repair of RAAA carries a high morbidity and mortality. Future improvements will depend on prevention with early diagnosis and elective AAA repair, improvements in endovascular repair, and strategies to prevent postoperative organ injury after prolonged states of malperfusion.

References

1. Khaw H, Sottiurai VS, Craighead CC, Batson RC. Ruptured abdominal aortic aneurysm presenting as symptomatic inguinal mass: Report of six cases. J Vasc Surg 1986: 4, 384–9.
2. Marston WA, Ahlquist R, Johnson G Jr., Meyer AA. Misdiagnosis of ruptured abdominal aortic aneurysms. J Vasc Surg 1992: 16, 17–22.
3. Wakefield TW, Whitehouse WM Jr, Wu SC, et al. Abdominal aortic aneurysm rupture: Statistical analysis of factors affecting outcome of surgical treatment. Surgery 1982: 91, 586–96.
4. Stine RJ, Trued SJ. Hiccups: An unusual manifestation of an abdominal aortic aneurysm. JACEP 1979: 8, 368–70.
5. Georgopoulos SE, Arvanitis DP, Tekerlekis P, et al. Rupture of an aortic anastomotic aneurysm into a ureter. Urol Int 2003: 71, 333–5.
6. Fetting JH, Eagan JW Jr., Hutchins GM. Hematuria due to an abdominal aortic aneurysm leaking into a urethral stump. Johns Hopkins Med J 1973: 133, 339–42.
7. Eckford SD, Gillatt DA. Abdominal aortic aneurysms presenting as renal colic. Br J Urol 1992: 70, 496–8.
8. Keripe S, Slavik S, Oshidi T. Primary aortoappendicular fistula arising from an infected, chronic, contained, ruptured abdominal aortic aneurysm. Ann Vasc Surg 2006: 20, 820–4.
9. Defraigne JO, Sakalihasan N, Lavigne JP. Chronic rupture of abdominal aortic aneurysm manifesting as crural neuropathy. Ann Vasc Surg 15: 2001, 405–11.
10. Fletcher HS, Frankel J. Ruptured abdominal aneurysms presenting with unilateral peripheral neuropathy. Surgery 1976: 79, 120–1.
11. Tejada E, Becker GJ, Waller BF. Two unusual manifestations of aortic aneurysms. Clin Cardiol 1990: 13, 132–5.
12. Politoske EJ. Ruptured abdominal aortic aneurysm presenting as an obstruction of the left colon. Am J Gastroenterol 1990: 85, 745–7.
13. Smith D, Campbell SM. Unruptured abdominal aortic aneurysm mimicking hip joint disease. J Rheumatol 1987: 14, 172–3.
14. Sufi PA. A rare case of leaking abdominal aneurysm presenting as isolated right testicular pain. CJEM 2007: 9, 124–6.
15. O'Keefe KP, Skiendzielewski JJ. Abdominal aortic aneurysm rupture presenting as testicular pain. Ann Emerg Med 1989: 18, 1096–8.
16. Abulafi AM, Mee WM, Pardy BJ. Leaking abdominal aortic aneurysm as an inguinal mass. Eur J Vasc Surg 1991: 5, 95–6.
17. Grabowski EW, Pilcher DG. Ruptured abdominal aortic aneurysm manifesting as symptomatic inguinal hernia. Am Surg 1981: 7, 11–12.
18. Duong C, Atkinson N. Review of aortoiliac aneurysms with spontaneous large vein fistula. Aust N Z J Surg 2001: 71, 52–5.

19. Woolley DS, Spence RK. Aortocaval fistula treated by aortic exclusion. J Vasc Surg 1995: 22, 639–42.

20. Hallett JW Jr, Marshall DM, Petterson TM, et al. Graft-related complications after abdominal aortic aneurysm repair: Reassurance from a 36-year population-based experience. J Vasc Surg 1997: 25, 77–86.

21. Brunkwall J, Hauksson H, Bengtsson H, et al. Solitary aneurysms of the iliac arterial system: An estimate of their frequency of occurrence. J Vasc Surg 1989: 10, 381–4.

22. Bernhard VM, Mitchell RS, Matsumura JS, et al. Ruptured abdominal aortic aneurysm endovascular repair. J Vasc Surg 2002: 35, 155–62.

23. Schaub TA, Upchurch GR, Jr. Pulsatile Abdominal Mass. In: Souba W (ed.), ACS Surgery. 5th Edition, New York, Web MD, Inc., pp. 778–93, 2005.

24. Borrero E, Queral LA. Symptomatic abdominal aortic aneurysms misdiagnosed as nephroureterolithiasis. Ann Vasc Surg 1988: 2, 145–9.

25. Valentine RJ, Barth MJ, Myers SI, et al. Nonvascular emergencies presenting as ruptured abdominal aortic aneurysms. Surgery 1993: 113, 86–9.

26. Sullivan CA, Rohrer MJ, Cutler BS. Clinical management of the symptomatic but unruptured abdominal aortic aneurysm. Surgery 1990: 11, 799–803.

27. Loughran CF. A review of the plain abdominal radiograph in acute rupture of abdominal aortic aneurysms. Clin Radiol 1986: 37, 383–7.

28. LaRoy LL, Cormier PJ, Matalon TA, et al. Imaging of abdominal aortic aneurysms. AJR Am J Roentgenol 1989: 152, 785–92.

29. Shuman WP. Suspected leaking abdominal aortic aneurysm: Use of sonography in the emergency room. Radiology 1988: 168, 117–9.

30. Weinbaum FI, Dubner S, Turner JW, Pardes JG. The accuracy of computed tomography in the diagnosis of retroperitoneal blood in the presence of abdominal aortic aneurysm. J Vasc Surg 1987: 6, 11–16.

31. Ratika D, Newatia A, Hines JJ, Spectrum of CT findings in rupture and impending rupture of abdominal aortic aneurysms. Radiographics 2007: 27, 497–507.

32. Lloyd GM, Bown MJ, Norwood MGA, et al. Feasibility of preoperative computer tomography in patients with ruptured abdominal aortic aneurysm: A time-to-death study in patients without operation. J Vasc Surg 2004: 39, 788–91.

33. Reichart M, Geelkerken RH, Huisman AB, et al. Ruptured abdominal aortic aneurysm: Endovascular repair is feasible in 40% of patients. Eur J Vasc Endovasc Surg, 2003: 26, 479–86.

34. Laukontaus SJ , Aho P, Pettilä V et al. Decrease of Mortality of Ruptured Abdominal Aortic Aneurysm after Centralization and In-Hospital Quality Improvement of Vascular Service. Ann Vasc Surg 2007: 21, 580–8.

35. Holmes JF, Sakles JC, Lewis G, Wisner DH. Effects of delaying fluid resuscitation on an injury to the systemic arterial vasculature. Acad Emerg Med 2002: 9, 267–74.

36. Bickell WH, Wall MJ Jr, Pepe PE, et al. Immediate versus delayed fluid resuscitation for hypotensive patients with penetrating torso injuries. N Engl J Med 1994: 331, 1105–9.

37. Crawford ES. Ruptured abdominal aortic aneurysm [editorial]. J Vasc Surg 1991: 13, 348–50.

38. Tang T, Lindop M, Munday I, et al. A cost analysis of surgery for ruptured abdominal aortic aneurysm. Eur J Vasc Endovasc Surg 2003: 26, 299–302.

39. Johansen K, Kohler TR, Nicholls SC, et al. Ruptured AAA: The Harborview experience. J Vasc Surg 1991: 13, 240–7.

40. Tambyraja AL, Murie JA, Chalmers RTA. Prediction of outcome after abdominal aortic aneurysm rupture. J Vasc Surg 2008: 47, 222–30.

41. Hardman DTA, Fisher CM, Patel MI, et al. Ruptured abdominal aortic aneurysms who should be offered surgery? J Vasc Surg 1996: 23, 123–9.

42. Boyle JR, Gibbs PJ, King D. et al. Predicting outcome in ruptured abdominal aortic aneurysms prospective study of 100 consecutive cases. Eur J Vasc Endovasc Surg 2003: 26, 607–11.

43. Prance SE, Wilson YG, Cosgrove CM, et al. Ruptured abdominal aortic aneurysms selecting patients for surgery. Eur J Vasc Endovasc Surg 1999: 17, 129–32.

44. Neary WD, Crow P, Foy C, Prytherch D. et al. Comparison of Possum scoring and the Hardman Index in selection of patients for repair of ruptured abdominal aortic aneurysm. Br. J Surg 2003: 90, 421–5.

45. Calderwood R, Halka T, Haji-Micheal P, et al. Ruptured abdominal aortic aneurysm. Is it possible to predict outcome? Int Angiol 2004: 23, 47–53.

46. Tambyraja AL, Fraser SC, Murie JA, et al. Validity of the Glasgow Aneurysm Score and Hardman Index in predicting outcome after ruptured abdominal aortic aneurysm repair. Br J Surg 2005: 92, 570.

47. Sharif MA, Arya N, Soong CV, et al. Validity of the hardman index to predict outcome in ruptured abdominal aortic aneurysm. Ann Vasc Surg 2007: 21, 34–8.

48. Samy AK, Murray G, MacBain G. Glasgow aneurysm score. Cardiovasc Surg 1994: 2, 41–4.

49. Copland GP, Jones D, Walters M. POSSUM: A scoring system for surgical audit. Br. J Surg 1991: 78, 356–60.

50. Harris JR, Forbes TL, Steiner SH, et al. Risk-adjusted analysis of early mortality after ruptured abdominal aortic aneurysm repair. J Vasc Surg 2005: 42, 387–91.

51. Prytherch DR, Ridler BM, Beard JD, et al. On behalf of the Audit and Research Committee of the Vascular Surgical Society of Great Britain and Ireland. A model for national outcome audit in vascular surgery. Eur J Vasc Endovasc Surg 2001: 21, 477–83.

52. Prytherch DR, Sutton GL, Boyle JR. Portsmouth POSSUM models for ruptured aortic aneurysm surgery. Br. J Surg 2001: 88, 958–63.

53. Lazarides MK, Arvanitis DP, Drista H, et al. POSSUM and APACHE II scores do not predict the outcome of ruptured infrarenal aortic aneurysms. Ann Vasc Surg 1997: 11, 155–8.

54. Chen JC, Hildebrand HD, Salvian AJ, et al. Predictors of death in nonruptured and ruptured abdominal aortic aneurysms. J Vasc Surg 1996: 24, 614–23.

55. Hsiang YN, Tumbull RG, Nicholls SC, et al. Predicting death from ruptured abdominal aortic aneurysms. Am J Surg 2001: 181, 30–5.

56. Johnston KW: Ruptured abdominal aortic aneurysm: Six-year follow-up results of a multicenter prospective study. Canadian Society for Vascular Surgery Aneurysm Study Group. J Vasc Surg 1994: 19, 888–900.

57. Maziak DE, Lindsay TF, Marshall JC, Walker PM. The impact of multiple organ dysfunction on mortality following ruptured abdominal aortic aneurysm repair. Ann Vasc Surg 1998: 12, 93–100.

58. Patel ST, Korn P, Haser PB, et al. The cost-effectiveness of repairing ruptured abdominal aortic aneurysms. J Vasc Surg 2000: 32, 247–57.

59. Coppi G, Silingardi R, Gennai S, et al. A single-center experience in open and endovascular treatment of hemodynamically unstable and stable patients with ruptured abdominal aortic aneurysms. J Vasc Surg 2006: 44, 1140–7.

60. Posacio H, Apaydin A Z, Islamo F, et al. Adverse effects of cell saver in patients undergoing ruptured abdominal aortic aneurysm repair. Ann Vasc Surg 2002: 16, 450–5.

61. Arthurs Z, Sohn V, Starnes B. Ruptured abdominal aortic aneurysms: Remote aortic occlusion for the general surgeon. Surg Clin N Am 2007: 87, 1035–45.

62. Islamoglu F, Apayd n AZ, Posacoglu H, et al. Effects of thoracic and hiatal clamping in repair of ruptured abdominal aortic aneurysms. Ann Vasc Surg 2007: 21, 423–32.

63. Ohki T, Veith FJ. Endovascular grafts and other image-guided catheter-based adjuncts to improve the treatment of ruptured aortoiliac aneurysms. Ann Surg 2000: 232, 466–79.

64. Chang BB, Shah DM, Paty PS, et al. Can the retroperitoneal approach be used for ruptured abdominal aortic aneurysms? J Vasc Surg 1990: 11, 326–30.

65. Nguyen AT, de Virgilio C. Transperitoneal approach should be considered for suspected ruptured abdominal aortic aneurysms. Ann Vasc Surg 2007: 21, 129–32.
66. Mulcare RJ, Royster TS, Weiss HJ, et al. Disseminated intravascular coagulation as a complication of abdominal aortic aneurysm repair. Ann Surg 1974: 18, 343–9.
67. Ernst C. Ruptured aortic aneurysm repair. In: Ernst C and Stanley JC (eds.), Current Therapy in Vascular Surgery (4th Edition). St. Louis: Mosby, pp. 233–235, 2000.
68. Frank SM, Fleisher LA, Breslow MJ, et al. Perioperative maintenance of normothermia reduces the incidence of morbid cardiac events: A randomized clinical trial. JAMA. 1997: 277, 1127–34.
69. Lindsay TF. Ruptured Abdominal Aortic Aneurysms. In Rutherford RB (ed.), Vascular Surgery, 6th Edition, Elsevier Saunders, Philadelphia, PA, pp. 1476–90, 2005.
70. Oelschlager BK, Boyle EM Jr., Johansen K, et al. Delayed abdominal closure in the management of ruptured abdominal aortic aneurysms. Am J Surg 1997: 172, 411–415.
71. Chew HF, You CK, Brown MG, et al. Mortality, morbidity, and costs of ruptured and elective abdominal aortic aneurysm repairs in Nova Scotia, Canada. Ann Vasc Surg, 2003: 17, 171–9.
72. Dardik A, Burleyson GP, Bowman H, et al. Surgical repair of ruptured abdominal aortic aneurysms in the state of Maryland: Factors influencing outcome among 527 recent cases. J Vasc Surg 1998: 28, 413–20.
73. Kazmers A, Perkins AJ, Jacobs LA. Aneurysm rupture is independently associated with increased late mortality in those surviving abdominal aortic aneurysm repair. J Surg Res 2001: 95, 50–3.
74. Laukontaus SJ, Pettila V, Kantonen I, et al. Utility of surgery for ruptured abdominal aortic aneurysm. Ann Vasc Surg 2006: 20, 42–8.
75. Tambyraja AL, Fraser SCA, Murie JA. Functional outcome after open repair of ruptured abdominal aortic aneurysm. J Vasc Surg 2005: 41, 758–61.

Chapter 13

Endovascular Repair of Ruptured Abdominal Aortic Aneurysm

Paul J. Riesenman and Mark A. Farber

Abstract Ruptured abdominal aortic aneurysm (rAAA) is a highly lethal condition with an overall mortality rate of approximately 90%. Patients who survive to present to the hospital require an intervention to reestablish aortic integrity, otherwise hospital mortality is certain. Traditional open surgery, with placement of an interposition graft under general anesthesia, is a durable form of repair. Despite advancements in surgical technique and post-operative critical care, the mortality associated with this form of treatment in the setting of rAAA remains high.

Endovascular aneurysm repair (EVAR) has emerged as an alternative to open surgery for the elective treatment of AAAs with short- and long-term advantages in aneurysm-related mortality. This form of therapy is more commonly being applied to the treatment of rAAAs. The application of EVAR to rAAAs has several inherent advantages over open surgical reconstruction, which may translate into improved patient outcomes. Several challenges inherent to EVAR must be addressed in order to successfully apply this form of treatment to rAAAs in the acute setting. Early reported outcomes of utilizing EVAR for rAAAs have demonstrated the technical feasibility of this approach, and several studies have suggested a mortality advantage over conventional open surgery.

Keywords Operative mortality RAAA, EVAR candidacy, Aortic occlusion, Endoleak follow RAAA, Vascular anatomy and RAAA

Endovascular Aneurysm Repair of Ruptured Abdominal Aortic Aneurysms

The relatively recent application of endovascular aneurysm repair (EVAR) to ruptured abdominal aortic aneurysms (rAAAs) has partially been driven by persistently poor outcomes associated open repair since the development of operative reconstruction in the 1950s.[1,2] A meta-analysis of open repair of rAAAs over the last 50 years by Brown et al. demonstrated a reduction in operative mortality of only 3.5% per decade, with an estimated mortality rate of 41% for the year 2000.[2] In a review of 6223 patients from the National

G. Upchurch and E. Criado (eds.) *Aortic Aneurysms, Contemporary Cardiology*
DOI: 10.1007/978-1-60327-204-9_13, © Humana Press, a part of
Springer Science+Business Media, LLC 2009

Hospital Discharge Survey database between 1985 and 1994, an operative mortality rate of 68% was reported.[3] Recent single institution series have demonstrated comparable outcomes with reported 30-day or operative mortality rates of 33–54%.[4-7]

Much of the operative mortality associated with open surgery may be attributed to the additional physiological insult the patient sustains from the operative intervention. Open surgical repair necessitates operative exposure through a transabdominal or retroperitoneal approach. Either approach necessitates the use of general anesthesia which impairs sympathetic tone, potentially precipitating hemodynamic collapse in these often hypotensive and hypovolemic patients. Similarly, sudden decompression of intra-abdominal pressure following opening of the abdomen may also result in an acute drop in blood pressure. Dissection in the retroperitoneum may potentially precipitate free rupture of the contained hematoma. Operative exposure potentiates hypothermia and blood loss, both of which may contribute to coagulopathy. Cross clamping of the aorta interrupts outflow to the pelvis and lower extremities, and places significant stress on the heart especially in patients who are hemodynamically unstable, or have preexisting cardiac disease. Additionally, clamping and unclamping may also subject the patient to ischemia reperfusion injuries, as well as potentiating the fibrinolytic state.

The application of EVAR to rAAAs largely avoids the aforementioned physiological stress associated with open surgery. Remote access to the aorta through the femoral vessels is largely a minimally invasive procedure which can often be performed without the need for a general anesthetic. Adequate availability of personal and institutional resources are necessary to successfully provide this form of treatment. Additionally, the patient's candidacy for EVAR must be evaluated with sufficient imaging studies in a limited amount of time.

Preoperative Evaluation and Management

Patients who survive to present to the hospital with rAAAs usually have contained ruptures with slow bleeds into the retroperitoneum, or arrested hemorrhage secondary to tamponade from the periaortic tissues. These patients require hemodynamic management to minimize propagation of the retroperitoneal hematoma, and risk of free rupture. Control of blood pressure through limited fluid resuscitation and intravenous antihypertensives should be utilized to maintain the systolic blood pressure at approximately 100 mmHg during evaluation and transfer to the operating room. For patients who present hypotensive, a systolic blood pressure as low as 80 mmHg may be tolerated without intervention. The patient's mental status can be utilized as a clinical assessment of end organ perfusion and guide for resuscitation in this setting. Appropriate hemodynamic management will often allow time for a dedicated computed tomographic (CT) arteriogram of the abdomen and pelvis to be obtained. CT evaluation will allow for rapid confirmation of the diagnosis, define the extent of aneurysm involvement, provide detailed vascular anatomic information, and may potentially define other etiologies for the patient's symptoms when the diagnosis is uncertain. When a patient's renal function is prohibitive to intravenous contrast administration, a CT without IV contrast can be obtained and will still yield valuable information about the vascular anatomy such as the proximal aortic neck length and external diameter. If the patient's condition precludes obtaining cross-sectional imaging studies, anatomic information to evaluate for EVAR candidacy may still be performed in the operating room through an aortogram and/or intravascular ultrasound.

Although profound hypotension and/or an expanding abdomen are clear indications to forgo CT evaluation and proceed emergently to the operating room, concern has been raised about the risk of delaying intervention in order to obtain preoperative imaging in stable patients. In a review of 56 patients who did not undergo intervention following admission to the hospital for rAAA by Lloyd et al., the majority of patients (87.5%) survived longer than 2 hours after admission.[8] Additionally, in a series of patients who underwent open rAAA repair reported by Boyle et al., operative mortality was not affected by the length of delay to surgery, or by obtaining a preoperative CT scan.[4] These reports would suggest that in institutions with readily available access to modern spiral CT scans, there is enough time for data acquisition, multiplanar reconstruction, and evaluation of EVAR candidacy in the majority of these patients.

Anatomic Canadacy for EVAR

The appropriate application of specific endovascular components is defined by the device-specific manufacture's instructions for use. Currently available Food and Drug Administration (FDA)-approved devices allow for the off-label treatment of rAAAs with a proximal aortic neck length of ≥10 mm, neck diameter of ≤32 mm, neck angulation ≤60°, iliac artery diameter ≤22 mm, and access vessels of adequate diameter to accommodate the delivery sheaths to be utilized based on these anatomic guidelines. Expanding the anatomic criteria beyond these guidelines allows for the treatment of a greater number of patients, but may compromise technical success and long-term durability. Anatomic EVAR eligibility for patients who present with rAAAs are often dependent upon institutional criteria, and reported rates vary between 34% and 100%.[9] The majority of patients who are excluded as candidates for EVAR most commonly have contraindications based upon aortic neck morphology (length, angulation, and/or diameter).[10–12]

The anatomic parameters for EVAR candidacy will also be dependent on the institutional availability of abdominal aortic endograft components. Maintaining a wide range of components in stock will prevent device availability from being a limiting factor. In a retrospective review of CT scans performed on patients who underwent emergent or elective EVAR by Lee et al., patients emergently treated for rAAAs or symptomatic nonruptured AAAs had significantly larger mean proximal aortic necks diameters,[11] suggesting that in order to treat this patient population, larger components must be readily available. Institutions with a substantial annual volume in treating elective AAAs with a variety of devices are best suited for maintaining adequate endograft stocks for emergent EVAR.

The majority of US FDA-approved abdominal aortic endografts are in a bifurcated modular configuration. Utilization of these devices adds minimal additional procedure time both with contralateral groin exposure and endograft limb placement. Additionally, aneurysm exclusion is not obtained until placement of the contralateral limb following deployment of the main body, and this may allow for persistent perfusion of the aneurysm sac and bleeding through the aortic defect. The utilization of aortouniiliac configured endografts have been advocated due to the ability to rapidly exclude the aneurysm from aortic blood flow.[13] Additionally this configuration expands candidacy to patients with contralateral access vessel stenosis, occlusion, or tortuosity. However, it must also be recognized that by employing advanced endovascular techniques, bifurcated devices can be converted to an aortouniiliac configuration. The application of aortouniiliac devices necessitates the placement of a femoral–femoral bypass graft and an iliac occlusion device.

Technical Considerations

The choice of anesthetic is the first consideration upon proceeding to the operative intervention. Local anesthesia can be rapidly administered, and maintains abdominal wall and sympathetic tone, which may be lost with the induction of general anesthesia. The use of a local anesthetic as primary anesthesia management can often be maintained throughout the entire procedure without the need to convert to general anesthesia.[14,15] Reasons for conversion to general anesthetic include loss of consciousness, hemodynamic deterioration, respiratory distress, and patient discomfort. Patient discomfort and the inability to remain motionless during the procedure may contribute to movement artifact and maldeployment of the endograft.[15] Additionally, conversion to general anesthesia may be necessary when aortouniiliac devices are utilized due to the ischemic rest pain, which may develop following endograft deployment, and preceding completion of the femoral–femoral bypass graft,[16,17] although this is rarely necessary in our experience.

The use of endovascular occlusive aortic balloons has been commonly described as a way to rapidly obtain proximal control of hemorrhage in hemodynamically unstable patients with rAAAs.[14,18,19] Placement of an aortic occlusive balloon may be performed through a transbrachial or transfemoral approach under local anesthesia. Additionally, prepositioning of an occlusive balloon may be a useful adjunctive procedure in patients who will undergo conversion from local to general anesthesia due to the anticipated acute drop in blood pressure following induction. When supraceliac aortic occlusion is performed, care should be taken to minimize the ischemic time to the renal and mesenteric vessels. Several different techniques have been described that either minimize or avoid loss of proximal hemodynamic control by coordinating aortic occlusion and endograft deployment.[14,19] We utilize occlusive balloons from a transfemoral approach delivered through a 16 French sheath. By lodging the balloon against the top of the sheath, additional structural support is provided to resist dislodgement with restoration of the patient's blood pressure. The utility of aortic occlusive balloons has been questioned by some authors who advocate rapidly obtaining definitive hemorrhage control through endograft deployment over performing this additional adjunctive procedure.[15,17,20,21] Aortic balloon occlusion does add time to the intervention, and it appears to facilitate stabilization in hemodynamically unstable patients unresponsive to other resuscitative efforts. In our experience, aortic occlusive balloons have been necessary in approximately one-third of patients who underwent EVAR for rAAA.

Complications

Despite the minimally invasive approach of EVAR, patients treated for rAAAs may experience many complications during their recovery secondary to the physiological insults sustained during the rupture. Systemic complications have been reported to occur in 28% of patients following EVAR in this setting.[22] Preexisting comorbidities in this patient population makes them particularly susceptible to developing these complications. Additionally, the treating physician should be aware of some specific complications associated with EVAR of rAAAs.

Postoperative renal complications are a recognized complication of emergent EVAR.[15,18,23] Patients presenting with rAAAs may have baseline renal insufficiency and a depleted intravascular volume. Additionally, renal perfusion pressure may be impaired by elevated intra-abdominal pressures from the retroperitoneal hematoma. These patients are also exposed to significant volumes of iodinated contrast both during CT evaluation and intraprocedurally (Fig. 1). Furthermore, the complex vascular anatomy encountered in these patients may require larger volumes of contrast than is typically required during an elective endovascular procedure. All of these factors may contribute to an increased risk of contrast-induced nephropathy and subsequent renal failure, although no data exists to support this observation.

Abdominal compartment syndrome can occurs in patients following open surgery or EVAR for rAAAs. This complication has been observed in up to 18% of patients following EVAR for rAAAs,[13,18,21,24–27] and has been associated with a higher hospital mortality.[28] The etiology of this condition is largely a result of the retroperitoneal hematoma that develops following aortic rupture. Unlike with open surgery, EVAR does not afford the opportunity to evacuate the retroperitoneal hematoma during the primary procedure. At the conclusion of the endovascular intervention, patients with obvious signs of abdominal compartment syndrome, such as a tense distended abdominal wall and elevated airway pressures, should undergo immediate surgical decompression (Fig. 2). Despite successful exclusion of the aortic defect following endograft deployment, retrograde perfusion of the aneurysm sac from aortic branch vessels may contribute to further expansion of the retroperitoneal hematoma especially in the setting of coagulopathy. For patients who develop evidence of physiological compromise following EVAR, abdominal compartment syndrome

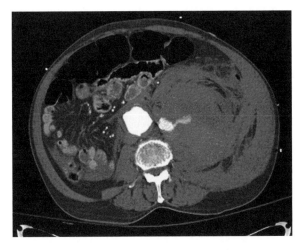

Fig. 1 Contrast-enhanced computed tomographic scan demonstrates an abdominal aortic aneurysm with active contrast extravagation into a large left-sided retroperitoneal hematoma

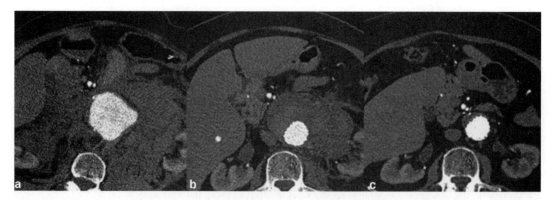

Fig. 2 Seventy-year-old female who underwent EVAR for a 6.4 cm ruptured abdominal aortic aneurysm. (**a**) Computed tomographic angiography scan demonstrates a large infrarenal abdominal aortic aneurysm with a focal outpouching along the left anteriolateral boarder. Extensive retroperitoneal hematoma displacing the abdominal viscera is appreciated. (**b**) One-month following EVAR, there has been a significant resolution of the retroperitoneal hematoma. (**c**) One-year following EVAR, there is near complete resolution of the retroperitoneal hematoma and a significant reduction in aneurysm sac size

must be a primary consideration. Expectant management utilizing supportive measures may be initially employed depending upon the severity of intra-abdominal hypertension, and may avoid surgical decompression,[13,14,18,21,24–27] otherwise laparotomy to evacuate the hematoma remains the definitive form of treatment. Successful hematoma evacuation can often be performed through a limited retroperitoneal incision, unless free rupture has occurred into the peritoneal cavity.[18]

Failure to successfully deploy the endograft and obtain aneurysm exclusion necessitating intraoperative conversion has been reported in several institutional series. Intraoperative conversion rates have ranged from 0 to18%[15–17,20,21,24–26,29,30] with reported indications for conversion including persistent blood loss,[30] difficult access,[21] endograft migration,[29] coverage of the renal arteries,[26] endograft thrombosis,[16] inability to attach to a short proximal neck,[21] and failure to deploy the contralateral limb.[17,24] Late surgical conversion has been reported to occur in 1.7–2.1% of patients who have undergone EVAR for nonruptured AAAs.[31–33] The risk of late conversion following EVAR for rAAAs is undefined due to a lack of reported long-term follow-up. Among 33 survivors following EVAR for rAAA, Mehta et al. reported only 1 (3%) late open conversion through a mean follow-up of 19 months.[25] This observation was slightly better then the 9% late conversion rate reported by Hechelhammer et al. through a mean follow-up of 24 months.[26]

Endoleaks are a well-defined complication following elective EVAR of AAAs, and result in an incomplete exclusion of the aneurysm sac from the systemic circulation. Endoleaks have been reported to occur in approximately 26% of electively treated EVAR patients with long-term follow-up, and this complication has been associated with subsequent rupture.[32] Endoleaks of all types (I, II, and III) are the most common indication for reintervention following EVAR of nonruptured AAAs,[34] as well as rAAAs.[26] Given the more complex aortic neck anatomy encountered in several patients with rAAAs, it would be expected that there may be a greater risk of developing a proximal type Ia endoleak following EVAR in this setting, although this risk is presently undefined. In a midterm follow-up report by Hechelhammer et al., the overall freedom from type I, II, or III endoleak was 57% at 1 year, and 49% at 2 years.[26] Of the 22 endoleaks observed, none were proximal type Ia endoleaks, and half (11/22; 50%) were type II. The absence of type Ia endoleaks among 36 patients who successfully received endografts may have been a result of strict adherence to anatomic EVAR candidacy including a minimal proximal neck length of 15 mm. Additionally, the absence of secondary aneurysm rupture among patients with type II endoleaks would suggest that this complication can be managed expectantly as they are following EVAR of nonruptured AAAs.

In addition to a potential for a greater frequency of endoleaks, complex vascular anatomy may also increase the risk for other complications such as endograft migration, limb occlusion, or thrombosis. More of these complications would result in a greater number of secondary interventions in patients who underwent EVAR for rAAAs compared with electively treated AAAs. One study by Oranen et al. compared the rate of secondary interventions following elective and emergent EVAR.[35] No significant difference in the rate of secondary interventions was observed between these groups through midterm follow-up, although the emergent group did include nonruptured asymptomatic AAAs (22/56; 39%). Although the reported risk of secondary intervention among the rAAA subgroup was 5.1% at 1 year and 16.2% at 2 and 3 years, these observations are considerably lower then the secondary intervention rates reported by Hechelhammer et al. (35.7% and 44.6% at 2 and 3 years, respectively).[26] Both studies had similar EVAR anatomic candidacy criteria, and comparable mean durations of follow-up.

Published Outcomes

Minimizing the physiological insult from the aortic intervention is largely the reason that EVAR has been advocated over conventional open surgery for rAAAs. The minimally invasive nature of EVAR should therefore, at the very least, translate into improved short-term outcomes in hospital morbidity and mortality. These potential benefits are, at present, difficult to assess. EVAR in this setting has been criticized in that it tends to subselect the more stable patients with less complex aortic anatomy largely due to the imaging requirements and anatomic limitations of the endovascular intervention. Many of the reported outcomes are from single institution case series greatly limited by sample size. Studies comparing EVAR to open surgery for rAAAs often lack randomization, and some have included symptomatic AAAs in their emergent cohorts. Despite these limitations, outcomes are encouraging, and there appears to be a general consensus that EVAR is feasible, and at least equivalent to open surgery for patients with rAAA and suitable vascular anatomy.

One prospective randomized controlled trial comparing EVAR with open surgery for rAAAs has been reported.[16] In this single-institution study reported by Hinchliffe et al., all randomized patients were assessed to be candidates for open surgery with a total of 32 patients recruited ($n = 15$ EVAR; 17 open surgery). Thirty-day mortality was reported on an intention-to-treat basis and demonstrated no difference between EVAR (53%) and open surgical groups (53%). Additionally, among survivors in both groups, there was no difference in the overall number of moderate or severe postoperative complications (EVAR 77%; open surgery 80%). Although the study design represents a significant improvement over nonrandomized retrospective case series, the low number of patients randomized to both study arms makes conclusions unreliable. Additionally the mortality rates for both interventions were surprisingly high despite the exclusion of high risk patients.

Harkin et al. performed a systematic review of the literature for studies relevant to EVAR of rAAAs.[9] Of the 34 published reports identified, 17 compared EVAR and open surgery. The overall procedure-related mortality was 18% for EVAR and 34% for open surgery (not subjected to statistical analysis). Additionally, of the studies reporting secondary outcomes, the majority reported significant reductions in length of intensive care unit stay, length of procedure, blood loss, and transfusion requirements in favor of EVAR.

In another systematic review by Visser et al., the inclusion criteria limited the analysis to ten studies directly comparing EVAR and open surgery.[22] In this review, a total of 148 patients underwent EVAR and 330 underwent open surgical procedures. Although an advantage in favor of EVAR was observed for the pooled 30-day mortality (22% vs 38%) and systemic complications (28% vs 56%), the mortality benefit was not significant when adjusting for hemodynamic condition at presentation.

Greco et al. performed a review of public discharge data sets from four states (California, Florida, New Jersey, and New York) from 2000 through 2003.[23] Patients who underwent EVAR or open surgery for rAAA were identified through International Classification of Diseases, 9th revision (ICD-9) diagnosis and procedure codes. The analysis consisted of 290 EVAR and 5508 open surgery patients. A significant overall mortality advantage in favor of EVAR was observed when combining data from all four states (39.3% vs 47.7%), although this observation was not consistent when analyzing outcomes in individual states. Additionally, EVAR was found to be associated with significantly lower rates of pulmonary, bleeding, and renal complications, as well as a shorter overall length of stay.

Conclusions

EVAR is a technically feasible form of treatment for rAAAs in patients with suitable vascular anatomy. Patient candidacy for EVAR in this setting is largely dependant upon anatomic considerations. Despite the minimally invasive approach of this form of therapy, postprocedure complications are common mainly due to the physiological insult sustained from the rupture, although additional procedure-related complications can occur. Although endograft-related complications would be expected to be high given the complex vascular anatomy encountered in this patient population, the long-term durability and risk of secondary intervention in these patients appear relatively limited. EVAR for rAAA has become the standard of care at many major vascular centers and appears to be at least equivalent to conventional open surgery in the short-term.

References

1. Ernst CB. Abdominal aortic aneurysm. N Engl J Med 1993;328(16):1167–72.
2. Bown MJ, Sutton AJ, Bell PR, Sayers RD. A meta-analysis of 50 years of ruptured abdominal aortic aneurysm repair. Br J Surg 2002;89(6):714–30.
3. Lawrence PF, Gazak C, Bhirangi L, et al. The epidemiology of surgically repaired aneurysms in the United States. J Vasc Surg 1999;30(4):632–40.

 4. Boyle JR, Gibbs PJ, Kruger A, Shearman CP, Raptis S, Phillips MJ. Existing delays following the presentation of ruptured abdominal aortic aneurysm allow sufficient time to assess patients for endovascular repair. Eur J Vasc Endovasc Surg 2005; 29(5):505–9.

 5. Harris JR, Forbes TL, Steiner SH, Lawlor DK, Derose G, Harris KA. Risk-adjusted analysis of early mortality after ruptured abdominal aortic aneurysm repair. J Vasc Surg 2005;42(3):387–91.

 6. Noel AA, Gloviczki P, Cherry KJ, Jr., et al. Ruptured abdominal aortic aneurysms: the excessive mortality rate of conventional repair. J Vasc Surg 2001;34(1):41–6.

 7. May J, White GH, Stephen MS, Harris JP. Rupture of abdominal aortic aneurysm: concurrent comparison of outcome of those occurring after endovascular repair versus those occurring without previous treatment in an 11-year single-center experience. J Vasc Surg 2004;40(5):860–6.

 8. Lloyd GM, Bown MJ, Norwood MG, et al. Feasibility of preoperative computer tomography in patients with ruptured abdominal aortic aneurysm: a time-to-death study in patients without operation. J Vasc Surg 2004;39(4):788–91.

 9. Harkin DW, Dillon M, Blair PH, Ellis PK, Kee F. Endovascular ruptured abdominal aortic aneurysm repair (EVRAR): a systematic review. Eur J Vasc Endovasc Surg 2007;34(6):673–81.

10. Wilson WR, Fishwick G, Sir Peter RFB, Thompson MM. Suitability of ruptured AAA for endovascular repair. J Endovasc Ther 2004;11(6):635–40.

11. Lee WA, Huber TS, Hirneise CM, Berceli SA, Seeger JM. Eligibility rates of ruptured and symptomatic AAA for endovascular repair. J Endovasc Ther 2002;9(4): 436–42.

12. Rose DF, Davidson IR, Hinchliffe RJ, et al. Anatomical suitability of ruptured abdominal aortic aneurysms for endovascular repair. J Endovasc Ther 2003;10(3):453–7.

13. Hinchliffe RJ, Braithwaite BD, European Bifab Study C. A modular aortouniiliac endovascular stent-graft is a useful device for the treatment of symptomatic and ruptured infrarenal abdominal aortic aneurysms: one-year results from a multicentre study. Eur J Vasc Endovasc Surg 2007;34(3):291–8.

14. Lachat ML, Pfammatter T, Witzke HJ, et al. Endovascular repair with bifurcated stent-grafts under local anaesthesia to improve outcome of ruptured aortoiliac aneurysms. Eur J Vasc Endovasc Surg 2002;23(6):528–36.

15. Gerassimidis TS, Papazoglou KO, Kamparoudis AG, et al. Endovascular management of ruptured abdominal aortic aneurysms: 6-year experience from a Greek center. J Vasc Surg 2005;42(4):615–23; discussion 23.

16. Hinchliffe RJ, Bruijstens L, MacSweeney ST, Braithwaite BD. A randomised trial of endovascular and open surgery for ruptured abdominal aortic aneurysm - results of a pilot study and lessons learned for future studies. Eur J Vasc Endovasc Surg 2006;32(5):506–13; discussion 14–5.

17. Alsac JM, Desgranges P, Kobeiter H, Becquemin JP. Emergency endovascular repair for ruptured abdominal aortic aneurysms: feasibility and comparison of early results with conventional open repair. Eur J Vasc Endovasc Surg 2005;30(6):632–9.

18. Ohki T, Veith FJ. Endovascular grafts and other image-guided catheter-based adjuncts to improve the treatment of ruptured aortoiliac aneurysms. Ann Surg 2000;232(4):466–79.

19. O'Donnell ME, Badger SA, Makar RR, Loan W, Lee B, Soong CV. Techniques in occluding the aorta during endovascular repair of ruptured abdominal aortic aneurysms. J Vasc Surg 2006;44(1):211–5.

20. Yilmaz N, Peppelenbosch N, Cuypers PW, Tielbeek AV, Duijm LE, Buth J. Emergency treatment of symptomatic or ruptured abdominal aortic aneurysms: the role of endovascular repair. J Endovasc Ther 2002;9(4):449–57.

21. Coppi G, Silingardi R, Gennai S, Saitta G, Ciardullo AV. A single-center experience in open and endovascular treatment of hemodynamically unstable and stable patients with ruptured abdominal aortic aneurysms. J Vasc Surg 2006;44(6):1140–7.

22. Visser JJ, van Sambeek MR, Hamza TH, Hunink MG, Bosch JL. Ruptured abdominal aortic aneurysms: endovascular repair versus open surgery – systematic review. Radiology 2007;245(1):122–9.

23. Greco G, Egorova N, Anderson PL, et al. Outcomes of endovascular treatment of ruptured abdominal aortic aneurysms. J Vasc Surg 2006;43(3):453–9.

24. Scharrer-Pamler R, Kotsis T, Kapfer X, Gorich J, Sunder-Plassmann L. Endovascular stent-graft repair of ruptured aortic aneurysms. J Endovasc Ther 2003;10(3):447–52.

25. Mehta M, Taggert J, Darling RC, 3rd, et al. Establishing a protocol for endovascular treatment of ruptured abdominal aortic aneurysms: outcomes of a prospective analysis. J Vasc Surg 2006;44(1):1–8; discussion 8.

26. Hechelhammer L, Lachat ML, Wildermuth S, Bettex D, Mayer D, Pfammatter T. Midterm outcome of endovascular repair of ruptured abdominal aortic aneurysms. J Vasc Surg 2005;41(5):752–7.

27. Resch T, Malina M, Lindblad B, Dias NV, Sonesson B, Ivancev K. Endovascular repair of ruptured abdominal aortic aneurysms: logistics and short-term results. J Endovasc Ther 2003;10(3):440–6.

28. Mehta M, Darling RC, 3rd, Roddy SP, et al. Factors associated with abdominal compartment syndrome complicating endovascular repair of ruptured abdominal aortic aneurysms. J Vasc Surg 2005;42(6):1047–51.

29. Larzon T, Lindgren R, Norgren L. Endovascular treatment of ruptured abdominal aortic aneurysms: a shift of the paradigm? J Endovasc Ther 2005;12(5):548–55.

30. Visser JJ, Bosch JL, Hunink MG, et al. Endovascular repair versus open surgery in patients with ruptured abdominal aortic aneurysms: clinical outcomes with 1-year follow-up. J Vasc Surg 2006;44(6):1148–55.

31. Ohki T, Veith FJ, Shaw P, et al. Increasing incidence of midterm and long-term complications after endovascular graft repair of abdominal aortic aneurysms: a note of caution based on a 9-year experience. Ann Surg 2001;234(3):323–34; discussion 34–5.

32. Brewster DC, Jones JE, Chung TK, et al. Long-term outcomes after endovascular abdominal aortic aneurysm repair: the first decade. Ann Surg 2006;244(3):426–38.

33. Drury D, Michaels JA, Jones L, Ayiku L. Systematic review of recent evidence for the safety and efficacy of elective endovascular repair in the management of infrarenal abdominal aortic aneurysm. Br J Surg 2005;92(8):937–46.

34. Endovascular aneurysm repair versus open repair in patients with abdominal aortic aneurysm (EVAR trial 1): randomised controlled trial. Lancet 2005; 365(9478):2179–86.

35. Oranen BI, Bos WT, Verhoeven EL, et al. Is emergency endovascular aneurysm repair associated with higher secondary intervention risk at mid-term follow-up? J Vasc Surg 2006;44(6):1156–61.

Chapter 14

Complications After Endovascular Ruptured Abdominal Aortic Aneurysm Repair

Jonathan L. Eliason and Todd E. Rasmussen

Abstract Abdominal aortic aneurysm (AAA) rupture is an event with very high associated morbidity and mortality. Perioperative mortality rates in the United States for open repair of ruptured AAA have averaged around 45% since the late 1980s. Although elective aneurysm repair is four to five times more common than emergent repair, and despite aggressive programs to screen at-risk populations, the incidence of ruptured AAA continues to increase. There is a great need for improvement in early aneurysm detection, which could lead to improved outcomes. However, even with improved methods of detection, due to patient-related factors, a sizeable number of patients with AAA can be anticipated to remain undiagnosed. Improved outcomes with respect to repair of ruptured AAA are therefore vital. Endovascular aneurysm repair (EVAR) has steadily gained in popularity since the first report of its successful application to human patients in 1991 by Parodi et al. Indeed, recent estimates in the United States suggest that elective EVAR is now utilized more commonly than open AAA repair. Because randomized controlled trials (RCTs) have shown perioperative morbidity and mortality advantages for EVAR over open AAA repair in the elective setting, there have been many proponents of using EVAR preferentially for aneurysm patients with the highest mortality, those with rupture. In fact, reports of using EVAR for ruptured AAA can be found in the literature as early as 1994. This chapter will provide an overview of the complications specifically associated with using EVAR for ruptured AAAs. Complications will be categorized into two groups, those that occur in the perioperative setting (early) and those that occur thereafter (late).

Keywords EVAR complications, Ruptured AAA repair, Perioperative morbidity, endoleak, colonic ischemia, ACS, Postimplant syndrome, Graft thrombosis

G. Upchurch and E. Criado (eds.) *Aortic Aneurysms, Contemporary Cardiology*
DOI: 10.1007/978-1-60327-204-9_14, © Humana Press, a part of
Springer Science+Business Media, LLC 2009

Early Complications

Mortality

The most important endpoint for evaluating the efficacy of EVAR in treating ruptured abdominal aortic aneurysm (AAA) is mortality. As stated earlier, only minimal mortality reductions have been seen over the last 20–30 years using open surgical repair of ruptured AAA. Conversely, the literature has included a growing number of reports suggesting improved survival after ruptured AAA utilizing EVAR.[1–10] Inclusion of symptomatic nonruptured patients, the selection of patients with a more stable hemodynamic profile and the variability in control groups make the interpretation of these data difficult.

In 2005, data generated from the state of Illinois Department of Public Health-accredited hospitals was published which used the increased power available with administrative data to compare open surgical repair with EVAR. In the ruptured cohort, no significant difference in mortality between EVAR and open surgical repair was seen in patients grouped by age.[11]

An RCT of endovascular and open surgery for ruptured AAA was finally reported in 2006.[12] Of 103 patients admitted with suspected ruptured AAA over a 2-year study period, 32 were enrolled in the study. Thirty-day mortality rates for both the EVAR and the open surgery groups were 53%. Additionally, other single and multicenter reports have reported no difference in mortality between these groups.[13–16]

Because of the paucity of randomized data and some ambiguity in the non-randomized data, several reviews have been performed in an attempt to obtain a consensus. The first, by Larzon et al., searched the English language literature from January 1994 until March 2006. Ten studies including 148 endovascular repairs and 330 open repairs met their inclusion criteria. After pooling the mortality data and adjusting for heterogeneity in patients' hemodynamic condition, a trend was seen toward decreased mortality with EVAR for ruptured AAA, although this did not reach statistical significance.[17] The Cochrane Peripheral Vascular Diseases Group then searched their trial register through October 2006, and like the first review, at that time, no RCTs had been reported on this subject. Their assessment of evidence from prospective controlled studies without randomization, prospective studies, and retrospective studies was that EVAR for rupture is feasible, with outcomes comparable to best conventional open surgical repair for the treatment of ruptured AAA.[18] These findings were supported by an additional review from the same authors which included the interval publication of the single RCT in the analysis.[19] In summary, although EVAR for rupture may have some advantages; at this time, there is no definitive report demonstrating superiority in mortality over conventional open surgical repair.

Technical Failure

Complete technical failure to deploy an endovascular graft is rare in the elective setting, with rates less than 2% even in clinical trial data.[20–22] In the best of circumstances, such as elective EVAR, however, the need for acute conversion to open repair still carries with it considerable risk. Causes of technical endovascular failure in the acute setting include access problems, failed deployment, graft thrombosis, acute endograft migration, aortic rupture, and postoperative suspicion of rupture.[23,24] The EUROSTAR data registry recording at least eight different endograft device types demonstrates that primary conversion during the initial procedure is associated with an 18% mortality rate.[24]

Applying these data to ruptured AAA, it is intuitive that the incidence of technical failure would be higher with EVAR for rupture than for elective EVAR. Theoretical factors include suboptimal imaging, limited shelf-stock, "on-call" staffing unfamiliar with EVAR, and technical imprecision due to the urgency of the procedure. In actuality, technical failure is reported infrequently, with many single centers reporting technical success rates at or near 100%.[4,5,8,25] High technical success rates are likely in part a reflection of centers developing ruptured AAA EVAR protocols, thereby creating systems in which these patients can be safely and efficiently triaged.[10]

Endoleak

Endoleaks are complications unique to EVAR and can be divided into five basic types. Type I endoleaks occur due to inadequate graft seal resulting in perigraft flow (Fig. 1). These can be proximal (Ia) or distal (Ib). Type II endoleaks occur when branch arteries such as the inferior mesenteric artery or lumbar artery backbleed into the aneurysm (Fig. 2). Type III endoleaks occur when flow persists between the segments of a modular graft. Type IV endoleaks result from flow of blood through the endograft material (graft porosity). Type V endoleaks, or "endotension," occur when there is pressurization of the aneurysm sac in the absence of demonstrable type I–IV endoleak.

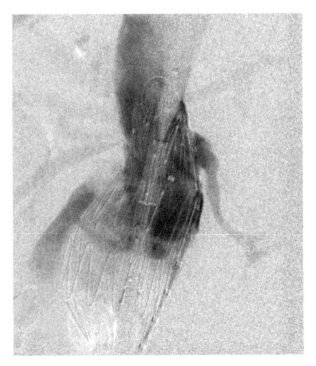

Fig 1 Aortogram after endovascular aneurysm repair (*EVAR*) for ruptured abdominal aortic aneurysm (*AAA*) demonstrating right renal artery stenosis and immediate Type Ia endoleak. The aneurysm sac blush is noted adjacent to the endograft body

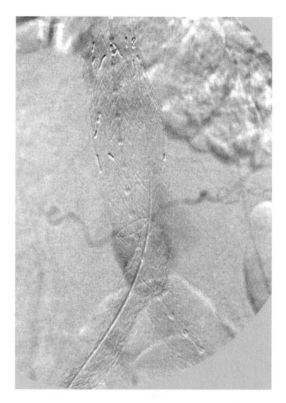

Fig. 2 Late-phase aortogram after endovascular aneurysm repair (*EVAR*) for ruptured abdominal aortic aneurysm (*AAA*) demonstrating a type II endoleak arising from paired lumbar arteries. The aneurysm sac blush is noted behind the endograft

The absence of type I and type III endoleaks on completion angiography are essential components of a technically successful EVAR.[26] In the setting of EVAR for aneurysm rupture, however, even type II endoleaks can be associated with ongoing hemorrhage.[27] The incidence of acute type I and type III endoleaks range from 0 to 16%, and the majority have been successfully treated with endovascular techniques.[2,5,8,15,25,28-30] However, as demonstrated in the subsequent section, inability to treat these can result in the need for open surgical conversion.

Acute Conversion to Open Repair

Although technical success is surprisingly high, acute conversion to open repair does occur. Inadvertent coverage of both renal arteries has been reported as an indication for acute conversion.[2,13] Inability to deliver the endograft due to iliac diameter or aortoiliac tortuosity has also resulted in conversion to open surgery.[5,13,31] Similarly, inability to access the contralateral limb of a bifurcated endograft has been implicated.[29] Persistent type I endoleak with inability to achieve seal using endovascular techniques most commonly occurs in the setting of a short infrarenal neck, and can result in loss of seal or acute migration.[5,30,32] Finally, antegrade and retrograde aortic dissection from the proximal seal zone has also been reported.[32] In the 10 patients reflected by the above-described acute conversions, a 40% perioperative mortality rate was observed.

Visceral Ischemia/Bowel Infarction

Colonic ischemia is a known complication of AAA repair. The inferior mesenteric artery and hypogastric arteries may each be affected during open repair or EVAR. EVAR has been associated with lower rates of colonic ischemia than open repair, but mortality rates remain greater than 50% for either group when severe ischemia is encountered.[33] When mandatory postoperative flexible sigmoidoscopy is performed following EVAR for ruptured AAA, the incidence of colonic ischemia is 23%, although the majority of cases are considered mild.[34] Reports of EVAR for ruptured AAA that include colonic ischemia requiring resection demonstrate that this complication is often fatal, and commonly includes interruption of one or both hypogastric arteries.[1,5,6,15]

Abdominal Compartment Syndrome

Abdominal compartment syndrome (ACS) is caused by increased intra-abdominal pressures and results in decreased intra-abdominal organ perfusion and increased airway pressures. It was first reported as a complication of ruptured AAA in the late 1980s.[35] Since the recognition of ACS as a significant cause of morbidity and mortality following repair of ruptured AAA, strategies have been specifically aimed at temporarily increasing the abdominal domain following open repair in order to prevent this complication.[36,37] There is no easy mechanism for increasing abdominal domain with EVAR. As such, ACS is frequently reported as a complication in cases of EVAR for AAA rupture.[1–3,5,6,28,30–32] Mehta et al. reported successful EVAR for ruptured AAA in 40 patients between 2002 and 2004.[6] Seven of these patients developed ACS, reflecting an 18% incidence. When comparing mortality rates in this series [without ACS 3/33 (9%); with ACS 4/7 (57%)], the severity of this complication is underscored. When this complication is associated with EVAR for rupture, decompressive laparotomy, percutaneous drainage, and incisional lumbar drainage techniques have all been employed to increase abdominal domain or decrease the source of intra-abdominal pressure, namely, a large retroperitoneal hematoma (Fig. 3).

Postimplant Syndrome

Postimplant syndrome is exceedingly rare with open repair of AAA, but is a well-described complication of EVAR.[38] It is characterized by fever, leukocytosis, backache, and an increase in nonspecific markers of inflammation. It is generally thought to be a benign complication with no lasting sequelae, but can sometimes result in a diagnostic dilemma if not considered. In a report including 30 patients treated emergently with EVAR from Italy, Lagana et al. reported postimplant syndrome occurred "in all cases."[4] In other reported series using EVAR to treat ruptured AAA, this syndrome is often left unreported or with a much lower frequency.[8]

Paresis/Paraplegia

One of the most feared and devastating complications of aortic surgery is spinal cord ischemia resulting in paresis or paraplegia. This complication in the context of EVAR for ruptured AAA was analyzed in a multicenter study from the Netherlands and Belgium.[39] The 3-year study period included 35 patients

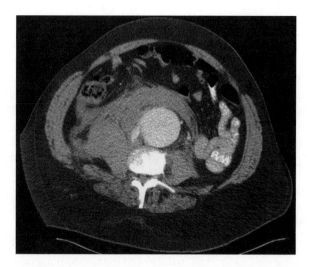

Fig. 3 CT image of ruptured abdominal aortic aneurysm (*AAA*) resulting in laparotomy and temporary vacuum-assisted abdominal closure due to large retroperitoneal hematoma. Active extravasation of contrast to the patient's right is noted on this image

treated emergently with EVAR. Four patients (11.5%) developed paraplegia postoperatively. Factors significantly associated with paraplegia included hypogastric artery occlusion and prolonged functional aortic occlusion time. Reports of this complication are otherwise rare.[30]

Acute Renal Failure

Renal failure associated with endovascular repair of ruptured AAA is common. Renal failure rates of 20% have been reported following EVAR for rupture when defined by an increase in serum creatinine of 2 mg/dl or more.[32] Renal injury is often multifactorial. Contrast nephropathy, hypotension, shock, atheroembolic, or thromboembolic events, and even renal artery coverage by the endograft are all contributors. The utilization of temporary aortic occlusion balloons for hemodynamic instability is another theoretical concern, as this may prolong the period of absolute renal ischemia and promote embolic injury. Reports of bilateral renal artery occlusion following EVAR suggest that this complication results in permanent renal failure, but may be successfully treated by acute conversion to open repair if recognized promptly.[25,28]

Late Complications

Endoleaks

Like in the acute period, secondary endoleak following EVAR for rupture is a very commonly reported complication. Type I and III endoleaks are typically treated using endovascular techniques, rarely result in conversion to open repair, and are almost never followed without intervention.[1,2,4,6,15,25,40] Similar to the elective setting, type II endoleaks are generally treated with coil embolization in the setting of aneurysm enlargement.[2,4,6,8,15] If the aneurysm size remains stable or shrinks, secondary type II endoleaks are observed.

Delayed Conversion to Open Repair

The mortality associated with conversion to open aneurysm repair in the delayed setting is not felt to be as high as when these procedures are performed acutely.[41,42] The reported causes necessitating conversion in the chronic setting are variable. Persistent type I endoleak not amenable to endovascular repair, endograft migration, and infection are some examples.[2,5] Persistent endoleak does not necessarily mean that the patient requires endograft explantation, however. Techniques such as wrapping the proximal neck with a synthetic band to decrease the diameter, or placing aortic sutures externally to fix the endograft in place have also been described.[5]

Graft Thrombosis

Endograft-associated thrombotic complications are reported rarely after EVAR for AAA rupture, but have been seen both early and late. The most severe complication is endograft thrombosis. This has been reported with the aortounifemoral graft configuration in two reports involving three patients, two within 30-days of graft implantation, and one late presentation at 240 days. One patient with acute thrombosis and one with delayed thrombosis were treated with emergent axillobifemoral bypass, while the other acute thrombosis was treated with endograft thrombectomy and angioplasty.[5,25] Limb thrombosis of bifurcated endografts has also been described in the early and late time periods. These were treated with femoro–femoral bypass.[5,8]

Graft Infection

Graft infection is a serious complication for both open and endovascular repair of AAA. Emergency surgery is also a known independent predictor of increased rates of infection.[43] However, retrospective analyses of graft infection rates following open and endovascular repair of ruptured AAA do not seem to reflect the same risk.[44,45] This does not mean that reports of graft-related infectious complications after ruptured EVAR cannot be found in the literature. Alsac et al. reported early graft-related sepsis as a cause of death in 1/37 patients undergoing EVAR for rupture, while Hechelhammer et al. reported graft-related infection as a late complication resulting in conversion to open repair in a series of 37 patients.[1,2] Still, similar to graft thrombosis, this complication is noted infrequently.

Table 1 Randomized trial data of endovascular and open surgery for ruptured abdominal aortic aneurysm (Eur J Vasc Endovasc Surg 2006;32:506–13)

Repair Type	Patient #	Died Prior to Repair	Crossover to Other Group Prior to Repair	Acute Conversion to Open Repair	Number Receiving Intended Treatment	30-Days Mortality Rate (%)*
Open	17	3			14	9/17 (53%)
Endovascular	15	1	1	2	13	8/15 (53%)

*Intention to treat

Conclusion

Currently there is no definitive 30-day mortality data demonstrating superiority of EVAR for AAA rupture over open repair. As detailed in this chapter, EVAR for AAA rupture carries with it the potential for significant morbidity as well. Nevertheless, a careful review of the literature from the early 1990s to the present reveals incredible growth and improvement in endograft technology, in the clinical experience of practitioners, and in outcomes for elective EVAR. It is therefore a reasonable hope and expectation that patient survival and complication rates can be improved in the setting of EVAR for rupture by ongoing clinical research and the implementation of protocols for the emergent endovascular treatment of ruptured AAA.

References

1. Alsac JM, Desgranges P, Kobeiter H, Becquemin JP. Emergency endovascular repair for ruptured abdominal aortic aneurysms: feasibility and comparison of early results with conventional open repair. Eur J Vasc Endovasc Surg 2005;30:632–9.
2. Hechelhammer L, Lachat ML, Wildermuth S, Bettex D, Mayer D, Pfammatter T. Midterm outcome of endovascular repair of ruptured abdominal aortic aneurysms. J Vasc Surg 2005;41:752–7.
3. Veith FJ, Ohki T, Lipsitz EC, Suggs WD, Cynamon J. Endovascular grafts and other catheter-directed techniques in the management of ruptured abdominal aortic aneurysms. Semin Vasc Surg 2003;16:326–31.
4. Lagana D, Carrafiello G, Mangini M, et al. Emergency endovascular treatment of abdominal aortic aneurysms: feasibility and results. Cardiovasc Intervent Radiol 2006;29:241–8.
5. Coppi G, Silingardi R, Gennai S, Saitta G, Ciardullo AV. A single-center experience in open and endovascular treatment of hemodynamically unstable and stable patients with ruptured abdominal aortic aneurysms. J Vasc Surg 2006;44:1140–7.
6. Mehta M, Taggert J, Darling RC, 3rd, et al. Establishing a protocol for endovascular treatment of ruptured abdominal aortic aneurysms: outcomes of a prospective analysis. J Vasc Surg 2006;44:1–8; discussion.
7. Brandt M, Walluscheck KP, Jahnke T, Graw K, Cremer J, Muller-Hulsbeck S. Endovascular repair of ruptured abdominal aortic aneurysm: feasibility and impact on early outcome. J Vasc Interv Radiol 2005;16:1309–12.
8. Castelli P, Caronno R, Piffaretti G, et al. Ruptured abdominal aortic aneurysm: endovascular treatment. Abdom Imaging 2005;30:263–9.
9. Lee WA, Hirneise CM, Tayyarah M, Huber TS, Seeger JM. Impact of endovascular repair on early outcomes of ruptured abdominal aortic aneurysms. J Vasc Surg 2004;40:211–5.
10. Moore R, Nutley M, Cina CS, Motamedi M, Faris P, Abuznadah W. Improved survival after introduction of an emergency endovascular therapy protocol for ruptured abdominal aortic aneurysms. J Vasc Surg 2007;45:443–50.
11. Leon LR, Jr., Labropoulos N, Laredo J, Rodriguez HE, Kalman PG. To what extent has endovascular aneurysm repair influenced abdominal aortic aneurysm management in the state of Illinois? J Vasc Surg 2005;41:568–74.
12. Hinchliffe RJ, Bruijstens L, MacSweeney ST, Braithwaite BD. A randomised trial of endovascular and open surgery for ruptured abdominal aortic aneurysm - results of a pilot study and lessons learned for future studies. Eur J Vasc Endovasc Surg 2006;32:506–13; discussion 14–5.
13. Hinchliffe RJ, Yusuf SW, Macierewicz JA, MacSweeney ST, Wenham PW, Hopkinson BR. Endovascular repair of ruptured abdominal aortic aneurysm – a

challenge to open repair? Results of a single centre experience in 20 patients. Eur J Vasc Endovasc Surg 2001;22:528–34.

14. Peppelenbosch N, Geelkerken RH, Soong C, et al. Endograft treatment of ruptured abdominal aortic aneurysms using the Talent aortouniiliac system: an international multicenter study. J Vasc Surg 2006;43:1111–23; discussion 23.

15. Ockert S, Schumacher H, Bockler D, Megges I, Allenberg JR. Early and midterm results after open and endovascular repair of ruptured abdominal aortic aneurysms in a comparative analysis. J Endovasc Ther 2007;14:324–32.

16. Resch T, Malina M, Lindblad B, Dias NV, Sonesson B, Ivancev K. Endovascular repair of ruptured abdominal aortic aneurysms: logistics and short-term results. J Endovasc Ther 2003;10:440–6.

17. Visser JJ, van Sambeek MR, Hamza TH, Hunink MG, Bosch JL. Ruptured abdominal aortic aneurysms: endovascular repair versus open surgery – systematic review. Radiology 2007;245:122–9.

18. Dillon M, Cardwell C, Blair PH, Ellis P, Kee F, Harkin DW. Endovascular treatment for ruptured abdominal aortic aneurysm. Cochrane Database Syst Rev 2007: CD005261.

19. Harkin DW, Dillon M, Blair PH, Ellis PK, Kee F. Endovascular ruptured abdominal aortic aneurysm repair (EVRAR): a systematic review. Eur J Vasc Endovasc Surg 2007;34:673–81.

20. Greenberg RK, Chuter TA, Sternbergh WC, 3rd, Fearnot NE. Zenith AAA endovascular graft: intermediate-term results of the US multicenter trial. J Vasc Surg 2004;39:1209–18.

21. Carpenter JP. The Powerlink bifurcated system for endovascular aortic aneurysm repair: four-year results of the US multicenter trial. J Cardiovasc Surg (Torino) 2006;47:239–43.

22. Curci JA, Fillinger MF, Naslund TC, Rubin BG. Clinical trial results of a modified gore excluder endograft: comparison with open repair and original device design. Ann Vasc Surg 2007;21:328–38.

23. May J, White GH, Yu W, et al. Conversion from endoluminal to open repair of abdominal aortic aneurysms: a hazardous procedure. Eur J Vasc Endovasc Surg 1997;14:4–11.

24. Cuypers PW, Laheij RJ, Buth J. Which factors increase the risk of conversion to open surgery following endovascular abdominal aortic aneurysm repair? The EUROSTAR collaborators. Eur J Vasc Endovasc Surg 2000;20:183–9.

25. Gerassimidis TS, Papazoglou KO, Kamparoudis AG, et al. Endovascular management of ruptured abdominal aortic aneurysms: 6-year experience from a Greek center. J Vasc Surg 2005;42:615–23; discussion 23.

26. Chaikof EL, Blankensteijn JD, Harris PL, et al. Reporting standards for endovascular aortic aneurysm repair. J Vasc Surg 2002;35:1048–60.

27. Hartung O, Vidal V, Marani I, Saran A, Bartoli JM, Alimi YS. Treatment of an early type II endoleak causing hemorrhage after endovascular aneurysm repair for ruptured abdominal aortic aneurysm. J Vasc Surg 2007;45:1062–5.

28. Hinchliffe RJ, Braithwaite BD, European Bifab Study C. A modular aortouniiliac endovascular stent-graft is a useful device for the treatment of symptomatic and ruptured infrarenal abdominal aortic aneurysms: one-year results from a multicentre study. Eur J Vasc Endovasc Surg 2007;34:291–8.

29. Scharrer-Pamler R, Kotsis T, Kapfer X, Gorich J, Sunder-Plassmann L. Endovascular stent-graft repair of ruptured aortic aneurysms. J Endovasc Ther 2003;10:447–52.

30. Van Herzeele I, Vermassen F, Durieux C, Randon C, De Roose J. Endovascular repair of aortic rupture. Eur J Vasc Endovasc Surg 2003;26:311–6.

31. Kapma MR, Verhoeven EL, Tielliu IF, et al. Endovascular treatment of acute abdominal aortic aneurysm with a bifurcated stentgraft. Eur J Vasc Endovasc Surg 2005;29:510–5.

32. Larzon T, Lindgren R, Norgren L. Endovascular treatment of ruptured abdominal aortic aneurysms: a shift of the paradigm? J Endovasc Ther 2005;12:548–55.

33. Becquemin JP, Majewski M, Fermani N, et al. Colon ischemia following abdominal aortic aneurysm repair in the era of endovascular abdominal aortic repair. J Vasc Surg 2008;47:258–63; discussion 63.

34. Champagne BJ, Lee EC, Valerian B, Mulhotra N, Mehta M. Incidence of colonic ischemia after repair of ruptured abdominal aortic aneurysm with endograft. J Am Coll Surg 2007;204:597–602.

35. Fietsam R, Jr., Villalba M, Glover JL, Clark K. Intra-abdominal compartment syndrome as a complication of ruptured abdominal aortic aneurysm repair. Am Surg 1989;55:396–402.

36. Ciresi DL, Cali RF, Senagore AJ. Abdominal closure using nonabsorbable mesh after massive resuscitation prevents abdominal compartment syndrome and gastrointestinal fistula. Am Surg 1999;65:720–4; discussion 4–5.

37. Rasmussen TE, Hallett JW, Jr., Noel AA, et al. Early abdominal closure with mesh reduces multiple organ failure after ruptured abdominal aortic aneurysm repair: guidelines from a 10-year case-control study. J Vasc Surg 2002;35:246–53.

38. May J, White GH, Harris JP. Complications of aortic endografting. J Cardiovasc Surg (Torino) 2005;46:359–69.

39. Peppelenbosch N, Cuypers PW, Vahl AC, Vermassen F, Buth J. Emergency endovascular treatment for ruptured abdominal aortic aneurysm and the risk of spinal cord ischemia. J Vasc Surg 2005;42:608–14.

40. Veith FJ, Ohki T, Lipsitz EC, Suggs WD, Cynamon J. Treatment of ruptured abdominal aneurysms with stent grafts: a new gold standard? Semin Vasc Surg 2003;16:171–5.

41. de Vries JP, van Herwaarden JA, Overtoom TT, Vos JA, Moll FL, van de Pavoordt ED. Clinical outcome and technical considerations of late removal of abdominal aortic endografts: 8-year single-center experience. Vascular 2005;13:135–40.

42. Jimenez JC, Moore WS, Quinones-Baldrich WJ. Acute and chronic open conversion after endovascular aortic aneurysm repair: a 14-year review. J Vasc Surg 2007;46:642–7.

43. Neumayer L, Hosokawa P, Itani K, El-Tamer M, Henderson WG, Khuri SF. Multivariable predictors of postoperative surgical site infection after general and vascular surgery: results from the patient safety in surgery study. J Am Coll Surg 2007;204:1178–87.

44. Cho JS, Gloviczki P, Martelli E, et al. Long-term survival and late complications after repair of ruptured abdominal aortic aneurysms. J Vasc Surg 1998;27:813–9; discussion 9–20.

45. Sharif MA, Lee B, Lau LL, et al. Prosthetic stent graft infection after endovascular abdominal aortic aneurysm repair. J Vasc Surg 2007;46:442–8.

Chapter 15

Treatment of Mycotic Abdominal Aortic Aneurysms and Infected Aortic Grafts

J. Gregory Modrall

Abstract Mycotic aortic aneurysms and infection of aortic grafts are dreaded complications of aortic disease that have been associated with high rates of major morbidity and mortality. Improved outcomes reported in recent years have been predicated on arriving at a timely diagnosis and developing an appropriate treatment plan after consideration of all options. This chapter will provide data to support a rational algorithm for the diagnosis of these challenging conditions. The various treatment options will be discussed, ranging from antibiotic therapy alone to complete resection of the infected aneurysm or graft with *in situ* or remote arterial reconstruction of the resected aortic segment. Various adjuncts to *in situ* repair of the aorta, such as antibiotic-impregnated grafts and omental flap coverage of prosthetic grafts, will be outlined. The relative advantages and pitfalls of each approach and their outcomes are reviewed. The goal of this chapter is to aid clinicians in the diagnosis and treatment of these difficult complications in order to minimize the risk of major morbidity or mortality.

Keywords Infected aortic aneurysm, Prosthesis-related infections

Introduction

Mycotic aneurysms and infected aortic grafts are among the most challenging conditions that clinicians who treat aortic disease will face in clinical practice. Without proper treatment, these conditions are often lethal. Despite advances in treatment, the mortality for both conditions remains substantial. The challenges posed by these conditions lie both in their diagnosis and treatment. To aid clinicians in optimizing outcomes for these conditions, this chapter will review the pathogenesis, diagnosis, treatment, and outcomes of these vexing clinical problems. Mycotic aneurysms and aortic graft infections will be addressed separately, although similar principles guide treatment of both conditions. The diagnosis and management of aortoenteric fistulas are addressed in a separate chapter.

G. Upchurch and E. Criado (eds.) *Aortic Aneurysms, Contemporary Cardiology*
DOI: 10.1007/978-1-60327-204-9_15, © Humana Press, a part of
Springer Science+Business Media, LLC 2009

Mycotic Aneurysms

Pathogenesis

The term *mycotic aneurysm* was initially introduced by Osler to denote infected aneurysms associated with endocarditis.[1] Today the term is broadly applied to any infected aneurysm, regardless of etiology. For the purposes of this discussion, mycotic aneurysms will include primary arterial infections causing aneurysm formation, arteritis related to contiguous spread of infection, and preexisting aneurysms that become secondarily infected.

Primary arterial infections are believed to result either from hematogenous seeding of the arterial wall during episodes of bacteremia or contiguous spread of local infections. Since the intima of an artery provides a relative barrier to infection, intimal injury related to atherosclerosis is usually required as a cofactor in the development of arteritis.[2] Histopathology of involved sections of artery typically shows transmural acute inflammation with focal microabscesses superimposed on a diffuse intimal atherosclerosis in the wall of mycotic aneurysms.[3] Since wall destruction is a critical element in the pathogenesis of aneurysms related to bacterial arteritis, it should be recognized that many aneurysms related to bacterial arteritis are actually *pseudoaneurysms*.

In the era prior to the introduction of antibiotics, the causative organisms were those associated with endocarditis, including *Streptococcal* species, *Staphylococcal* species, and *Pneumococcus*.[4] In a contemporary series from the Mayo Clinic,[3] Gram-positive cocci were responsible for 50% of cases (*Staphylococcus* in 30% and *Streptococcus* in 20%) and Gram-negative bacilli were cultured in 35% (*Salmonella* in 20% and *Escherichia coli* in 15%).

Bacterial arteritis may also result from contiguous spread from adjacent infected tissues, such as vertebral osteomyelitis or suppurative lymphadenitis. Alternatively, preexisting aortic aneurysms may become secondarily infected by hematogenous seeding due to infection of the atherosclerotic intima or mural thrombus within an aneurysm.[2,3]

Clinical Presentation

The clinical presentation of patients with mycotic aortic aneurysms ranges from overt aortic rupture and systemic inflammatory response syndrome (SIRS) to asymptomatic findings on radiological imaging studies. Between 46% and 61% of patients have a history of a recent or ongoing septic illness.[5,6] Comorbid conditions associated with relative immunosuppression are present in more than two-thirds of patients, including diabetes (33%), chronic renal failure (30%), chronic steroid use (16%), and chronic illnesses (16%).[6] Ninety-three percent of patients in a recent series from the Mayo Clinic were symptomatic, and the average duration of symptoms was 38 days.[6] Symptoms may be broadly categorized as septic symptoms, pain syndromes, and hemodynamic symptoms. Fever (77%), chills (51%), and sweats (28%) were typical septic symptoms.[6] Abdominal or back pain was present in 65% of patients.[6] Hemodynamic instability was present in only 7% of patients, despite aortic rupture in 21% of cases.[6] Laboratory abnormalities typically include elevated sedimentation rate (86%) or C-reactive protein (79%) and leukocytosis

(54%).[5,6] Seventy percent of patients with mycotic aneurysms of the aorta meet the clinical criteria for SIRS syndrome at initial presentation.[7,8]

Diagnosis and Imaging

Imaging tests are often helpful in ascertaining the diagnosis of a mycotic aneurysm. Computed tomography (CT) scan is the mainstay of imaging tests for the diagnosis of a mycotic aneurysm. The entire aorta should be imaged since mycotic aneurysms are found throughout the aorta: ascending aorta (6%), descending thoracic aorta (23%), paravisceral aorta (6%), juxtarenal aorta (10%), and infrarenal aorta (32%). A key element in the diagnosis of mycotic aneurysms is the aneurysm morphology. Mycotic aneurysms are characteristically saccular in 93% of cases.[9] Secondary signs of infection on CT scan include the presence of a para-aortic soft tissue mass, stranding, or fluid, which are seen nearly half of cases (Fig. 1).[9] Thirty percent of patients have CT evidence of aortic rupture.[8] Retroperitoneal gas in the context of a saccular aneurysm is rare (7% of cases), but pathognomonic for a mycotic aneurysm (Fig. 1).[9] Vertebral body destruction with psoas abscess adjacent to an aortic aneurysm is another ominous finding on CT scan.[9] Among patients with serial CT scans available for comparison, periaortic edema and interval development or expansion of an aneurysm are highly suspicious for the presence of an infected aneurysm.[9] Overall, 75% of CT scans will have findings consistent with a mycotic aneurysm in surgically proven cases of mycotic aneurysm.[3]

Arteriography may demonstrate the presence of a saccular aneurysm with lobulated contour (Fig. 2), which was found to correlate with the diagnosis of a mycotic aneurysm in 77% of cases.[9] However, the various secondary signs of a mycotic aneurysm discussed above will not be visualized on arteriography,

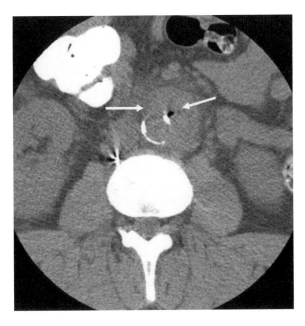

Fig. 1 CT of mycotic aneurysm. Periaortic fluid is evident anterior and lateral to the aorta with gas noted within the fluid collection (*arrows*)

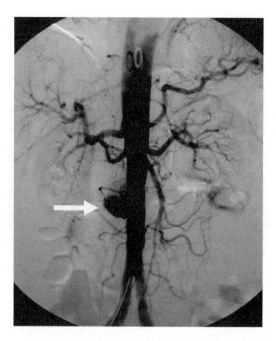

Fig. 2 Aortogram of saccular aneurysm. A lobulated saccular aneurysm (*arrow*) typical of a mycotic aneurysm is noted

relegating arteriography to answering specific anatomic questions in most cases. Nuclear imaging often shows increased activity in the vicinity of the aneurysm, consistent with an infection.[9] Magnetic resonance imaging (MRI) may show a saccular aneurysm. Since most cases may be diagnosed by clinical presentation and CT, other imaging studies such as MRI, arteriography, and nuclear imaging should be reserved for stable patients in whom the diagnosis remains uncertain.

Treatment

The first priority after the presumptive diagnosis of a mycotic aneurysm is initiation of appropriate antibiotic therapy. A history of recent septic episodes or invasive procedures will guide the choice of antibiotics based on the likely organisms.[5,6] Without such a history, broad-spectrum antibiotics are appropriate since both Gram-positive cocci and Gram-negative bacilli have been isolated from mycotic aneurysms.[3] It must be understood, however, that the role of antibiotics is simply to limit the septic complications until definitive surgical therapy may be undertaken. Without surgery to address the mycotic aneurysm, the patient is certain to progress to frank aneurysm rupture or overwhelming sepsis.

The guiding principle of surgical treatment of mycotic aneurysms is surgical debridement of the infected aortic tissue and periaortic tissue, followed by appropriate revascularization to reestablish distal perfusion. Many series include a subset of patients in whom a contained aneurysm rupture was noted at surgery,[6,8,10] so proximal and distal aortic control should be obtained well away from the inflamed segment of aorta (Fig. 3) in order to avoid inadvertent entry into a contained rupture. An important goal of surgical therapy is complete debridement of the grossly infected aorta and surrounding periaortic tissues. The aorta should be debrided back to healthy tissue (Fig. 4) which should be ascertained by direct visual inspection rather than intraoperative Gram stain or histopathology.

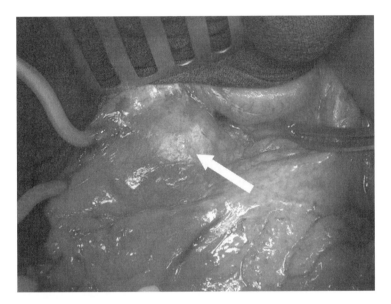

Fig. 3 Mycotic aneurysm. A bulge representing a mycotic aneurysm of the aorta is evident in the retroperitoneum (*arrow*). To the right, an aortic cross-clamp is occluding the aorta proximal to the mycotic aneurysm. To the left, tourniquets are occluding the common iliac arteries distal to the infected aneurysm

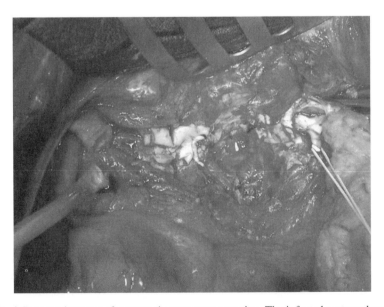

Fig. 4 Retroperitoneum after mycotic aneurysm resection. The infected aorta and peri-aortic tissues from Fig. 3 have been debrided, leaving a large defect in the aorta and proximal iliac arteries (*See Color Plates*)

After debridement, distal flow may be reconstituted by either *in situ* graft placement or aortic ligation with extra-anatomic bypass. The choice of approaches will be dictated by several factors. First, the location of the mycotic aneurysm is a primary determinant. Extra-anatomic bypass of the thoracic or paravisceral aorta is difficult and fraught with problems, so *in situ* repair is usually necessary for mycotic aneurysms in these segments of the aorta. For the infrarenal aorta, either form of aortic reconstruction (*in situ* vs extra-anatomic bypass) has been described. In this location, additional variables may dictate the approach. For instance, instability of the patient may dictate an expeditious *in situ* repair as the more appropriate strategy. The relative virulence of the organisms may also play a role in the decision-making. Intraoperative Gram stain of the resected tissue should be performed if an *in situ* repair is contemplated on a relatively stable patient, as the presence of Gram-negative rods or probable anaerobes would mitigate against an *in situ* repair in a stable patient. Conversely, the presence of Gram-positive cocci consistent with staphylococcal species is suggestive of a relatively low-grade infection that may be amenable to *in situ* repair. Cases in which there is substantial aortic destruction and the aortic wall adjacent to the aneurysm demonstrates a "tissue-paper" consistency are indicative of a high-grade infection with a relatively virulent organism, which would favor an extra-anatomic repair. In the final analysis, neither approach is appropriate for all cases, so the surgeon should be well versed in the technical aspects of both approaches.

The classic approach to treatment of infected aneurysms is aggressive debridement of the infected aortic tissue, followed by closure of the aortic stump in three layers.[10] Meticulous closure with a two layers of nonabsorbable polypropylene suture followed by reinforcement of the closure with either omentum, ligamentum flavum, or other retroperitoneal tissue is critical to minimizing the risk of stump blowout – a highly lethal complication of this operation. Distal revascularization is then performed using a prosthetic bypass through uninvolved tissue planes (extra-anatomic bypass), such as axillofemoral bypass to the lower extremities. If the diagnosis of a mycotic aneurysm is known preoperatively, the extra-anatomic bypass should be performed prior to resection of the infected aneurysm. This approach minimizes the risk of cross-contamination of the extra-anatomic bypass graft and lessens the duration of distal ischemia. The results of aortic resection with extra-anatomic bypass are reported below (in Section *Outcomes*).

In situ aortic reconstruction after resection of a mycotic aneurysm may seem contrary to the established principle of performing a bypass in an uncontaminated field whenever possible. However, several modifications to the operative technique have been introduced to minimize the risk of graft infection after *in situ* aortic repair in an infected or contaminated field. These modifications include the use of omental flap coverage of a prosthetic polyester graft, antibiotic-impregnated grafts, cryopreserved human allografts, and autogenous vein as the conduit for *in situ* repair.[6,8,11–14] Each of these approaches merits further discussion.

Omental flap coverage was described as a means of providing a vascularized pedicle flap to cover a dacron graft used for *in situ* repair in an infected operative field.[11,15] The technique for omental flap coverage involves mobilization of the omentum from the transverse colon to create a long flap that remains attached at its origin on the transverse colon, followed by transposition to the infrarenal retroperitoneal space through an opening of the transverse mesocolon to wrap the prosthetic graft and fill the infected space.[15]

The use of antibiotic-impregnated grafts was initially described as an approach for the treatment of infected aneurysms of the paravisceral aorta, where it is difficult to perform an extra-anatomic bypass. Preliminary studies by Bandyk's group found that bonding of Rifampin (1200 mg in 20 cc sterile water, >30 min) to a gelatin-impregnated dacron graft produced prolonged antistaphylococcal activity *in vivo*.[16] This group described its clinical use in two patients, and both patients survived without evidence of graft infection at 10 months. Others have adopted this approach as an alternative to extra-anatomic bypass.[8]

The use of cryopreserved allograft was initially described for *in situ* repair of an infected aneurysm of the infrarenal aorta.[17] The purported advantage of allograft is its relative resistance to reinfection, compared to Dacron grafts. Several centers in Europe preferentially use cryopreserved allograft as first-line therapy for repair of mycotic aneurysms.[5,12,13,18,19] Late aneurysmal degeneration and rupture have been described with these grafts, however.[13]

A more recent modification for *in situ* repair of the aorta involves the use of autogenous superficial femoral vein (SFV; Fig. 5). This approach was based on the experience using SFV for *in situ* aortoiliac reconstruction after excision of infected aortic grafts.[20–22] SFV offers resistance to reinfection and excellent long-term patency. The use of SFV for *in situ* repair will be described in greater detail below (see Section *Infected Aortic Grafts*). Fillmore and Valentine described the use of SFV in four patients with infected infrarenal aortic aneurysms with acceptable clinical results.[8]

With the recent advances in endovascular approaches to the treatment of aortic aneurysms, it is not surprising that aortic stent grafting has emerged as

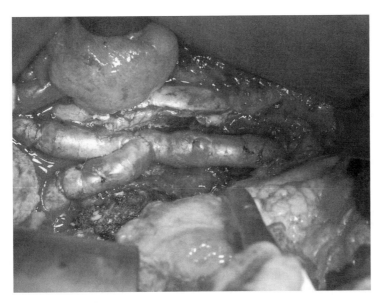

Fig. 5 *In situ* aortic repair with superficial femoral vein (*SFV*). The SFV has been used to reconstruct the aorta and iliac segments after debridement of the mycotic aneurysm pictured in Figs. 3 and 4 (*See Color Plates*)

an option for the treatment of mycotic aneurysms. The risks of placing a prosthetic graft in an infected field are obvious. However, there is precedent for this concept in the form of *in situ* repair of mycotic aneurysms using a prosthetic graft. There are significant differences in the two operations that should be recognized. The open surgical approach to *in situ* repair offers the advantage of permitting aggressive debridement of infected aorta and periaortic tissue, removing necrotic and infected tissues and decreasing the bacterial counts. In addition, the open surgical approach affords the surgeon the opportunity to use adjunctive measures to decrease the risk for reinfection, such as using an antibiotic-impregnated graft or omental flap. Nonetheless, there are potential advantages of endografting. First, endografting lessens the magnitude of the operation for patients who are usually profoundly ill. Second, endografting provides an opportunity to temporize, even definitively treat, contained ruptures in unstable patients. The results of endografting of mycotic aneurysms are discussed below (see Section *Outcomes*). Postoperative management of the treated mycotic aneurysm will entail long-term antibiotic therapy and imaging for recurrent infection. The appropriate duration of antibiotic therapy is not known. The durations of therapy described in the literature are highly variable, but most series report using 6 week of antibiotics or longer. Some authors advocate lifelong suppressive antibiotic therapy.[6,10] No studies have systematically addressed the appropriate duration of antibiotic therapy in patients with mycotic aneurysms, so all current recommendations are empiric. Surveillance of grafts placed into infected fields mandates CT scans for regular intervals. Signs of infection would include a pseudoaneurysm adjacent to a surgical repair, fluid, or air persisting around a graft more than 4 months postoperatively, or inflammatory stranding that persists beyond the perioperative period.

Outcomes

The outcomes for the treatment of mycotic aneurysms of the aorta are predictably associated with marked morbidity and mortality. Operative mortality rates for aneurysm resection range from 15% to 40% in reported series.[6,8,10,12,14,19] Reports that utilized both anatomic (*in situ*) and extra-anatomic repairs failed to show any influence of the type of reconstruction on outcomes.[6,8,19] Factors associated with increased perioperative mortality include the presence of a ruptured mycotic aneurysm, suprarenal aneurysm location, preoperative hemodynamic instability, and preoperative SIRS.[6,8,10,14]

Late reinfection of the aorta or aortic graft is surprisingly uncommon after open repair of mycotic aneurysms, occurring in 0–5% of cases regardless of the approach to aortic reconstruction.[6,10,11] The highest reported incidence of recurrent sepsis was 15%.[23] In that series, two patients died of sepsis and pneumonia after *in situ* repair.[23]

The results after endovascular stent graft repair of mycotic aneurysms of the aorta have been mixed. There have been fewer than 40 cases reported in the literature to date. Among these, there are reports of success with this form of treatment.[24–29] However, there are also cautionary tales of recurrent infection, mycotic aneurysm formation, and death due to sepsis or aneurysm rupture.[30–32] It is notable that in the five reports accounting for the majority of world-wide experience (25 patients) with endografting of mycotic aneurysms, there was a 32% incidence of recurrent sepsis or bleeding.[24,30–33] Until further data are available, endografting should be viewed as an option to temporize the patient with a ruptured or rapidly expanding mycotic aneurysm until a more definitive surgery may be performed. Endografting may be an option for patients who are too ill to undergo a more definitive repair, understanding that it may be palliative, rather than curative treatment.

Infected Aortic Grafts

Pathogenesis

Graft infection is an uncommon, but not rare, complications after aortic surgery, occurring in 1–5% of cases.[34,35] The pathogenesis of graft infection is likely multifactorial. Since *Staphylococcal* species are the most common organisms isolated from infected grafts, most authorities have concluded that the majority of graft infections occur through seeding from the patient's skin flora at the time of graft implantation.[36] Operative factors may increase the risk of an aortic graft infection. Aortic operations that require a groin incision, such an aortobifemoral bypass, increase the risk of graft infection severalfold, which probably relates the bacterial milieu of the groin. The groin is known to harbor high surface concentrations of *Staphylococcus* species.[37] Furthermore, a groin dissection to expose the femoral vessels disrupts the rich network of lymphatics that drain the leg, which may potentially release bacteria draining from the lower leg into the wound. Finally, persistent leakage of lymph fluid in the groin after a groin incision may cause a lymphocutaneous fistula, or lymphorrhea, which provides a ready portal of entry for bacterial influx from the skin and increases the risk of graft infection.

Graft contamination may also occur months or years later due to reoperation or percutaneous access of a graft for an unrelated procedure. Patients with infected aortobifemoral grafts will often relate a history of multiple procedures performed via a graft limb that presents with evidence of infection months or years later. These procedures may inadvertently expose the graft to skin flora despite topical antiseptic preparation of the skin.

Clinical Presentation

The presentation for aortic graft infections varies according to the time frame after surgery. Bandyk defined *early* graft infections as those occurring within 4 months of surgery, while *late* graft infections presented after 4 months.[36] He further subdivided graft infections based on their presentation as perigraft infection, graft-enteric erosion, and graft-enteric fistula. The latter two categories will be addressed in a separate chapter. The remainder of this section will be devoted to perigraft infections. Early perigraft infections usually present as a surgical site infection or wound complication with graft exposure. Purulent drainage and signs of sepsis are the most common findings. Less-frequent manifestations of a perigraft infection are pseudoaneurysm formation or anastamotic disruption with hemorrhage. Early infection of an aortic graft confined to the abdomen usually presents with relatively nonspecific findings such as an ileus, persistent low-grade fever, or leukocytosis. The most common organism isolated from early graft infections is *Staphyloccus aureus*.

Late graft infections (>4 months after surgery) may present as a persistent sinus tract, anastamotic pseudoaneurysm or rupture, graft occlusion, or sepsis. There is also a subset of patients who remain asymptomatic. A graft infection in the latter subset is discovered incidentally during an imaging study for an unrelated indication. Most late graft infections present more than 1 year after graft implantation. The most common organism for late graft infections is *Staphylococcus epidermidis*. *S. epidermidis* produces a glycocalyx slime layer, or biofilm, that coats the graft, shielding the organisms from phagocytosis. This biofilm produces the "unincorporated" appearance of a graft that is characteristic of a perigraft infection at operative exploration. This finding has been associated with positive cultures in 71% of cases.[38]

Diagnosis and Imaging

Early graft infections involving aortic grafts confined to the abdomen present a particular challenge for diagnosis. These infections produce nonspecific signs, such as a persistent ileus, fever, or leukocytosis. As will be discussed below, imaging is rarely helpful in the early postoperative period unless a pseudoaneurysm or rupture is visualized. If there is a high index of suspicion, operative exploration and examination of the graft for purulence may be necessary to ascertain the diagnosis. Fortunately infections of aortic grafts confined to the abdomen are rare.

The vast majority of *early* graft infections involve aortic grafts that include a groin incision. An early graft infection in this circumstance will manifest as a wound infection in the groin overlying the graft. While cellulitis may be treated initially with empiric antibiotics, any significant drainage or partial dehiscence of the postoperative wound overlying a wound mandate operative exploration. The goal of operative exploration is to ascertain the full extent and depth of involvement of the wound in any infectious process. If there is viable, uninfected tissue overlying the graft, the likelihood of graft infection is low. If the infectious process extends to the graft, however, the graft itself is assumed to be infected and definitive therapy should be planned. Any graft that develops an early postoperative pseudoaneurysm or hemorrhage should be considered infected.

Late graft infections are usually more subtle in presentation. Any aortic graft that presents with a persistent wound or sinus tract overlying a graft, anastamotic pseudoaneurysm, or graft thrombosis should be investigated further with an imaging study. Anastamotic pseudoaneurysms may be caused by late degeneration of the arterial to which a graft is sutured, but 60% of anastamotic pseudoaneurysms are culture positive.[39] There are several choices for imaging for possible graft infection, including CT, MRI, radionuclide scanning, ultrasound, and arteriography. The utility of each modality will be discussed.

CT provides excellent visualization of the various secondary signs of a *late* graft infection, including ectopic gas, perigraft fluid, increased perigraft inflammatory changes ("stranding"), anastomotic pseudoaneurysm, and thickening of adjacent bowel (Fig. 6).[40–43] CT scan has a sensitivity of 94% for the diagnosis of late graft infection.[44] In his series of 12 patients, Low et al. found that the presence of perigraft fluid, increased perigraft soft tissue, or ectopic gas identified all cases of graft infections, providing a sensitivity

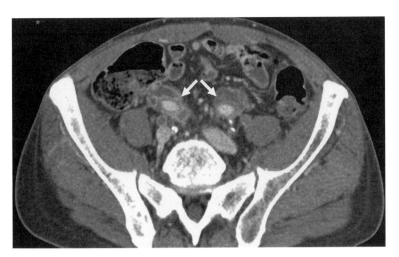

Fig. 6 Perigraft fluid. Note the loculated fluid surrounding the two limbs (*arrows*) of an aortobifemoral bypass graft

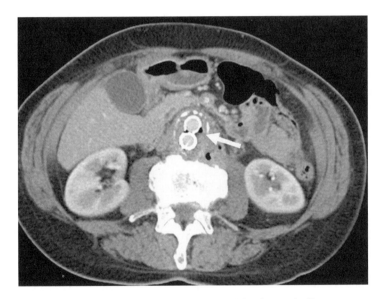

Fig. 7 Gas adjacent to aortic endograft. Gas (*arrow*) is observed adjacent to an aortic endograft years after graft implantation

100%.[44] Ectopic gas is the only single finding that is diagnostic of a late graft infection, but it is present in a minority of cases (Fig. 7).[44]

In contrast, CT offers little assistance in the diagnosis of *early* graft infections because perigraft hematoma and retained ambient gas are normal findings in the early postoperative period. Serial scanning of postoperative aortic grafts found that perigraft hematoma should resolve within 3 months, and no ectopic gas should be present beyond 3–4 weeks after surgery.[45] By 3 months after graft implantation, hematoma should resorb, perigraft tissue planes should normalize, and perigraft fluid should be minimal (<5 mm) or

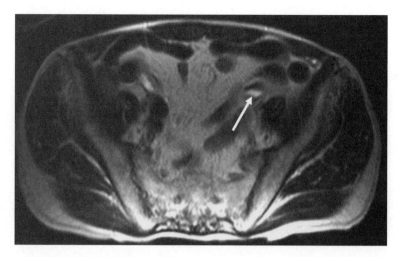

Fig. 8 MRI with T2-weighted image. This heavily weighted T2 image shows high-intensity signal (*arrow*) posterior to the left limb of an aortobifemoral bypass graft

absent.[40,44,45] After 3 months, CT scanning is considered the diagnostic test of choice in most cases.

MRI is an alternative modality for imaging-suspected aortic graft infections. On MRI, the perigraft fluid of a graft infection is characterized by a low-to-medium intensity signal on T1-weighted images and high intensity on T2-weighted images (Fig. 8).[46] The characteristic T1- and T2-weighted images will also permit differentiation of perigraft fluid soft tissue inflammation from subacute or chronic hematoma, which is a distinction that is difficult on CT.[47] Using operative exploration as the gold standard for comparison, Auffermann et al. found that MRI had a sensitivity of 85% and a specificity of 100%.[46] A shortcoming of MRI is its inability to distinguish perigraft gas from calcification in the remnant aorta.[47] Because the characteristic high-intensity signal on T2-weighted images permits visualization of even small amounts of fluid, MRI remains an important modality for imaging of graft infections and is often used when CT findings are equivocal for graft infection.

Radionuclide scanning using [111]indium-labeled white blood cells (WBCs; Fig. 9) is the favored approach of many infectious disease specialists. The advantage of this approach is its high sensitivity, which approaches 100% in some centers.[48–50] The primary shortcoming of radionuclide scanning has been a propensity for yielding false positive results, producing relatively low specificity (80–82%).[48–50] It has been suggested that inadvertent radiolabeling and inclusion of platelets in the [111]indium-labeled WBC preparation may result in nonspecific adherence of the platelets to pseudointima of a vascular grafts, leading to a false positive results. This phenomenon is particularly evident in the early postoperative period when there is active adherence of platelets to a prosthetic graft. Sedwitz et al. found that [111]indium-labeled WBC scans are positive in 80% of grafts imaged within 4 months of implantation.[51] Thus, indium scanning offers no help in the diagnosis of a suspected *early* graft infection. For the diagnosis of *late* graft infections, the utility of radionuclide scanning remains a subject of debate. The combination of high sensitivity and specificity for CT and MRI has supplanted indium scanning in most centers.

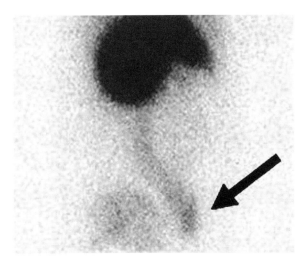

Fig. 9 [111]Indium-labeled WBC scan. Increased activity (*arrow*) indicative of a possible graft infection is noted on lateral view of an aortobifemoral bypass graft

Ultrasonography offers few advantages for the diagnosis of graft infection. Imaging of intra-abdominal portions of an aortic graft with ultrasonography is difficult, and the resolution is usually insufficient to provide adequate information. Arteriography plays an equally limited role in the diagnosis of graft infections. While anastamotic pseudoaneurysms are well visualized by arteriography, the majority of extraluminal manifestations of a graft infection will not be imaged by arteriography. The primary role of arteriography is to provide anatomic information for planning definitive therapy after the diagnosis of a graft infection is secure.

Some authors have proposed using CT guidance for percutaneous aspiration of perigraft fluid to confirm the diagnosis of a graft infection.[52,53] The pitfall to this technique is the risk of seeding a sterile perigraft fluid collection while performing the aspiration. Considering the exceptional sensitivity and specificity of CT and MRI, this risk cannot be justified in most cases. Belair et al. tested percutaneous drainage as a therapeutic modality for the treatment of confirmed aortic graft infections.[53] In 11 patients, 4 were successfully treated with percutaneous drainage and antibiotics alone. Of the remaining seven patients, six ultimately proceeded to surgery for surgical drainage or graft excision, and one died of procedure-related hemorrhage. Percutaneous drainage should be reserved for patients who cannot survive a more definitive procedure.

Treatment

The guiding principles in the surgical management of infected aortic grafts are analogous to the principles outlined for management of mycotic aneurysms. Surgical dogma has traditionally dictated the standard of care to be complete graft excision, ligation of the aorta, and extra-anatomic bypass through uninfected tissue planes. This approach remains a viable option in many cases. Recognizing the magnitude of this operation and its physiological impact on patients, the University of California at San Francisco group recommended a staged approach to this operation. They proposed performing the extra-anatomic bypass first, followed in 1–2 days by the definitive graft excision. This approach not only separated the clean and contaminated components of surgical management, but it produced better physiological outcomes.[54] Other groups have adopted this approach with reasonable outcomes.[55] However, this approach is not without significant potential pitfalls, such as a risk of aortic stump blowout, late infection of the prosthetic extra-anatomic bypass, and poor long-term graft patency of extra-anatomic bypasses.[34,54,55]

In situ replacement of an infected graft has been proposed as an alternative to aortic ligation with extra-anatomic bypass. The appeal of this approach lies in its direct revascularization of the lower extremities and avoidance of an extra-anatomic bypass with inferior long-term patency. Moreover, the predominance of relatively low virulence organisms, such as *S. epidermidis*, is probably the optimal circumstance for *in situ* repair. Various conduits have been proposed for *in situ* repair. Antibiotic-impregnated prosthetic graft replacement, adjunctive omental flap coverage of prosthetic grafts, and the use of arterial allografts were discussed previously (see Section *Mycotic Aneurysms*). The use of SFV for *in situ* graft replacement was described by Clagett et al.[20] Clagett described the creation of a neo-aortoiliac system with SFV to reconstruct the aortoiliac segments after complete graft excision. The purported advantages of SFV are its relative resistance to infection, excellent long-term patency, and avoidance of stump blowout. The technique for harvest is described in detail elsewhere.[56] Harvesting SFV for aortic reconstruction causes surprisingly little venous morbidity in the harvested limbs.[57–59] The primary disadvantage of this approach is the length and magnitude of this operation. Two teams of surgeons are optimal for this operation, and the mean duration of this operation is 8 h.[34]

In cases in which the entire graft is not infected, partial graft excision is an option. The advantage of this approach is the ability to minimize the extent of operation in relatively infirmed patients. The concern with this approach relates to the risk of recurrent infection in the residual graft. The results for each approach to aortic graft infection are described below (see Section *Outcomes*).

Outcomes

Total graft excision with extra-anatomic bypass has been associated with 11–12% operative mortality.[55,60] Seeger reported that only one aortic stump blowout occurred in his series of 36 patients.[55] The rate of reinfection of the prosthetic extra-anatomic bypass was equally low (1 in 36 grafts) in that series. Others have reported higher rates of reinfection of the extra-anatomic bypass, ranging from 10% to 20%.[34,61] Seeger found that the long-term patency of the extra-anatomic bypass was dependent on the type of bypass performed. The 5-year primary patency rates were 75% and 64% for axillofemoral–femoral bypass and axillofemoral bypasses, respectively, whereas none of the axillo-popliteal bypasses were patent beyond 7 months.[55]

The operative mortality rate for *in situ* repair varies between 4% and 18%.[62,63] This approach is associated with an inherent risk of reinfection of the prosthetic graft, which complicates 10–11% of cases.[62–64] A nonrandomized cohort study from the Mayo Clinic compared *in situ* repair using either antibiotic impregnated grafts or omental flap coverage (or both adjuncts), compared with traditional aortic ligation with extra-anatomic bypass.[65]*In situ* repair provided superior 5-year primary patency (89%) versus axillofemoral bypass (48%).[65] Moreover, major morbidity or procedure-related mortality were twofold higher after graft excision with axillofemoral bypass compared with *in situ* reconstruction.[65] Operative mortality, limb salvage, and reinfection rates were not statistically different between groups, although all trends favored *in situ* repair.[65] These data argue strongly that *in situ* repair with omental flap coverage or antibiotic impregnated grafts is superior to extra-anatomic reconstructions.

In situ graft replacement with human allograft has yielded mixed results. Leseche reported a series of 28 patients in whom there were no recurrent infections over a mean follow-up of 35 months.[66] Kieffer et al. reported a series of 179 patients operated for aortic graft infections or secondary aortoenteric fistulas.[67] In that series, the operative mortality was 20.1%. Early and late allograft ruptures occurred in 2.8% and 2.1% cases, respectively. Vogt et al. described a series of mycotic aneurysms and aortic graft infections in which there was a 16% incidence of allograft-related technical complications.[13] The US cryopreserved aortic allograft registry reported a 20% incidence of allograft-related complications, including 9% rate of reinfection.[68] Based on these reports, there appears to be a propensity for reinfection or rupture of allografts. The role of allograft in the management of infected aortic grafts remains undefined.

In the original series reported by Clagett on the use of SFV for *in situ* aortic reconstruction, the operative mortality was 10%.[20] No grafts became infected, and there was 100% patency at a mean follow-up of 22 months. In that series, a separate cohort of patients underwent reconstruction using saphenous vein, but those grafts universally failed. In a follow-up study of 41 patients by the same group, the mortality for SFV reconstruction after infected graft excision was 7.3% and the primary patency was 83%.[21] Similar results have been reported by other groups. A report from Belgium described an 8% operative mortality and a 5-year primary patency of 91%.[69] With expanded indications for the use of SFV, potential pitfalls have emerged. Graft-related hemorrhage has been observed in 11 of 364 patients (3%).[70] Although 3 of the 11 episodes of bleeding were caused by technical errors, 8 of the 11 patients experienced hemorrhage as a consequence of infection of the vein graft. Despite this report, it is apparent that reinfection is relatively infrequent event compared to the alternative approaches to *in situ* aortic reconstruction. Venous morbidity after SFV harvest includes a 17% incidence of fasciotomy and a 15% incidence of minor venous insufficiency (CEAP Class C_3, leg edema, or less). These data indicate that *in situ* reconstruction with SFV offers the greatest opportunity for a definitive repair without mortality, graft occlusion, or graft infection. However, this approach may not appropriate for all patients.

For grafts in which preoperative imaging suggests that only a portion is infected, such as a femoral limb of aortobifemoral bypass, partial excision is a viable option. A critical prerequisite for this approach is meticulous care to avoid cross-contaminating uninfected portions of the graft. Separate studies by Towne and Calligaro found that 86–92% of grafts will remain free of infection during follow-up using this approach.[71,72] If partial excision is attempted, careful long-term surveillance with CT is an important component of the follow-up of these patients.

Summary

Mycotic aneurysms of the aorta and aortic graft infections are dreaded complications of aortic disease. A thoughtful plan for treatment that is tailored to each case will minimize the risk of major morbidity or mortality. For mycotic aneurysms *in situ* and extra-anatomic approaches are both viable options, while endovascular repair should be reserved for patients unable to tolerate more definitive procedures. For infected aortic grafts, evidence suggests that *in situ* repair offer significant advantages over traditional extra-anatomic approaches. Clearly, however, no single approach is appropriate for all patients, so a thorough understanding of the various options and their utility will permit the clinician to optimize outcomes.

References

1. Osler W. Gulstonian lectures on malignant endocarditis. Br Med J 1985;1: 467–470.
2. Hawkins J, Yeager G. Primary mycotic aneurysm. Surgery 1956;40:747–756.
3. Miller DV, Oderich GS, Aubry M-C, Panneton JM, Edwards WD. Surgical pathology of infected aneurysms of the descending thoracic and abdominal aorta: Clinicopathologic correlations in 29 cases (1976 to 1999). Hum Pathol 2004;35:1112–1120.
4. Revell STRJr . Primary mycotic aneurysms. Ann Intern Med 1945;22:431–440.
5. Muller BT, Wegener OR, Grabitz K, Phillny M, Thomas L, Sandmann W. Mycotic aneurysms of the thoracic and abdominal aorta and iliac arteries: Experience with anatomic and extra-anatomic repair in 33 cases. J Vasc Surg 2001;33:106–113.
6. Oderich GS, Panneton JM, Bower TC, Cherry KJJr, Rowland CM, Noel AA, Hallett JWJr , Gloviczki P. Infected aortic aneurysms: Aggressive presentation, complicated early outcome, but durable results. J Vasc Surg 2001;34:900–9008.
7. Muchart DJ, Bhagwanjee S. American College of Chest Physicians/Society of Critical Care Medicine Consensus Conference definitions of systemic inflammatory response syndrome and allied disorders in relation to critically injured patients. Crit Care Med 1997;25:1281–1286.
8. Fillmore AJ, Valentine RJ. Surgical mortality in patients with infected aortic aneurysms. J Am Coll Surg 2003;196:435–441.
9. Macedo TA, Stanton AW, Oderich GS, Johnson CM, Panneton JM, Tie ML. Infected aortic aneurysms: Imaging findings. Radiology 2004;231:250–257.
10. Moneta GL, Taylor LM, Jr., Yeager RA, Edwards JM, Nicoloff AD, McConnell DB, Porter JM. Surgical treatment of infected aortic aneurysm. Am J Surg 1998;175:396–399.
11. Fichelle JM, Tabet G, Cormier P, Farkas JC, Laurian C, Gigou F, Marzelle J, Acar J, Cormier JM. Infected infrarenal aortic aneurysms: When is in situ reconstruction safe? J Vasc Surg 1993;17:635-645.
12. Arbatli H, DeGeest R, Demirsoy E, Wellens F, Degrieck I, VanPraet F, Korkut AK, Vanermen H. Management of infected grafts and mycotic aneurysms of the aorta using cryopreserved homografts. Cardiovasc Surg 2003;11:257–263.
13. Vogt PR, Brunner-LaRocca HP, Lachat M, Ruef C, Turina MI. Technical details with the use of cryopreserved arterial allografts for aortic infection: Influence on early and midterm mortality. J Vasc Surg 2002;35:80–86.

14. Ihaya A, Chiba Y, Kimura T, Morioka K, Uesaka T. Surgical outcome of infectious aneurysm of the abdominal aorta with or without SIRS. Cardiovasc Surg 2001;9:436–440.

15. Yokoyama H, Maida K, Takahashi S, Tanaka S. Purulently infected abdominal aortic aneurysm: In situ reconstruction with transmesocolic omental transposition technique. Cardiovasc Surg 1994;2:78–80.

16. Gupta AK, Bandyk DF, Johnson BL. In situ repair of mycotic abdominal aortic aneurysms with rifampin-bonded gelatin-impregnated Dacron grafts: A preliminary case report. J Vasc Surg 1996;24:472–476.

17. Alonso M, Caeiro S, Cachaldora J, Segura R. Infected abdominal aortic aneurysm: In situ replacement with cryopreserved arterial homograft. J Cardiovasc Surg 1997;38:371–375.

18. Kerzmann A, Ausselet N, Daenen G, Linder JL. Infected abdominal aortic aneurysm treated by in situ replacement with cryopreserved arterial homograft. Acta Chir Belg 2006;106:447–449.

19. Muller BT, Wegener OR, Grabitz K, Pillny M, Thomas L, Sandmann W. Mycotic aneurysms of the thoracic and abdominal aorta: Experience with anatomic and extra-anatomic repair in 33 cases. J Vasc Surg 2002;33:106–113.

20. Clagett GP, Bowers BL, Lopez-Viego MA, Rossi MB, Valentine RJ, Myers SI, Chervu A. Creation of a neo-aortoiliac system from lower extremity deep and superficial veins. Ann Surg 1993;218:239–249.

21. Clagett GP, Valentine RJ, Hagino RT. Autogenous aortoiliac/femoral reconstruction from superficial femoral-popliteal veins: Feasibility and durability. J Vasc Surg 1007;25:255–270.

22. Gordon LL, Hagino RT, Jackson MR, Modrall JG, Valentine RJ, Clagett GP. Complex aortofemoral prosthetic infections: The role of autogenous superficial femoropopliteal vein reconstruction. Arch Surg 1999;134:615–621.

23. Ting AC, Cheng SW, Ho P, Poon JT, Tsu JH. Surgical treatment of infected aneurysms and pseudoaneurysms of the thoracic and abdominal aorta. Am J Surg 2005;189:150–154.

24. Semba CP, Sakai T, Slonim SM, Razavi MK, Kee ST, Jorgensen MJ, Hagberg RC, Lee GK, Mitchell RS, Miller DC, Dake MD. Mycotic aneurysms of the thoracic aorta: Repair with use of endovascular stent-grafts. J Vasc Interv Radiol, 1998;9:33–40.

25. Kinney EV, Kaebnick HW, Mitchell RA, Jung MT. Repair of mycotic paravisceral aneurysm with a fenestrated stent-graft. J Endovasc Ther 2000;7:192–197.

26. Madhavan P, McDonnell CO, Dowd MO, Sultan SA, Doyle M, Colgan MP, McEniff N, Molloy M, Moore DJ, Shanik GD. Suprarenal mycotic aneurysm exclusion using a stent with a partial autologous covering. J Endovasc Ther 2000;7:404–409

27. Bond SE, McGuinness CL, Reidy JF, Taylor PR. Repair of secondary aortoesophageal fistula by endoluminal stent-grafting. J Endovasc Ther 2001;8:597–601.

28. Bell RE, Taylor PR, Aukett M, Evans GH, Reidy JF. Successful endoluminal repair of an infected thoracic pseudoaneurysm caused by methicillin-resistant Staphylococcus aureus. J Endovasc Ther 2003;10:29–32.

29. Koeppel TA, Gahlen J, Diehl S, Prosst RL, Dueber C. Mycotic aneurysm of the abdominal aorta with retroperitoneal abscess: Successful endovascular repair. J Vasc Surg 2004;40:164–166.

30. Forbes TL, Harding GEJ. Endovascular repair of Salmonella-infected abdominal aortic aneurysms: A word of caution. J Vasc Surg 2005;44:198–200.

31. Jones KG, Bell RE, Sabharwal T, Aukett M, Reidy JF, Taylor PR. Treatment of mycotic aortic aneurysms with endoluminal grafts. Eur J Vasc Endovasc Surg 2005;29:139–144.

32. Lee KH, Won JY, Lee DY, Choi D, Shim WH, Chang BC, Park SJ. Stent-graft treatment of infected aortic and arterial aneurysms. J Endovasc Ther 2006;13:338–345.

33. Stanley BM, Semmens JB, Lawrence-Brown MMD, Denton M, Grosser D. Endoluminal repair of mycotic thoracic aneurysms. J Endovasc Ther 2003;10: 511–515.

34. Valentine RJ. Diagnosis and management of aortic graft infection. Sem Vasc Surg 2001;14:292–301.
35. Hallett JWJr , Marshall DM, Petterson TM, Gray DT, Bower TC, Cherry KJ Jr., Glovicski P, Pairolero PC. Graft-related complications after abdominal aortic aneurysm repair: Reassurance from a 36-year population-based experience. J Vasc Surg 1997; 25:277–284.
36. Bandyk DF, Esses GE. Aortic graft infection. Surg Clin North Am 1994;74:571–590.
37. Seabrook GR. Pathobiology of graft infections. Sem Vasc Surg 1990;3:77–80.
38. Padberg FT, Jr, Smith SM, Eng RH. Accuracy of disincorporation for identification of vascular graft infection. Arch Surg 1995;130:183–187.
39. Seabrook GR, Schmitt DD, Bandyk DF, Edmiston CE, Krepel CJ, Towne JB. Anastamotic femoral pseudoaneurysms: An investigation of occult infection as an etiologic factor. J Vasc Surg 1990;11:629–634.
40. Hilton S, Megibow AJ, Naidich DP, Bosniak MA. Computed tomography of the postoperative abdominal aorta. Radiology 1982;145:403–407.
41. Mark A, Moss AA, Lusby R, Kaiser JA. CT evaluation of complications of aortic surgery. Radiology 1982;145:409–414.
42. Mark AS, Moss AA, McCarthy S, McCowin M. CT of aortoenteric fistulas. Invest Radiol 1985;20:272–275.
43. Haaga JR, Baldwin GN, Reich NE, Beven E, Weinstein A, Havrilla TR, Seidelmann FE, Namba AH, Parrish CM. CT detection of infected synthetic grafts: Preliminary report of a new sign. Am J Roentgenol 1978;131:317–320.
44. Low RN, Wall SD, Jeffrey RBJr , Sollitto RA, Reilly LM, Tierney LMJr . Aortoenteric fistula and perigraft infection. Radiology 1990;175:157–162.
45. Qvafordt PG, Reilly LM, Mark AS, Goldstone J, Wall SD, Ehrenfeld WK, Stoney RJ. Computerized tomographic assessment of graft incorporation after reconstruction. Am J Surg 1985;150:227–231.
46. Auffermann W, Olofsson PA, Rabahie GN, Tavares NJ, Stoney RJ, Higgins CB. Incorporation versus infection of retroperitoneal aortic grafts: MR imaging features. Radiology 1989;172:359–362.
47. Orton DF, LeVeen RF, Saigh JA, Culp WC, Fidler JL, Lynch TJ, Goertzen TC, McCowan TC. Aortic prosthetic graft infections: Radiologic manifestations and implications for management. RadioGraphics 2000;20:977–993.
48. Brunner MC, Mitchell RS, Baldwin JC, James DR, Olcott C 4th, Mehigan JT, McDougall IR, Miller DC. Prosthetic graft infections: Limitations of indium white blood cell scanning. J Vasc Surg 1986;3:42–48.
49. Lawrence PF, Dries DJ, Alazraki N, Albo DJr . Indium 111-labeled leukocyte scanning for detection of prosthetic vascular graft infection. J Vasc Surg 1985;2:165–173.
50. Reilly DT, Grigg MJ, Cunningham DA. Vascular graft infection: The role of indium scanning. Eur J Vasc Surg 1989;3:393–397.
51. Sedwitz MM, Davies RJ, Pretorisu HT, Vasquez TE. Indium 111-labeled white blood cell scans after vascular prosthetic reconstruction. J Vasc Surg 1987;6:476–481.
52. Harris KA, Kozak R, Carroll SE, Meads GE, Sweeney JP. Confirmation of infection of an aortic graft. J Cardiovasc Surg 1989;30:230–232.
53. Belair M, Soulez G, Oliva VL, Laperriere J, Gianfelice D, Blair JF, Sarrazin J, Therasse E. Aortic graft infections: The value of percutaneous drainage. Am J Roentgenol 1998;171:119–24.
54. Reilly LM, Stoney RJ, Goldstone J, Ehrenfeld WK. Improved management of aortic graft infection: The influence of operation sequence and staging. J Vasc Surg 1987;5:421–431.
55. Seeger JM, Pretus HA, Welborn MB, Ozaki CK, Flynn TC, Huber TS. Long-term outcome after treatment of aortic graft infection with staged extra-anatomic bypass grafting and aortic graft removal. J Vasc Surg 2000;32:451–459.
56. Valentine RJ. Harvesting the superficial femoral vein as an autograft. Sem Vasc Surg 2000;13:257–264.

57. Modrall JG, Sadjadi J, Ali AT, Anthony T, Welborn MBIII , Valentine RJ, Hynan LS, Clagett GP. Deep vein harvest: Predicting need for fasciotomy. J Vasc Surg 2004;39:387–394.

58. Wells JK, Hagino RT, Bargmann KM, Jackson MR, Valentine RJ, Kakish HB, Clagett GP. Venous morbidity after superficial femoral-popliteal vein harvest. J Vasc Surg 1998;29:282–291.

59. Modrall JG, Hocking JA, Rosero E, Timaran CH, Arko FAIII , Valentine RJ, Clagett GP. Late incidence of chronic venous insufficiency after deep vein harvest. J Vasc Surg 2007;46:520–525.

60. Yeager RA, Taylor LM, Jr., Moneta GL, Edwards JM, Nicoloff AD, McConnell DB, Porter JM. Improved results with conventional management of infrarenal aortic infection. J Vasc Surg 1999;30:76–83.

61. Reilly LM, Altman H, Lusby RJ, Kersh RA, Ehrenfeld WK, Stoney RJ. Late results following surgical management of vascular graft infection. J Vasc Surg 1984;1:36–44.

62. Bandyk DF, Novotney ML, Back MR, Johnson BL, Schmacht DC. Expanded application of in situ replacement for prosthetic graft infection. J Vasc Surg 2001;34:411–419.

63. Hayes PD, Nasim A, London NJ, Sayers RD, Barrie WW, Bell PR, Naylor AR. In situ replacement of infected aortic grafts with rafampicin-bonded prostheses: The Leicester experience (1992 to 1998). J Vasc Surg 1999;30:92–98.

64. Young RM, Cherry KJJr , Davis PM, Glovicski P, Bower TC, Panneton JM, Hallet JWJr . The results of in situ prosthetic replacement for infected aortic grafts. Am J Surg 1999;178:136–140.

65. Oderich GS, Bower TC, Cherry KJJr , Panneton JM, Sullivan TM, Noel AA, Carmo M, Cha S, Kalra M, Glovicski P. Evolution from axillofemoral to in situ prosthetic reconstruction for the treatment of aortic graft infections at a single center. J Vasc Surg 2006;43:1166–1174.

66. Leseche G, Castier Y, Petit MD, Bertrand P, Kitzis M, Mussot S, Besnard M, Cerceau O. Long-term results of cryopreserved arterial allograft reconstruction in infected prosthetic grafts and mycotic aneurysms of the abdominal aorta. J Vasc Surg 2001;34:616–622.

67. Kieffer E, Gomes D, Chiche L, Fleron MH, Koskas F, Bahnini A. Allograft replacement for infrarenal aortic graft infection: Early and late results in 179 patients. J Vasc Surg 2004;39:1009–1017.

68. Noel AA, Glovicski P, Cherry KJJr , Safi H, Goldstone J, Morasch MD, Johansen JH. Abdominal aortic reconstruction in infected fields: Early results of the United States cryopreserved aortic allograft registry. J Vasc Surg 2002;35:847–852.

69. Daenens K, Fourneau I, Nevelsteen A. Ten-year experience in autogenous reconstruction with the femoral vein in the treatment of aortofemoral prosthetic infection. Eur J Vasc Endovasc Surg 2003;25:240–245.

70. Ali AT, Bell C, Modrall JG, Valentine RJ, Clagett GP. Graft-associated hemorrhage from femoropopliteal vein grafts. J Vasc Surg 2005;42:667–672.

71. Towne JB, Seabrook GR, Bandyk DF, Freischlag JA, Edmiston CE. In situ replacement of arterial prosthesis infection by bacterial biofilms: Long-term follow-up. J Vasc Surg 1994;19:226–233.

72. Calligaro KD, Veith FJ, Valladares JA, McKay J, Schindler N, Dougherty MJ. Prosthetic patch remnants to treat infected arterial grafts. J Vasc Surg 2000;31:245–252.

Chapter 16

Evaluation and Management of Aortoenteric Fistula

Martin J. Carignan and Marc A. Passman

Abstract Aortoenteric fistula is a life-threatening problem presenting either as a primary disease process of the aorta and alimentary tract or as a secondary aortic graft-related complication. A high index of suspicion and diagnostic testing are essential for prompt identification. Nonoperative management carries 100% mortality. Once diagnosis of an aortoenteric fistula has been made, there is no role for conservative medical management, and prompt surgical treatment is mandatory. Even with the most appropriate treatment, the outcome for operative treatment of aortoenteric fistula carries high morbidity and mortality rates.

Keywords Aortoenteric fistula, Aortic graft infection

Definition

An aortoenteric fistula is an uncommon, but potentially serious and life-threatening communication between the aorta and the gastrointestinal tract. A *primary aortoenteric fistula*, first described by Sir Astley Cooper in 1829, is a consequence of either aortic or gastrointestinal pathology which causes an inflammatory or erosive reaction leading to a communication between these two adjacent structures.[1] Because of the anatomic relationship between the infrarenal aorta and the duodenal–jejunal junction, a primary aortoenteric fistula usually occurs between an infrarenal abdominal aortic aneurysm and the third or fourth portion of the duodenum, but can occur less frequently with other aortic diseases and other bowel segments. Primary aortoenteric fistulae are rare with a reported incidence in the general population of approximately 0.04–0.07% based on autopsy studies, and 0.1–0.8% in patients with aortic aneurysm, although it is likely that many of these cases go underreported.[2] A *secondary aortoenteric fistula*, as described by Brock in 1953, is a communication between a previously reconstructed aorta and the gastrointestinal tract.[3] These can occur after prior endarterectomy, prosthetic graft or homograft, or more recently endovascular stent graft.[4] Secondary aortoenteric

G. Upchurch and E. Criado (eds.) *Aortic Aneurysms, Contemporary Cardiology*
DOI: 10.1007/978-1-60327-204-9_16, © Humana Press, a part of
Springer Science+Business Media, LLC 2009

fistula is more common than primary, with a previously reported incidence of 10% after aortic repairs, which has decreased to 1% with improvements in surgical technique, suture, and graft material over the last few decades.[5,6]

Although aortoenteric fistula is uncommon, when present, potential for morbidity and mortality is significant. A high index of suspicion along with rapid diagnosis is critical for patient survival. The surgical correction of this life-threatening and complex problem requires an operative team well-versed in the management of these difficult patients with multiple medical problems often presenting in hemorrhagic or septic shock. In the acute setting, the gastrointestinal tract and the aorta require reconstruction while controlling sepsis and ongoing hemorrhage. The following text will review the pathophysiology, clinical presentation, diagnostic algorithm, treatment options, and outcomes for both primary and secondary aortoenteric fistulae.

Pathophysiology

For aortoenteric fistula formation, there is usually an underlying inflammatory process in either the aorta or the gastrointestinal tract that causes the formation of the fistula. Mechanical forces related to aortic pulsation may also lead to erosion of the aorta into adjacent structures. The anatomic proximity of the anterior surface of the infrarenal aorta and relatively fixed third and fourth portions of the duodenum within the retroperitonum explains this most common location. Eighty-three percent of aortoenteric fistulae are between the infrarenal aorta and the duodenum, while a smaller percentage will occur elsewhere including the esophagus, stomach, jejunum, ileum, appendix, and colon.[7–10] An association with infection also exists, including mycotic aneurysms, tuberculosis, and syphilis for primary aortoenteric fistula and graft infection for secondary fistula, although it is unclear whether the infection is the initial cause or a consequence of the process. For primary aortoenteric fistula, aortic pathology that may cause fistulization with the intestinal tract may include aneurysmal degeneration of the aorta, ruptured abdominal aorta, mycotic aortic aneurysm, inflammatory aneurysm, and primary aortitis. For secondary aortoenteric fistula, additional factors may include aortic graft suture line failure with proximal anastomotic disruption, and pseudoaneuysm formation with subsequent erosion into adjacent bowel. The pathogenesis of secondary aortoenteric fistula is unknown, but technical problems at initial aortic operation, repetitive mechanical trauma from aortic pulsation leading to erosion of the graft into the intestine, suture or graft material fatigue over time, inadvertent bowel injury and delayed indolent graft infection have been implicated. While the indication for initial aortic repair, aneurysm versus occlusive disease does not seem to predispose to aortic graft enteric fistula formation, repair of ruptured aortic aneurysm is associated with a higher potential for aortoenteric fistula than elective aneurysm repair, with an incidence of 1.7% and 0.7%, respectively. Prevention of secondary aortoenteric fistula is best at the time of initial aortic graft placement with measures consisting of strict aseptic technique, perioperative antibiotics, hemostasis at the suture line, complete covering of prosthetic material with retroperitonum, graft bolsters over the suture line, and a retroperitoneal approach having been suggested to reduce fistula formation.[11] Less commonly, pathological processes in the gastrointestinal tract such as esophagitis, peptic ulcer disease, ingested foreign body, cholecystitis, pancreatitis, appendicitis, diverticulitis, pancreatic pseudocyst, radiation injury, and malignancy have also been implicated.[12]

Clinical Presentation

Symptoms and signs of an aortoenteric fistula are varied, but include gastrointestinal bleeding (84%), fever (30%), abdominal pain (33%), back pain (20%), and abdominal pulsatile mass (7%). For patients presenting with gastrointestinal bleeding, melena (41%) and hematemesis (47%) are seen most often. The diagnosis of secondary aortoenteric fistula should be suspected in any patient with symptoms of gastrointestinal bleeding and prior aortic bypass graft until proven otherwise. Most commonly, secondary aortoenteric fistula will present between 2 and 6 years after the implantation of the graft. Patients usually present with a "herald bleed," which is a brief and brisk episode of bleeding that stops. The normal clotting mechanism temporarily thromboses the fistula tract causing melena, hematochezia, hematemesis, and chronic anemia at the time of initial presentation. Although a mean duration of bleeding episode prior to diagnosis has been reported as long as 25 days, potential recurrent delayed life-threatening hemorrhage is possible, and when aortoenteric fistula is suspected, prompt diagnosis and treatment is important.[13] Once aortoenteric fistula has been excluded, other more common causes of upper gastrointestinal hemorrhage should be considered. The differential diagnosis of upper gastrointestinal hemorrhage includes peptic ulcer disease, erosive gastritis, esophageal varices, Mallory-Weiss tear, malignancy, and esophagitis.

Aortoenteric fistula can also present with low-grade sepsis and no evidence of bleeding. Symptoms can be nonspecific and include fever, generalized malaise, and leukocytosis of unknown etiology. For primary aortoenteric fistula, infection is less likely unless there is an underlying mycotic aneurysm or other infective aortic process, while secondary aortoenteric fistula findings will more often be associated with infection from a sinus or erosion between the aortic graft and gastrointestinal tract representing infected or colonized graft material, but not necessarily a direct hemorrhagic communication.

Diagnostic Evaluation

The urgency of evaluation is dependent on the acuity of the patient's hemodynamic status. In those patients who are unstable, emergent laparotomy may be required with intraoperative identification of the aortoenteric fistula. However, most clinical presentations will be more subacute thereby allowing further evaluation and diagnosis. Although only 50% of aortoenteric fistulae can be definitively diagnosed preoperatively, knowing this preoperatively is important for appropriate operative planning.[14,15] Undertaking a full evaluation of a patient with suspected gastrointestinal hemorrhage needs to also take into consideration the possibility of an aortoenteric fistula, when an abdominal aortic aneurysm is present or there has been any prior operative intervention on the aorta or its branches.

Physical findings which may prompt a heightened concern for aortoenteric fistula may include a pulsatile abdominal mass suggesting an abdominal aortic aneurysm or pseudoaneurysm, abdominal incisions from previous aortic surgery, groin incisions from endovascular repair, or generalized sepsis for unknown reasons. Blood work including complete blood count, erythrocyte sedimentation rate, and blood culture with Gram stain are often nonspecific, but in conjunction with the clinical history may be suggestive of an aortoenteric fistula. Lack of diagnostic yield with blood cultures may reflect a noninfectious etiology with only 54% of eventual operative Gram stains performed being positive. Operative cultures usually contain mixed organisms (43%), most commonly including Gram-positive cocci (*Streptococcus* and *Staphylococcus* species) (36%), *Escherichia coli* (11%), *Klebsiella* (2%), *Enterbacter* (2%), and *Candida* species (2%).[16] Although nonspecific, these findings should increase suspicion for aortoenteric fistula leading to more extensive diagnostic evaluation.

Given consideration for other more common causes of upper gastrointestinal bleeding, the preferred initial diagnostic test should be esophagogastroduodenoscopy (EGD). When aortoenteric fistula is suspected, complete EGD should include a thorough examination of the duodenum extending into the third and fourth portions, since most will be identified in this location. EGD should be performed by an experienced endoscopist and if an active bleeding source is seen in the third or fourth portion of the duodenum, direct and emergent operative treatment should be undertaken. If clot is visualized in the third or fourth portion of the duodenum, it should be left intact as any attempt to remove the clot can lead to uncontrollable hemorrhage. EGD only has a sensitivity of 24%, and failure to find a bleeding source does not eliminate aortoenteric fistula from the differential. Although most common in the third and fourth portion of the duodenum, aortoenteric fistula can occur in other locations of the gastrointestinal tract below the ligament of Treitz [duodenum (60%), jejunum (12%), ileum (18%), and cecum (8%)], and additional endoscopy may be required. There have also been reports of coincidental aortoenteric fistulas and other causes of upper gastrointestinal bleeding.

Contrast-enhanced computed tomography (CT) of the abdomen and pelvis should follow if EGD is nondiagnostic. The CT scan is most useful when performed with intravenous contrast. Oral contrast should not be given, but water as an alternative to oral contrast may improve visualization of the fistula. The presence of an abdominal aortic aneurysm or pseudoaneurysm may be suggestive of primary aortoenteric fistula, while the presence and location of prior aortic bypass graft may be suggestive of secondary aortoenteric fistula. Findings suspicious for aortoenteric fistula are associated retroperitoneal inflammation, periaortic gas or fluid, and bowel wall thickening (Fig. 1). Contrast entering the gastrointestinal tract through the fistulas tract is diagnostic, but rarely seen. CT scans have a sensitivity and specificity of 94% and 85%, respectively, for findings suggesting aortoenteric fistula, and has the advantage of providing additional diagnostic information for other potential causes of bleeding. Furthermore, additional information obtained from the CT scan can help with operative planning. This valuable diagnostic tool has continued to improve over time in data acquisition, image processing, and 3-D reformatting, which have helped improve image quality and timing of diagnosis, and has led to a shift in diagnostic decision making with CT scanning now the primary diagnostic test needed for surgical disposition.

In the current age of CT, there is no longer a role for contrast fluoroscopic imaging of the upper gastrointestinal tract (barium or water-soluble contrast) for diagnosis of aortoenteric fistula, and use of contrast will curtail the diagnostic

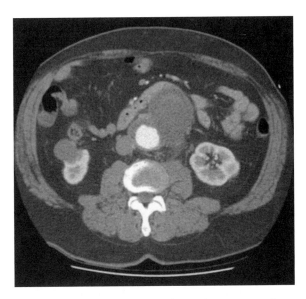

Fig. 1 CT angiogram revealing an abdominal aortic pseudoaneurysm at the proximal anastomosis of a prior aortofemoral graft with abutment of the fourth portion of the duodenum with associated periaortic fat stranding in a patient presenting with aortoenteric fistula

ability of CT scan or angiography. Findings described include a sinus tract from the bowel wall, contrast material around the graft, a defect in the bowel wall, partial intestinal obstruction, and bowel displacement. Upper gastrointestinal contrast imaging will rarely diagnosis aortoenteric fistula. Its diagnostic yield is better for other problems.

Angiography is usually not useful as a diagnostic test (sensitivity of 18%), but may be helpful for operative planning. Although aortographic documentation of extravasation of intravenous contrast into the bowel is diagnostic and may define the fistula site, this is rarely seen. There are other advantages beyond diagnosis including characterizing the abdominal aorta and additional lower extremity angiography, which helps plan any needed revascularization. As magnetic resonance angiography and CT angiography technology improve, these modalities have essentially replaced angiography.

Nuclear imaging such as Gallium 67 or Indium 111-labeled white blood cell scanning are sensitive for aortic and graft infections. Indium 111-labeled leukocyte scans have less nonspecific bowel uptake and a greater target-to-background ratio than Gallium 67 scans. The utility of these scans is in the stable patient with questionable aorta or graft infection. A positive scan suggests infection but is not diagnostic of aortoenteric fistula.

Treatment

Once diagnosis of an aortoenteric fistula has been made, there is no role for conservative medical management and prompt surgical treatment is mandatory. Important tenants included early diagnosis, appropriate antibiotic coverage, consideration of timing of operative repair, rapid control of bleeding with control of the aorta above and below the fistula, complete removal of all affected aortic tissue or prosthetic graft material, consideration of aortic reconstruction and/or lower extremity revascularization options, and prevention of future secondary aortic problems.

If the patient is hemodynamically unstable and/or active bleeding is present, operative repair should be performed immediately. Exploration begins with immediate proximal control of the supraceliac aorta with vascular clamp application. Alternatively, endoluminal balloon tamponade or aortic stent graft deployment for actively bleeding fistula may be an option depending on the location of the aortoenteric fistula and if technically feasible and timely. Because the objective is immediate control of bleeding independent of any infectious process, emergent operative treatment may include direct repair of the fistula or primary aortic graft repair of the aorta. This is just a temporizing solution to allow for stabilization of the patient and definitive treatment should be delayed until the patient has stabilized. If the extent of devitalized tissue and infection precludes immediate direct repair then definitive treatment will need to be performed in the emergent setting with debridement of involved aorta for primary aortoenteric fistula and/or excision of any infected aortic graft material for secondary aortoenteric fistula preceding reconstruction.

If the patient is stable, operative repair should not be delayed, but careful preoperative preparation is required to determine the best surgical options. Definitive planning should include revascularization prior to aortic exposure through a noncontaminated field if possible, control of the aorta and any other sources of potential hemorrhage, removal of nonviable or infected aorta and/or infected graft material if present with containment of any ongoing peritoneal sepsis, and repair of the gastrointestinal tract.

For primary aortoenteric fistula, treatment will depend on the underlying aortic disease process and will follow standard operative techniques based on the causal problem. Usually, this will involve treatment of an associated abdominal aortic aneurysm and the adjacent duodenum. Because infection is uncommon for primary aortoenteric fistula, repair is often accomplished using standard aortic reconstruction and primary intestinal repair or resection. Depending on extent of inflammatory reaction near the fistula, aortic control can be obtained in the infrarenal position if safe exposure is possible, otherwise it should be sought at the supraceliac level with the plan to relocate the clamp to the infrarenal location when appropriate. Once aortic control has been obtained, the duodenum is widely mobilized to allow exposure of the fistula tract and complete separation from the aorta. Any gross contamination or spillage of bowel contents should be controlled. After the duodenum has been exposed and the fistula tract divided, the involved duodenum should be repaired either primarily if possible, or resected with reanastomosis. Serosal or omental patching and duodenal decompression or diversion may be a consideration for complex and extensive duodenal involvement. Attention is then directed at debridement of any devitalized aorta and retroperitoneal tissue with tissue samples sent for culture. If primary aortic repair is not possible, standard aortic reconstruction with in situ graft is usually performed, unless there is extensive infection in which case extra-anatomic bypass may be more of a consideration.

For secondary aortoenteric fistula, the traditional approach has been extra-anatomic axillofemoral bypass. The decision of a staged or immediate approach is based on the clinical setting, the former reserved for patients with occult bleeding, expected significant infective contamination and significant comorbidities, the later for more urgent situations. The technique for axillofemoral bypass may involve use of a unilateral axillary artery with a crossover femoral to femoral bypass or separate grafts from bilateral axillary arteries. The femoral exposure may also need to be modified so as not to expose any prior aortofemoral graft at the groin level. The common femoral arteries are the preferred distal target if there has been no prior prosthetic material in the groins, otherwise exposure of the superficial femoral artery, lateral approach to the profunda femoral artery, or exposure of the popliteal artery may be required. Once extra-anatomic bypass is completed, incisions are closed prior to proceeding with aortic graft excision and bowel repair. If the infrarenal aortic segment is adequate, aortic closure is performed at this level, but if the devitalized infected tissue extends to the suprarenal level, hepatorenal and splenorenal bypass may be required prior to removal of the aortic graft. The aortic stump is closed in with a tension-free, double layer of monofilament suture. Coverage of the aortic stump with anterior spinal ligament, omental pedicle flap, or omentum is also recommended as an adjunct. Because of concern for delayed aortic stump blowout, in situ alternatives to extra-anatomic bypass have been suggested including neo-aortic reconstruction with femoral vein, cryopreserved graft, or antibiotic-soaked prosthetic material.

Outcomes

Traditional approach to aortoenteric fistula involving aortic debridement and/or total graft excision with extra-anatomic bypass is associated with high morbidity and mortality. Extra-anatomic bypass may proceed or follow complete graft excision. O'Hara et al. reviewing a 25-year experience with management of aortoenteric fistula obtained a 72% 30-day survival and a 42% 1-year survival, with a major amputation rate of 27%.[6] Overall, there is evidence to suggest that simultaneous excision of prosthesis followed by extra-anatomic bypass has 26% perioperative mortality and a 25% amputation rate, while staged extra-anatomic bypass followed by delayed graft excision has a survival benefit with 18% mortality and 11% amputation rate.[17,18]

More recently, neo-aortic reconstruction with femoral vein has become a preferred alternative to the traditional approach described above. Clagett et al. were able to demonstrate a reduction from 17% to 38% mortality experienced with other approaches to 10% with the use of autologous veins.[19] They also report a 5% amputation rate as well as compartment syndrome in 12%. Their group preferentially used the larger deep veins over superficial veins with minimal morbidity from venous insufficiency. The use of autogenous grafts has the advantage of being viable and nonantigenic. The disadvantage of this procedure is its technical difficulty and lengthy operative time. Most recent results reported on 240 patients for several complex aortic problems over a 15-year period have shown a graft stenosis requiring open or endovascular graft revision in 4.6% and graft occlusions in 3.8%, with an overall 5-year primary patency of 82% and assisted primary patency of 94%.[20] Although the above report includes several aortic related problems, the use of neo-aortic reconstruction with femoral vein has a clear role for treatment of aortoenteric fistula and may have some advantage over traditional approaches.

Other options include in situ replacement using antibiotic soaked prosthetic material or cryopreserved allograft, both of which have shown an increased resistance to reinfection. In situ replacement of infected aortic grafts with prosthetic materials carries an 8% mortality rate. Polytetrafluoroethylene (PTFE) grafts have a greater resistance to bacterial adherence and therefore have lower infection rate than polyester grafts. Towne et al. suggest that PTFE grafts may be used safely in patients with low virulence organisms such as *Staphylococcus epidermidis*,[21] while rifampin-soaked polyester in situ grafts may be safely used in the presence of low-grade infections.[22] Young et al. implanted 64% standard grafts and 36% rifampin-impregnated grafts, with an overall 8% mortality and 100% limb salvage rate, and reinfection occurring in 29% of the standard grafts and only 11% with rifampin-impregnated grafts.[23]

The use of cryopreserved arterial allograft has been used as another option, but has the disadvantage of antigenicity and nonviability. Kieffer et al. reported an operative mortality of 12%, although late deterioration may be expected and complete protection against persistent or recurrent infection was not achieved.[24] Zhou et al. reported 42 patients requiring aortoenteric fistula repair with allograft with a 30-day mortality of 21% and complication rate of 50%, while only one patient required graft revision for thrombosis and only six required amputation.[25]

With newer endovascular options, there has also been some consideration for use of stent grafts for aortoenteric fistula in selected situations. Baril et al. in a 9-year review of their experience evaluated open repair and endovascular repair. The overall 30-day mortality was 18%, perioperative complication rate was 50%.[26] Length of stay was 44 days in the open group compared with 19 days in the endovascular group. Eighty percent of the open group was discharged to a skilled nursing facility, while 87% of the endovascular group was discharged to home.

As is evident by the different options in which aortoenteric fistula can be managed, there is no one definitive treatment. Rather the patient's condition, associated comorbidites and the resources available to the surgeon will determine the best surgical options for the individual patient. What is most important in determining best outcomes is selecting the most appropriate operative plan for that particular situation with the proper technical expertise for implementation. Even with the most appropriate treatment measures, the operative care of aortoenteric fistula still carries significant morbidity and mortality.

References

1. Cooper A, Tyrrell F. The lectures of Sir Astley Cooper on the principles and practice of surgery. 5th American, from the last London ed. Philadelphia: Haswell, Barrington, and Haswell. 1839:580.
2. Voorhoeve R, Moll FL, Bast TJ. The primary aortoenteric fistula in The Netherlands– the unpublished cases. *Eur J Vasc Endovasc Surg*, 1996; 11(4):429–31.
3. Brock RC. Aortic homografting; a report of six successful cases. Guys Hosp Rep, 1953; 102(3):204–28.
4. Norgren L, Jernby B, Engellau L. Aortoenteric fistula caused by a ruptured stent-graft: a case report. *J Endovasc Surg*, 1998; 5(3):269–72.
5. Donovan TJ, Bucknam CA. Aorto-enteric fistula. Arch Surg, 1967; 95(5):810–20.
6. O'Hara PJ, Hertzer NR, Beven EG, Krajewski LP. Surgical management of infected abdominal aortic grafts: review of a 25-year experience. *J Vasc Surg*, 1986; 3(5): 725–31.
7. Dossa CD, Pipinos II, Shepard AD, Ernst CB. Primary aortoenteric fistula: Part I. *Ann Vasc Surg*, 1994; 8(1):113–20.

8. Reckless JP, McColl I, Taylor GW. Aorto-enteric fistulae: an uncommon complication of abdominal aortic aneurysms. *Br J Surg*, 1972; 59(6):458–60.

9. Dossa CD, Pipinos II, Shepard AD, Ernst CB. Primary aortoenteric fistula: Part II. Primary aortoesophageal fistula. *Ann Vasc Surg*, 1994; **8**(2):207–11.

10. Lorimer JW, Goobie P, Rasuli P, et al. Primary aortogastric fistula: a complication of ruptured aortic aneurysm. *J Cardiovasc Surg (Torino)*, 1996; 37(4):363–6.

11. Hayes PD, Nasim A, London NJ, et al. In situ replacement of infected aortic grafts with rifampicin-bonded prostheses: the Leicester experience (1992 to 1998). *J Vasc Surg*, 1999; 30(1):92–8.

12. Odze RD, Begin LR. Peptic-ulcer-induced aortoenteric fistula. Report of a case and review of the literature. *J Clin Gastroenterol*, 1991; 13(6):682–6.

13. Champion MC, Sullivan SN, Coles JC, et al. Aortoenteric fistula. Incidence, presentation recognition, and management. *Ann Surg*, 1982; 195(3):314–7.

14. Baker BH, Baker BS, van der Reis L, Fisher JH. Endoscopy in the diagnosis of aortoduodenal fistula. *Gastrointest Endosc*, 1977; 24(1):35–7.

15. Ott DJ, Kerr RM, Gelfand DW. Aortoduodenal fistula: an unusual endoscopic and radiographic appearance simulating leiomyoma. *Gastrointest Endosc*, 1978; 24(6):296–8.

16. Pipinos, I.I., Carr, J.A., Haithcock, B.E., et al. Secondary aortoenteric fistula. *Ann Vasc Surg*, 2000; 14(6):688–96.

17. Montgomery RS, Wilson SE. The surgical management of aortoenteric fistulas. *Surg Clin North Am*, 1996; 76:1147–57.

18. Kuestner LM, Reilly LM, Jicha DL, et al. Secondary aortoenteric fistula: contemporary outcome with use of extraanatomic bypass and infected graft excision. *J Vasc Surg*, 1995; 21:184–95; discussion 195–6.

19. Clagett GP, Bowers BL, Lopez-Viego MA, et al. Creation of a neo-aortoiliac system from lower extremity deep and superficial veins. *Ann Surg*, 1993; 218(3):239–49.

20. Beck AW, Murphy EH, Hocking JA, et al. Aortic reconstruction with femoral-popliteal vein: Graft stenosis incidence, risk and reintervention *J Vasc Surg* (in press); [epublished 30 November 2007, http://www.jvascsurg.org/home].

21. Towne JB, Seabrook JR, Bandyk D, et al. In situ replacement of arterial prosthesis infected by bacterial biofilms: long-term follow-up. *J Vasc Surg*, 1994; 19(2):226–35.

22. Bandyk DF, Novotney ML, Johnson BL, et al. Use of rifampin-soaked gelatin-sealed polyester grafts for in situ treatment of primary aortic and vascular prosthetic infections. *J Surg Res*, 2001; 95(1):44–9.

23. Young RM, Cherry Jr. KJ, Davis PM, et al. The results of in situ prosthetic replacement for infected aortic grafts. *Am J Surg*, 1999; 178(2):136–40.

24. Kieffer, E., Gomes, D., Chiche L., et al. Allograft replacement for infrarenal aortic graft infection: early and late results in 179 patients. *J Vasc Surg*, 2004; 39(5):1009–17.

25. Zhou, W., Linn, P.H., Bush, R.L., et al. In situ reconstruction with cryopreserved arterial allografts for management of mycotic aneurysms or aortic prosthetic graft infections: a multi-institutional experience. *Tex Heart Inst J*, 2006; 33(1):14–18.

26. Baril, D.T., Carroccio, A., Ellozy, S.H., et al. Evolving strategies for the treatment of aortoenteric fistulas. *J Vasc Surg*, 2006; 44(2):250–7.

Chapter 17

Management of Abdominal Aortic Aneurysm in the Setting of Coexistent Renal and Splanchnic Disease

Houman Tamaddon, Peter Ford, and Robert Mendes

Abstract By definition, an infrarenal abdominal aortic aneurysm (AAA) is located in the distal portion of the abdominal aorta, inferior to the renal arteries. The segment of aorta between the renal arteries and an infrarenal aneurysm is commonly referred to as the "neck" of the aneurysm. The anatomic characteristics of this area are of critical importance when considering therapeutic strategies for both open and endoluminal interventions. Prior to the endovascular era, optimal management of coexistent aortic aneurysmal disease and visceral pathology was somewhat controversial. While some centers advocated open endarterectomy for stenotic ostial lesions of the renal and visceral vessels at time of aneurysm repair, others preferred reimplantation or bypass for similar lesions. The choice of intervention was often individualized and based somewhat upon surgeon preference.

With the advent and the widespread uptake and utilization of endovascular techniques, it is readily evident that many infrarenal and thoracic aortic aneurysms can be repaired using intraluminal stent-graft devices. Furthermore, the successful deployment of fenestrated or branched stent-graft devices are expanding the limits of endoluminal aneurysm repair. Currently, the treatment of juxtarenal, suprarenal, or even thoraco-AAAs may now be performed solely via endoluminal techniques, albeit in clinical trials.

Optimal management of aortic aneurysm and coexisting arterial branch-vessel occlusive disease is predicated on a thorough knowledge of the anatomy, pathophysiology, clinical picture, natural history, and therapeutic options that are available for each of the underlying disease processes. A logical platform from which to commence evaluating these processes is to review the current understanding of stenotic lesions affecting the renal arteries, superior mesenteric artery, and the celiac artery.

Keywords Infrarenal AAA, Endoluminal intervention, Renal artery stenosis, Renovascular disease intervention, RAS and surgery, Aorto renal endarterectomy, juxtarenal AAA, Mesenteric artery stenosis

G. Upchurch and E. Criado (eds.) *Aortic Aneurysms, Contemporary Cardiology*
DOI: 10.1007/978-1-60327-204-9_17, © Humana Press, a part of
Springer Science+Business Media, LLC 2009

Introduction

Aortic aneurysms are characterized by localized or diffuse enlargement of the aorta. The aorta is considered aneurysmal when the aortic diameter is 50% greater than the "normal" vessel diameter.[1] Aneurysms have a predilection for the abdominal component of the aorta, occurring 3.7 times more frequently in the infrarenal segment compared with the thoracic segment.[2] By definition, an infrarenal abdominal aortic aneurysm (AAA) is located in the distal portion of the abdominal aorta, inferior to the renal arteries. The segment of aorta between the renal arteries and an infrarenal aneurysm is commonly referred to as the "neck" of the aneurysm. The anatomic characteristics of this area are of critical importance when considering therapeutic strategies for both open and endoluminal interventions. Juxtarenal aneurysms encroach on the renal arteries but do not involve the renal artery ostia, whereas suprarenal AAAs involve one or more renal vessels but spare the superior mesenteric artery (SMA). Aneurysmal aortic degeneration in the region of the mesenteric vessels may occur as a localized process or may occur in conjunction with aneurysmal changes in other portions of the aorta. In these circumstances, the most familiar classification system described by Crawford allows stratification of thoraco-AAAs into Types I, II, III, and IV.

When aneurysmal aortic disease involves the visceral portion of the aorta, the complexity of potential therapeutic options increases exponentially. A treacherous combination of limited end-organ redundancy and variable collateral communication between visceral vessels increases the clinical imperative of appropriate assessment and management. Furthermore, the presence of divergent pathological processes, such as branch-vessel ostial stenosis occurring in proximity to aortic aneurysmal disease, can compound the complexity of management algorithms.

Prior to the endovascular era, optimal management of coexistent aortic aneurysmal disease and visceral pathology was somewhat controversial. While some centers advocated open endarterectomy for stenotic ostial lesions of the renal and visceral vessels at time of aneurysm repair, others preferred reimplantation or bypass for similar lesions. The choice of intervention was often individualized and based somewhat upon surgeon preference.

With the advent and the widespread uptake and utilization of endovascular techniques, it is readily evident that many infrarenal and thoracic aortic aneurysms can be repaired using intraluminal stent-graft devices. Furthermore, the successful deployment of fenestrated or branched stent-graft devices are expanding the limits of endoluminal aneurysm repair. Currently, the treatment of juxtarenal, suprarenal, or even thoraco-AAAs may now be performed solely via endoluminal techniques, albeit in clinical trials.

The first challenge when dealing with the presence of an aortic aneurysm and coexisting branch-vessel stenosis is to accurately define the anatomic features of the aneurysmal process. This involves defining the size of the aneurysm, its location within the aorta, and proximity of the aneurysm to the renal or visceral vessels. Factors that influence candidacy for endovascular repair are specifically sought. Identification of appropriate "landing-zones" or "seal-zones" both proximal and distal to the aneurysm are fundamental considerations. Defining an appropriate proximal landing-zone for an aortic stent-graft device is a somewhat complex undertaking. The process requires device-specific consideration of landing-zone diameter, length, angulation, and geometry. This process also requires identification of mural thrombus or calcification within the landing-zone that may compromise integrity of the seal or fixation of the device. Further considerations include caliber and patency of access vessels in the ileofemoral segment. In situations of small caliber ileofemoral vessels, the possible requirement for placement of an iliac conduit to facilitate insertion of the endoluminal device may need to be considered.

If the patient is considered a candidate for endovascular intervention, the next challenge is to accurately identify and define the functional significance of any proximate branch-vessel pathology. This process incorporates conceptual stratification of lesions into those that meet requirement for intervention and those that may be managed conservatively. All these patients should be evaluated carefully with preoperative duplex scanning of the visceral vessels and mandatory high-resolution cross-sectional imaging, preferably CT angiography with at least 2.0 mm cuts augmented with reconstructions. At our institution, we use CT angiography with sagital and coronal cuts and augment this with three-dimensional reconstruction using the TeraRecon software package. This has allowed us to detail the exact relationships between the AAA and the visceral vessels. Only with this information at hand, can a clear plan be formulated. The final conceptual challenge involves determination of whether the branch-vessel stenosis is best treated in a synchronous, metachronous, or independent manner to the aneurysmal process. In some situations, there will be an absolute requirement for simultaneous intervention on the branch-vessel stenosis, whereas in other situations, a staged approach may be preferable.

Optimal management of aortic aneurysm and coexisting arterial branch-vessel occlusive disease is predicated on a thorough knowledge of the anatomy, pathophysiology, clinical picture, natural history, and therapeutic options that are available for each of the underlying disease processes. A logical platform from which to commence evaluating these processes is to review the current understanding of stenotic lesions affecting the renal arteries, SMA, and the celiac artery.

Renal Artery Stenosis and Aneurysms

History

Richard Bright of Guy's Hospital, London, called attention to the association between hypertension and renal disease in 1836. It was not until 1934 that Goldblatt's dog experiment demonstrated that constriction of a renal artery resulted in systemic hypertension and renal parenchymal atrophy.[3] These findings prompted further investigation and stimulated successful performance of nephrectomy for uncontrolled hypertension. It was not until 1954 that Freeman et al. performed aortorenal endarterectomy on a patient resulting in successful resolution of refractory hypertension.[4] Presently, renal artery stenosis (RAS) may be treated via endovascular or open surgical techniques.

Prevalence

RAS refers to narrowing of the renal artery. Variant pathological processes ranging from fibromuscular dysplasia to atherosclerosis may result in narrowing of the renal arteries, thereby providing partial explanation for the predilection of RAS to occur at the extremes of age.[5] Regardless of the underlying etiology, activation of the rennin–angiotensin system results in systemic hypertension. Hypertension has an estimated prevalence of 40–50 million in the United States and RAS is thought to be the underlying stimulus in 5–10% of these patients.[6]

It is generally accepted that atherosclerosis is a systemic disease. Patients who have atherosclerotic disease of their coronary arteries have a high incidence of atherosclerotic disease in remote arterial beds. In one study, 47% of hypertensive patients referred for coronary angiography for suspected ischemic heart disease had some degree of atherosclerotic renovascular disease when screened with abdominal aortography at the time of cardiac catheterization.[7] This population demonstrated greater than 50% unilateral RAS in 19.2% of patients, high-grade stenosis (>70%) was identified in 7%, and bilateral RAS in 3.7%.

The prevalence of renovascular disease is even greater in patients with aortoiliac disease. In one retrospective review, some degree of RAS was detected in 96 of 201 patients (48%) who underwent abdominal aortography for aortoiliac disease. In this study, 26% of the patients had a greater than 50% RAS, and 22% had greater than 70% stenosis. In this cohort, 40 patients (20%) had bilateral stenoses, including four with greater than 70% stenosis bilaterally.[8] Hansen et al. found a 50% incidence of RAS in patients older than 60 years of age and with diastolic blood pressure higher than 110 mmHg.[9] When severe hypertension and elevated serum creatinine exist in the elderly, approximately 70% of patients were found to have RAS, with half of these cases involving bilateral renal arteries.

There is also an established association between renovascular disease and infrarenal aortic aneurysms. Cher et al.[8,10] looked at the incidence of RAS in their surgically revascularized population and found 26% of their patients had a concomitant AAA. In a retrospective review of cases, Olin et al.[11] showed that RAS greater than 50% was present in nearly 40% of patients with AAA. They also found that bilateral RAS was present in approximately 13% of patients with AAA and totally occluded renal arteries occurred in 5% of the patients in this population. Valentine et al.[12] also found a 22% incidence of significant RAS (>50%) in a retrospective review of AAA patients. Interestingly, they also discovered a high correlation between the presence of RAS and mesenteric artery stenosis (MAS). Brewster et al.[13] in 1975 looked at the utility of angiography for planning of AAA repair and they noted a 20% incidence of RAS and 9% incidence of celiac or SMA stenosis.

The relatively high incidence of concomitant RAS and AAA (20–40%) mandates a clear understanding of management options, technical pitfalls, and a candid review of how each strategy affects clinical outcome measures.

Intervention on Renovascular Disease

Interventional management of renovascular occlusive disease remains a controversial topic. Hunt and Strong evaluated the progression of chronic kidney disease in patients who received medical or drug therapy and compared them with those receiving operative treatment for renovascular hypertension (RVH). Outcomes were followed for 14 years.[14] The results identified a significant difference in survival rates, with 84% survival noted in the patient group receiving operative therapy while 66% survived medical treatment (100 patients operative, 114 medical). They also showed that 93% of the patients in the operative group were cured or had improvement and 21% of the patients in the medical therapy group required crossover to surgical intervention for treatment of their RVH.

Dean et al. reported on 41 patients treated nonoperatively for RVH over a mean follow-up of 28 months. They found 19 patients had a decline in their serum creatinine clearance by 25–50%, glomerular filtration rates decreased 25–50% in 12 patients, a 10% reduction in renal parenchymal length occurred in 14 patients, progression to renal artery occlusion occurred in 4 patients, and a total of 17 patients had worsening of renal function that led to operation. Dean et al. also showed that in patients with hypertension, RAS progressed in the ipsilateral renal artery in 44% of the time, with a 12% rate of progression to renal artery occlusion. Of these occlusions, 3% had loss of revascularization options.[15]

Wollenweber et al.[16] and Schreiber et al.[17] have also shown a similar deteriorating relationship of RAS and renal function. They report an ipsilateral progression of RAS in 44% of patients with 16% progressing to occlusion. Renal artery revascularization has been demonstrated to result in significant improvement in renal function and hypertension control, especially when revascularization is performed after rapid decline in renal excretory function.

Hansen et al. make a distinction between prophylactic (no presence of hypertension or renal insufficiency) and empirical RAS repair (presence of hypertension or renal insufficiency).[18] They conclude that only 5% of patients with known RAS, and without hypertension, would benefit from prophylactic renal artery revascularization. They recently reported from the Cardiovascular Health Study cohort that only 4% of diseased renal arteries progressed to significant stenosis and concluded that progression of RAS is rare.

In order to provide a guide for planning endovascular therapies, endovascular treatment of RAS will have to be evaluated. The majority of the studies available are retrospective reviews of institutional experiences.

Primary percutaneous angioplasty (PTA) has not shown to be a durable therapy. Many reports have indicated that PTA enjoys only a 24–25% success rate and restenosis occurs in 15–42%.[19] Recently, Leertouwer et al.[20] have published a meta-analysis of renal artery stenting versus angioplasty. They accumulated data from 14 articles resulting in 678 patients receiving renal artery stents and 10 articles resulting in 644 patients published before 1998. They showed that renal stenting was technically successful in 98% of cases with an overall hypertension cure rate of 20% and clinical improvement in 49% of patients. In terms of renal function, they found a serum creatinine and glomerular filtration rate improvement in 30% of patients and stabilized function in 38% of the patients. They concluded based on statistical significance that the stent group had a higher technical success rate (98% vs 77%) and lower restenosis rate (17% vs 26%) than PTA.

Management Options for Aortic Aneurysm with Associated RAS

Open Surgical Options for Management of Aortic Aneurysm and Associated RAS

The approach to open surgical repair of an aortic aneurysm is influenced by several factors, including the anatomic location of the aneurysm, presence or absence of a hostile peritoneal cavity, and the requirement for exposure of the renal or visceral vessels. Common surgical approaches include midline celiotomy, retroperitoneal incision, and thoracoabdominal incision.

Infrarenal AAAs are typically repaired with prosthetic material such as Dacron, utilizing a tubular conduit or a bifurcated graft based upon the distal extent of the aneurysmal process. If significant RAS is present in the setting of an infrarenal AAA, and concomitant open surgical intervention is felt to be indicated, options can be broadly divided into aortorenal endarterectomy, renal artery bypass, and renal artery reimplantation.

Open aortorenal endarterectomy directly removes atherosclerotic plaque from the aorta and the ostia of the renal artery but requires suprarenal application of an aortic cross-clamp. An important concept to remember is that aortorenal endarterectomy should only be contemplated in a nonaneurysmal portion of the aorta. This concept significantly influences open surgical options in the management of suprarenal AAA.

Different techniques have been described for performing renal artery endarterectomy. Stoney et al.[21] described the transaortic technique in 1989. They performed aortic replacement surgery with renal artery endarterectomy in 44 patients with aortic disease and concomitant RAS in symptomatic (35) and asymptomatic (9) patients. To effectively treat the combined aortic and renal disease in these patients, a supraceliac aortic cross-clamp was necessary in three patients, supramesenteric clamp was applied in 20 patients, and a suprarenal clamp was applied in 21 patients. They reported a mean renal ischemic time of 30 min (range 17–81 min). Follow-up of 33 patients demonstrated that 79% had improved or stable renal function and 69% with preoperative hypertension had improved blood pressure control. Stoney et al. claim adequate visualization of the distal intimal flap and stand behind this technique for patients with combined aortic disease and RAS. However, most would agree that the major contraindication to the use of this technique is aneurysmal degeneration of the perirenal aorta or extensive distal renal artery atherosclerosis past the ostia. Hansen et al.[22] advocate a transaortic longitudinal aortotomy and endarterectomy when both renal arteries diseased. They recommend a transrenal approach for unilateral disease or when the renal arteries potentially need ostial expansion with the use of a patch. Mainly, the techniques are surgeon dependent.

Renal artery bypass is an alternative option which includes constructing a bypass that circumvents the stenotic renal artery lesion. This procedure has been successfully performed utilizing a variety of inflow sources (e.g., aortorenal, splenorenal, hepatorenal, ileorenal) and a variety of conduits ranging from autogenous material (vein) to prosthetic material (Daron, PTFE). Another frequently utilized technique involves mobilization of the renal artery and reimplantation onto the aorta or aortic graft.

Cherr et al.[10] retrospectively studied 500 patients who underwent both unilateral and bilateral surgical procedures. Techniques used for renal artery revascularization included aortorenal bypass graft (384, Vein 204, PTFE 159, Dacron 21), splanchnorenal bypass graft (13), reimplantation (56), and endarterectomy (267). Of note, 200 patients (41%) had renal revascularization combined with aortic or mesenteric reconstruction. Seventy-six patients underwent combined repair of clinically significant aortic occlusive disease, and 57 patients underwent concomitant repair of AAA. The authors stressed the increased complexity of the combined procedure indicating that renal artery revascularization in conjunction with aortic reconstruction resulted in all but one of their 23 perioperative deaths. Mortality rates after isolated renal artery repair (0.8%) differed significantly from the rates for combined aortic and bilateral repair (6.9%). Therefore, Cherr et al. conclude that caution should be used when considering concomitant renal artery and aortic aneurysm repair.

Juxtarenal AAA by definition encroaches upon at least one of the renal arteries. When open repair is undertaken, positioning of the proximal cross-clamp tends to be guided by individual patient anatomy. In situations where the renal arteries originate from the aorta at different levels, the proximal clamp can occasionally be applied at an oblique orientation preserving perfusion to the more cephalad renal artery at the time of clamp application. In many regards, the therapeutic options and considerations for open renal revascularization for RAS associated with juxtarenal AAA overlap the therapeutic considerations of RAS and infrarenal AAA.

If an AAA has a proximal extension that involves the bilateral renal arteries then the aneurysm may be classified as a suprarenal AAA. Although conceptually simplistic, it is technically challenging to repair a suprarenal AAA from a transabdominal approach. The principal challenge in this circumstance arises from obtaining safe suprarenal control in the retroperitoneum without injuring the pancreas or compromising arterial flow to the SMA. A left retroperitoneal approach provides appropriate exposure and control of the proximal aorta, however, repair of the right renal artery becomes somewhat challenging. These factors raise the specter of performing initial revascularization of the right renal artery (e.g., right hepatorenal bypass), followed by retroperitoneal or thoracoabdominal approach to repair the aneurysm and revascularize the left renal artery.

Endovascular Options for Management of Aortic Aneurysm and Associated RAS

The first endovascular aneurysm repair (EVAR) was performed by Parodi in 1991. This procedure utilized a handmade device consisting of a balloon expandable Palmaz stent surrounded by (and sutured to) Dacron[23] Since that time, significant advancements have been made in device design and the FDA has approved four devices for endovascular repair of infrarenal AAAs. These devices can be divided into those with suprarenal stent-graft fixation (Cook Zenith) and those without suprarenal fixation (Medtronic Aneurex, Gore Excluder, and Endologic Powerlink). Each device has its own unique "pros and cons." For patients with AAA and concomitant splanchnic artery disease, thoughtful consideration of device selection is required because proximally located suprarenal fixation stents may theoretically complicate or compromise options for endovascular intervention.

When evaluating a patient that meets criteria for EVAR, a couple of key concepts need to be addressed. First, the location of the aneurysm in relation to the renal arteries is critical (infrarenal, juxtarenal, and suprarenal). For all FDA-approved devices, at least a 15-mm neck is required for adequate proximal fixation. If this criterion is not met, then the planning for repair of coexistent RAS becomes more complex and involves either planning for a hybrid approach or a branched or fenestrated stent-graft approach (currently in trials only). In addition, severe neck angulations (>60°), reverse tapering, and presence of intramural thrombus in the neck provide for challenging proximal seal zones.

Once the anatomical considerations have been worked out, timing of renal artery stenting is of the next importance. Three scenarios can be categorized: (1) RAS before EVAR, (2) RAS during EVAR, and (3) RAS after EVAR.

Renal artery stent deployment followed by staged performance of EVAR can be a consideration in patients with significant renal insufficiency who need maximal protection from contrast nephropathy by staging the contrast loads. With this theory, patients that are at high risk for postoperative contrast nephropathy could potentially benefit from improved blood flow to the renal parenchyma. In patients with renovascular disease induced nephropathy, further benefit may be achieved secondary to reduction of antihypertensive medicines resulting in improved renal artery perfusion, and more stable blood pressure control. The major concern involves the placement of the EVAR device after renal stent placement. An appropriately placed renal stent protrudes 2–3 mm into the aorta, and can be displaced or kinked during the placement of the aortic stent-graft. Both the Zenith and Aneurex devices involve manipulation above the renal arteries. The Zenith has a suprarenal bare stent fixation while the Aneurex device is partially deployed above and then pulled down across the renal arteries. Both have high risk of renal stent displacement or kinking if the stent is placed prior to EVAR. To avoid this potential hazard, the authors prefer to angioplasty an RAS rather than stent placement. After repair of the AAA, a stent can be placed in the renal artery if or when restenosis occurs.

EVAR followed by staged placement of renal artery stent would likely be the sequence of choice in patients that have mild clinical indicators for treatment such as marginally controlled RVH or slowly declining renal function. In this scenario, the surgeon delays the repair of significant RAS to repair a clinically significant AAA. Multiple factors may influence this decision-making process. Complex aneurysm anatomy will increase operative time and increase contrast load, especially when coupled with renal stenting. The choice of EVAR device has not been found to inhibit future cannulation and stenting of a diseased renal artery. Whenever possible, the authors prefer to stage the procedure in this order.

Simultaneous renal artery stent deployment at time of EVAR would likely be the planning of choice in a patient with an uncomplicated infrarenal AAA who also has clinically significant RAS. While these procedures are performed in the same setting, the authors place the EVAR device prior to placing the renal artery stent to avoid the unwanted renal stent complications discussed above. In renal vessels with severe disease, brachial artery access with placement of a 0.014″ wire into the affected vessel prior to EVAR device deployment will potentially simplify the renal stent placement after EVAR (Figs. 1 and 2).

Combination Approaches for Management of Aortic Aneurysm and Associated RAS

Hybrid approach: Renal BPG followed by EVAR repair is generally applied in patients who are poor candidates for traditional open juxtarenal AAA repair secondary to the likely complications from aortic cross-clamping in the suprarenal aorta. These patients are generally elderly and have increased baseline creatinine making them especially high risk for open AAA repair. Multiple extra-anatomical approaches can be applied to this patient population. Restoration of perfusion to the renal arteries using hepatorenal, splenorenal,

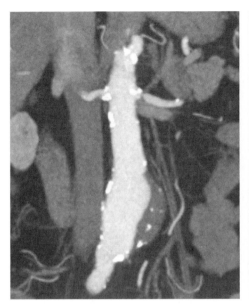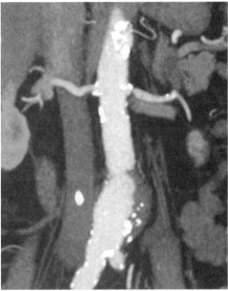

Fig. 1 Preoperative computed tomography angiogram (*CTA*) of 76-year-old male with symptomatic abdominal aortic aneurysm (*AAA*) and severe left renal artery stenosis (*RAS*) and renal insufficiency

or ileorenal conduits negates the need for manipulation and cross-clamping of a badly diseased aorta and offers the advantage of extending the proximal landing zone for a stent-graft device (Fig. 3). The results from these conduits have generally been exceptionally good. In an analysis of 222 patients treated more than 10 years earlier indicates that these procedures were performed with low mortality (2.2%) and low rates of restenosis (7.3%) and good long-term survival. The predictors of late mortality were age above 60 years, coronary disease, and previous vascular surgery.[24,25]

MAS and Aortic Aneurysms

Prevalence

The prevalence of MAS has not been as frequently reported in association to AAA. Likely, there is a similar association to aortic aneurysms as there is between RAS and AAA. Valentine et al.[12] retrospectively evaluated the incidence of MAS in patients with AAA. They found in their series that 55% of patients with AAA had celiac artery stenosis. Twenty-two percent had mild stenosis (0–49%), 29% had moderate or severe stenosis, and 4% were occluded. In this same group, the SMA was mildly occluded in 7% and only 4% had moderate stenosis. Four percent were found to have an occluded SMA. All of the patients with occluded or moderate SMA stenosis had moderate or greater celiac artery stenosis. They also pointed out the there was a significant correlation with hypertension and MAS.

As discussed earlier, Valentine et al. evaluated RAS rates in the AAA population and found that 22% of those patients had more than 50% stenosis.

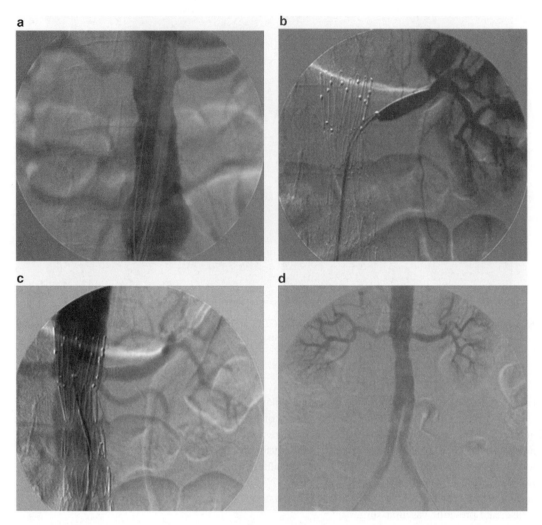

Fig. 2 (**a**) Intraoperative aortogram showing the severe left renal artery (*RA*) stenosis from the patient above. (**b**) Cook Zenith endovascular repair with suprarenal fixation allowing access to the left RA with a 6 French sheath and 014 Spartacore wire. (**c**) Balloon expandable Herculink 7-mm stent deployed with complete resolution of stenosis. (**d**) Completion aortogram after Cook Zenith abdominal aortic aneurysm (*AAA*) repair with iliac extensions and left RA stent

It was also reported that 50% of the severe RAS patients had concomitant celiac artery stenosis, suggesting that MAS is more prevalent in patients with known RAS.[12,15]

It is important to understand the time course of clinically relevant disease progression of MAS in the patient with aortic aneurysmal disease. AAAs frequently have intramural thrombus that can adversely affect the mesenteric blood supply by occluding the inferior mesenteric artery. Thomas et al.[26] reported the progression of asymptomatic mesenteric stenosis on approximately 1000 patients over a 6-year course. Eighty-two of these patients had SMA stenosis and 60 of these patients had significant stenosis (>50% diameter reducing).

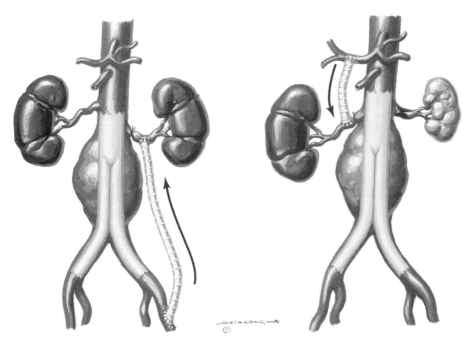

Fig. 3 Examples of iliorenal and hepatorenal bypass graft

Fifteen of these patients had three-vessel disease. Four (27%) patients of the 15 developed acute mesenteric ischemia during follow-up and 1 (7%) died. Each of these four patients had significant (>50%) stenosis or occlusion of the celiac artery, SMA, and inferior mesenteric artery. Four additional patients of the 15 died from coronary disease. Therefore, 8 of 15 patients with three-vessel disease died or developed MI in 2.6-year follow-up. They concluded that patients with significant three-vessel mesenteric arterial stenosis should be considered for prophylactic mesenteric arterial reconstruction.

For the general vascular patient with or without aortic disease, an occluded IMA is well tolerated and rarely if ever causes clinical manifestations of ischemia. This is not true for celiac or SMA stenosis or occlusion. For these patients, the risk of ischemia is high. Thomas et al.[27] showed that nearly 40% of patients with more than 50% mesenteric stenosis on abdominal angiogram died in 3 years and of the patients with three-vessel disease, about 30% developed symptomatic ischemia.

Intervention on Mesenteric Artery Disease

One fundamental question in mesenteric revascularization is the number of vessels to revascularize. In reports from the Mayo Clinic, it was first suggested that complete revascularization resulted in decreased symptomatic recurrence[28] and later that graft patency and survival in patients with three-vessel revascularization were improved compared with single-vessel revascularization.[29] Proponents of both celiac and SMA revascularization maintain that it may result in decreased symptomatic recurrence even if reocclusion of one of the grafts occurs.[28,29]

However, Foely et al.[30] demonstrated comparable durability with primary assisted 9-year patency rate of 79% in a series of 49 patients undergoing SMA reconstruction alone, and they concluded that multiple bypass grafts to other splanchnic vessels are unnecessary when adequate SMA reconstruction has been accomplished.

Farber et al.[31] provided a report on 18 patients with chronic mesenteric ischemia of which all had weight loss and chronic abdominal pain. Two of these patients had acute on chronic exacerbation of symptoms requiring urgent revascularization. Fourteen (78%) patients had both celiac and SMA disease, whereas three (17%) had only SMA involvement. All bypasses were performed from the descending thoracic aorta with PTFE grafts. Their results showed only one (6%) perioperative death from multisystem organ failure and three (17%) major complications (two myocardial infarctions and one reintubation). Graft durability was measured by survival rates and symptom relief, which were found to be 89%, 89%, and 76% at 1, 3, and 5 years, respectively. All grafts were found to be patent at 35-month follow-up.

Endovascular treatment of mesenteric ischemia has also been shown to be a safe and effective option. Kasirajan et al. in 2001[32] reported prospective data comparing endovascular treatment on CMI on patients from 1995 to 1998 with open repair on patients from 1977 to 1997. Twenty-eight patients received an endovascular treatment while 85 patients had a surgical bypass. Endovascular therapies included balloon expandable stents in 23 arteries, 3 self-expanding stents, and 6 angioplasties. Whereas surgical intervention included bypass grafting in 71% (retrograde 40%, antegrade 28%, reimplantation 30%) of the patients, eversion endarterectomy in 22%, and patch repair in 7%. No significant reduced length of stay could be appreciated in the endovascular group and the 3-year cumulative recurrent stenosis and mortality rates did not differ. However, patients receiving an endovascular therapy had a higher incidence of recurrent symptoms. Currently, the utility of endovascular revascularization of mesenteric vessels has been reserved for patients unfit for surgery and as a bridge to more definitive and durable open revascularization.[33]

Management Options for Aortic Aneurysm Repair with Associated MAS

Evaluation of Aortic Aneurysm and Associated MAS

Aside from the complex nature of AAA with concomitant RAS, MAS further adds to the complexity of the procedural and timing of visceral artery repair. For the vascular surgeon, it is imperative to identify patients that are at risk for mesenteric ischemia before and after AAA repair. The three abdominal aortic vessels and the internal iliac vessels become the focus of attention for open, endovascular, or a hybrid repair. Classically, the open repair of infrarenal AAA has the mandatory intraoperative evaluation of the inferior mesenteric artery. When the celiac and SMAs are without disease and the IMA has no back bleeding, there is no need to revascularize the IMA. Likewise, brisk back bleeding from the IMA with knowledge of widely patent celiac and SMAs does not require reimplantation of the IMA. However, the algorithm becomes immediately more complex in patients with stenotic celiac, SMA, or even diseased hypogastric arteries. It is in this population of patients that the vascular surgeon needs to heighten the awareness for mesenteric ischemia before and after AAA repair.

It becomes an important intraoperative decision to reimplant the IMA when the vessel has poor to moderate back bleeding, likely provided by mesenteric collaterals such as the Arc of Riolan, Marginal Artery of Drummond, or from branches of the hypogastric vessels. This potentially indicates poor collateral perfusion to the distal bowel, specifically, distal to the splenic flexure. Mesenteric stenosis is well tolerated in patients that have stenosis in one of the three vessels supplying the intestines. However, the risk of acute bowel ischemia increases as the number of stenotic vessels increases, and it is greatest if the SMA is critically stenosed and the hypogastric vessels are heavily diseased.

Therefore, it is our practice to address the issue of mesenteric perfusion before any AAA repair. Each patient gets a thorough workup for clinical signs and symptoms of mesenteric ischemia and this is complemented with a thin cut CT angiogram to evaluate the morphology of the AAA and, in symptomatic patients, noninvasive duplex scanning to obtain hemodynamic information-associated visceral stenosis. Since the notion of prophylactic repair of radiographic or duplex identified significant (50%) stenosis is controversial, the algorithm for intervention is dependent on the extent of the urgency for AAA repair and the extent of visceral disease.

In an asymptomatic patient with concomitant AAA and >50% diameter stenosis of the SMA or celiac, the authors prefer to evaluate the mesenteric vessels with an arteriogram. Selective injection of the three vessels gives an indication of dominant collateral blood supply and hints to the dominant vessel supplying the viscera. If the IMA is a large vessel, and selective injection with contrast shows reconstitution of the SMA, then the IMA is a critical vessel for blood supply. If there is competitive flow from the SMA, minimal filling of the Arc of Riolan, or Marginal Artery of Drummond, then collateral flow from the SMA is usually adequate.

Open Surgical Options for Management of Aortic Aneurysm and Associated MAS

It is very rare to consider an open approach to repair both mesenteric disease and AAAs simultaneously. However, if necessary, the authors prefer a thoracomesenteric bypass via a thoracoabdominal approach and subsequent retroperitoneal repair of the AAA. Other institutions may use a retrograde bypass from the iliac vessels or the aortic graft, while others describe an antegrade approach from the supraceliac aorta to supply the mesenteric vessels prior to a transabdominal repair of the aortic aneurysm. Simultaneous repair places significant stress on the patient and staging of the procedure would always be preferred.

Endovascular Options for Management of Aortic Aneurysm and Associated MAS

An endovascular approach to the repair is usually more appealing to the patient and some physicians. It should be reserved for the patient that is unable to tolerate an open procedure. The procedures are usually staged by first stenting the mesenteric vessels followed by EVAR of the aneurysm. This theoretically reduces the potential ischemic time of the viscera as an EVAR typically occludes inflow from the IMA.

Care must be taken when selecting the EVAR device. The Zenith device has a bare suprarenal fixation that may potentially extend to, or above, the SMA. This may cause a kink or even create a dislodgement of the SMA stent. Detailed preoperative planning avoids critical mistakes.

Combination Approaches for Management of Aortic Aneurysm and Associated MAS

Hybrid Approach: Mesenteric BPG followed by EVAR repair is generally applied in patients who are poor candidates for traditional open AAA repair secondary to the likely complications from aortic cross-clamping. These patients are generally elderly and have poor cardiac function, making them especially high risk for open AAA repair. Multiple extra-anatomical approaches can be applied to this patient population. Reconstruction of perfusion to the mesenteric arteries using thoracomesenteric, aortomesenteric (supraceliac origination), or ileomesenteric conduits negates the need for manipulation and cross-clamping of a diseased aorta in a high-risk patient.

The procedure is usually staged to reduce patient stress that is imposed with prolonged operative times. The endovascular repair of the aneurysm is performed several days later. Care must be taken to avoid coverage of the inflow source of the mesenteric bypass if an ileomesenteric bypass was performed. With current data leaning toward surgical bypass for treatment of mesenteric disease, due to lower recurrence of symptoms, the authors prefer this approach to the treatment of concomitant AAA and symptomatic mesenteric disease.

Conclusion

Management of AAA in the current era of open, endovascular, and hybrid procedures is a complex undertaking. Development of modern generation endovascular devices has opened the door for many high-risk patients who would otherwise have limited therapeutic options. Depending on neck length, size, angulation, and iliac anatomy, most of the available devices can be applied to complex aneurysm anatomy. In the population of AAA, those with concomitant visceral artery stenosis possess an even more complex treatment algorithm, due to simultaneous advances in endoluminal therapy for the management of diverse pathological processes affecting the renal and mesenteric vessels.

The historical paradigm of "hitting two birds with one stone" using open surgical techniques in patients with concomitant AAA and visceral vessel pathology have led to increased end-organ morbidity and patient mortality. An augmented understanding of the underlying data has leaned the pendulum toward an increased frequency of performing staged interventions. The planning of aortic aneurysm repair in patients with visceral vessel disease needs to be highly individualized based on the thorough understanding of visceral and aortic pathology, anatomy, and accessibility.

References

1. Johnston KW, Rutherford RB, Tilson MD, Shah DM, Hollier L, Stanley JC. Suggested standards for reporting on arterial aneurysms. Subcommittee on Reporting Standards for Arterial Aneurysms, Ad Hoc Committee on Reporting Standards, Society for Vascular Surgery and North American Chapter, International Society for Cardiovascular Surgery. J Vasc Surg 1991; 13(3):452–458.

2. Bickerstaff LK, Hollier LH, Van Peenen HJ, Melton LJ, III, Pairolero PC, Cherry KJ. Abdominal aortic aneurysms: the changing natural history. J Vasc Surg 1984; 1(1):6–12.

3. Goldblatt H, Lynch J, Hanzal RF, Summerville WW. Studies on experimental hypertension I. The production of persistent elevation of the systolic blood pressure by means of renal ischemia. J Exp Med 59, 347–379. 3–1–1934.

4. Freeman NE, Leeds FH, Elliott WG, Roland SI. Thromboendarterectomy for hypertension due to renal artery occlusion. J Am Med Assoc 1954; 156(11):1077–1079.

5. Lawson JD, Boerth R, Foster JH, Dean RH. Diagnosis and management of renovascular hypertension in children. Arch Surg 1977; 112(11):1307–1316.

6. Burt VL, Whelton P, Roccella EJ et al. Prevalence of hypertension in the US adult population. Results from the Third National Health and Nutrition Examination Survey, 1988–1991. Hypertension 1995; 25(3):305–313.

7. Rihal CS, Textor SC, Breen JF et al. Incidental renal artery stenosis among a prospective cohort of hypertensive patients undergoing coronary angiography. Mayo Clin Proc 2002; 77(4):309–316.

8. Iglesias JI, Hamburger RJ, Feldman L, Kaufman JS. The natural history of incidental renal artery stenosis in patients with aortoiliac vascular disease. Am J Med 2000; 109(8):642–647.

9. Hansen KJ. Renovascular disease: an overview. In: Robert B. Rutherford MD F, editor. Vascular Surgery. Denver, Colorado: Elsevier, Inc., 2005: 1763–1772.

10. Cherr GS, Hansen KJ, Craven TE et al. Surgical management of atherosclerotic renovascular disease. J Vasc Surg 2002; 35(2):236–245.

11. Olin JW, Melia M, Young JR, Graor RA, Risius B. Prevalence of atherosclerotic renal artery stenosis in patients with atherosclerosis elsewhere. Am J Med 1990; 88(1N):46N–51N.

12. Valentine RJ, Martin JD, Myers SI, Rossi MB, Clagett GP. Asymptomatic celiac and superior mesenteric artery stenoses are more prevalent among patients with unsuspected renal artery stenoses. J Vasc Surg 1991; 14(2):195–199.

13. Brewster DC, Retana A, Waltman AC, Darling RC. Angiography in the management of aneurysms of the abdominal aorta. Its value and safety. N Engl J Med 1975; 292(16):822–825.

14. Hunt JC, Strong CG. Renovascular hypertension. Mechanisms, natural history and treatment. Am J Cardiol 1973; 32(4):562–574.

15. Dean RH, Kieffer RW, Smith BM et al. Renovascular hypertension: anatomic and renal function changes during drug therapy. Arch Surg 1981; 116(11):1408–1415.

16. Wollenweber J, Sheps SG, Davis GD. Clinical course of atherosclerotic renovascular disease. Am J Cardiol 1968; 21(1):60–71.

17. Schreiber MJ, Pohl MA, Novick AC. The natural history of atherosclerotic and fibrous renal artery disease. Urol Clin North Am 1984; 11(3):383–392.

18. Hallett J, Mills J, Earnshaw J, Reekers J. Comprehensive vascular and endovascular surgery with CD-ROM. Mosby, 2008.

19. Blum U, Krumme B, Flugel P et al. Treatment of ostial renal-artery stenoses with vascular endoprostheses after unsuccessful balloon angioplasty. N Engl J Med 1997; 336(7):459–465.

20. Leertouwer TC, Gussenhoven EJ, Bosch JL et al. Stent placement for renal arterial stenosis: where do we stand? A meta-analysis. Radiology 2000; 216(1):78–85.

21. Stoney RJ, Messina LM, Goldstone J, Reilly LM. Renal endarterectomy through the transected aorta: a new technique for combined aortorenal atherosclerosis–a preliminary report. J Vasc Surg 1989; 9(2):224–233.

22. Hansen KJ, Ayerdi J, Edwards JM. Open surgical repair of renovascular diseaes. In: Robert B. Rutherford MD F, editor. Vascular Surgery. Elsevier, Inc., Denver, Colorado: 2005: 1851.

23. Parodi JC, Palmaz JC, Barone HD. Transfemoral intraluminal graft implantation for abdominal aortic aneurysms. Ann Vasc Surg 1991; 5(6):491–499.

24. Novick AC, Ziegelbaum M, Vidt DG, Gifford RW, Jr., Pohl MA, Goormastic M. Trends in surgical revascularization for renal artery disease. Ten years' experience. JAMA 1987; 257(4):498–501.
25. Steinbach F, Novick AC, Campbell S, Dykstra D. Long-term survival after surgical revascularization for atherosclerotic renal artery disease. J Urol 1997; 158(1):38–41.
26. Thomas JH, Blake K, Pierce GE, Hermreck AS, Seigel E. The clinical course of asymptomatic mesenteric arterial stenosis. J Vasc Surg 1998; 27(5):840–844.
27. Thomas JH, Blake K, Pierce GE, Hermreck AS, Seigel E. The clinical course of asymptomatic mesenteric arterial stenosis. J Vasc Surg 1998; 27(5):840–844.
28. Hollier LH, Bernatz PE, Pairolero PC, Payne WS, Osmundson PJ. Surgical management of chronic intestinal ischemia: a reappraisal. Surgery 1981; 90(6):940–946.
29. McAfee MK, Cherry KJ, Jr., Naessens JM et al. Influence of complete revascularization on chronic mesenteric ischemia. Am J Surg 1992; 164(3):220–224.
30. Foley MI, Moneta GL, bou-Zamzam AM, Jr. et al. Revascularization of the superior mesenteric artery alone for treatment of intestinal ischemia. J Vasc Surg 2000; 32(1):37–47.
31. Farber MA, Carlin RE, Marston WA, Owens LV, Burnham SJ, Keagy BA. Distal thoracic aorta as inflow for the treatment of chronic mesenteric ischemia. J Vasc Surg 2001; 33(2):281–287.
32. Kasirajan K, O'Hara PJ, Gray BH et al. Chronic mesenteric ischemia: open surgery versus percutaneous angioplasty and stenting. J Vasc Surg 2001; 33(1):63–71.
33. Biebl M, Oldenburg WA, Paz-Fumagalli R, McKinney JM, Hakaim AG. Endovascular treatment as a bridge to successful surgical revascularization for chronic mesenteric ischemia. Am Surg 2004; 70(11):994–998.

Chapter 18

Management of Abdominal Aortic Aneurysms in Patients with Renal Ectopia and Renal Fusion

Patrick J. O'Hara

Abstract Patients presenting with coexistent abdominal aortic aneurysm and renal ectopia or fusion abnormalities present a technical challenge to the vascular surgeon at the time of aortic aneurysm repair. The most common of these unusual renal conditions is horseshoe kidney, thought to occur in 0.25% of the population. Associated abnormalities in the number and distribution of renal arteries occur in three quarters of these patients and abnormalities of the renal collecting systems are also common. Because the renal blood supply may be asymmetric, division of the renal isthmus to allow aortic aneurysm exposure may be hazardous. Improvements in preoperative imaging modalities have facilitated the preoperative awareness of the aberrant renal anatomy. While endovascular aortic aneurysm exclusion may be feasible in some patients with appropriate renal anatomy and normal preoperative renal function, the sacrifice of renal arterial perfusion and the nephrotoxicity associated with contrast requirements may preclude this approach for others. However, using current open surgical techniques, including retroperitoneal exposure and renal preservation methods, safe aortic aneurysm repair with preservation of renal perfusion is now possible in the majority of patients with acceptable surgical risk.

Keywords Aneurysm, Aorta, Horseshoe kidney, Renal ectopia, Renal fusion

Background and Prevalence

Renal artery abnormalities, which can potentially complicate the repair of abdominal aortic aneurysms, are the most common congenital renal anomaly occurring in 25–40% of kidneys.[1] These are usually easily handled by the experienced vascular surgeon when encountered during abdominal aortic aneurysm repair. However, congenital anomalies of the upper urinary tract are much less common and can pose substantial technical challenges at the time of aneurysm repair, especially if their presence is not anticipated. Although upper urinary tract anomalies influencing abdominal aortic aneurysm repair have been generally categorized as those involving renal ascent, fusion, and rotation, they may also commonly be associated with coexisting anomalies of renal vasculature and

G. Upchurch and E. Criado (eds.) *Aortic Aneurysms, Contemporary Cardiology*
DOI: 10.1007/978-1-60327-204-9_18, © Humana Press, a part of
Springer Science+Business Media, LLC 2009

Table 1 Renal anomalies infrequently complicating aortic aneurysm repair.[2]

Agenesis
    Unilateral
    Bilateral

Ascent
    Simple ectopia
    Cephalad renal ectopia
    Thoracic kidney

Rotation
    Ventral
    Dorsal
    Lateral

the collecting system (Table 1).[2] The reported prevalence of renal ectopia ranges from 1 in 500 to 1 in 1200 in autopsy series, while horseshoe kidney is the most common renal fusion anomaly occurring in 0.25% of the population.[2]

Embryology

A review of the normal embryological development of the upper urinary tract is useful to allow visualization of the anatomic changes that may occur during abnormal development and provide perspective as to how they influence the approach to aortic reconstruction.

Three early kidneys, called the pronephros, the mesonephros, and the metanephros, develop from the mesoderm during the initial life of the embryo. The first two of these early structures regress, but by approximately the fourth week of gestation, the metanephros differentiates into the definitive fetal kidney, which forms in the sacral region. In this primitive single structure, a pair of ueteric buds develops and interacts with the metanephric mesenchyme to form a pair of fetal kidneys. It is thought that, during this process, the collecting system develops from each ureteric bud and the nephrons develop from the metanephric mesenchyme through reciprocal interaction. Between the sixth and ninth weeks of gestation, the two kidneys rotate and ascend from the pelvis to their usual anatomic position in the right and left side of the lumbar region, just below the adrenal glands. As the kidneys ascend, they receive their blood supply through a series of paired arteries arising in sequence from the primitive aorta and which degenerate as the kidneys migrate. The final result is usually a single pair of renal arteries, one for each kidney.[3]

Classification

Congenital anomalies of the kidneys and upper urinary tracts are categorized according to those resulting from problems with number, ascent, and rotation (Table 1),[2] as well as those resulting from problems with renal form and ascent (Table 2).[2] All can be associated with abnormalities in the renal vasculature as well as abnormalities

Table 2 Renal anomalies frequently complicating aortic aneurysm repair.[2]

Crossed renal ectopia without fusion
Solitary
Bilateral
Crossed renal ectopia with fusion
Inferior ectopic kidney
S-shaped (sigmoid) kidney
Lump kidney
L-shaped kidney
Disc kidney
Superior ectopic kidney
Horseshoe kidney

Table 3 Cold renal perfusate composition used by author.

1000 cc Ringer's lactate
1 ampoule (18 g) mannitol
500 mg methylprednisolone
2000 units heparin
Chill to 3°C

in the collecting system but the problems with renal form and ascent are the most troublesome for the vascular surgeon during aortic aneurysm repair.

If the kidney completely fails to ascend and remains in the pelvis, it is known as a pelvic kidney. However, if the renal ascent is only partially complete, the resulting kidney is known as an ectopic kidney. Because rotation is linked to ascent, pelvic and ectopic kidneys are usually also associated with some degree of malrotation. If the metanephric mass fails to separate in response to the development of two ureteric buds, a variety of fusion abnormalities may result, such as the development of a discoid or lump kidney (Table 2).[3] If one kidney fuses to the contralateral kidney and the fused kidneys ascend to the opposite side, crossed fused renal ectopia results. If the inferior poles of the two kidneys remain fused in the midline anterior to the aorta, the normal ascent of the fused renal mass may be blocked by the inferior mesenteric artery, resulting in the formation of a horseshoe kidney (Fig. 1).[3] Because the primitive renal unit fails to rotate medially, horseshoe kidneys and other forms of renal ectopia are often associated with abnormalities of the collecting system, such as the presence of multiple ureters, lying anterior to the renal isthmus in the case of horseshoe kidney, or a common renal pelvis, which can lie anterior to the abdominal aorta and, consequently, can complicate the exposure of an associated abdominal aortic aneurysm from the midline or transverse, transperitoneal approach.[4,5] Horseshoe kidneys are also often associated with multiple, abnormally located renal arteries (Fig. 2).[4,6] This feature probably arises because of disturbances in the appearance and regression of the sequential pairs of renal arteries that form during the normal ascent and rotation of the developing horseshoe kidney in the embryo. Only about one

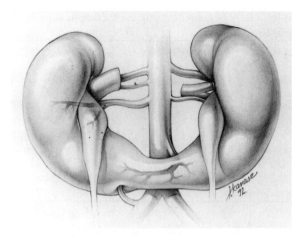

Fig. 1 Diagrammatic representation of horseshoe kidney anomaly and its relationship to the abdominal aorta. (Reprinted with permission from O'Hara et al.[4])

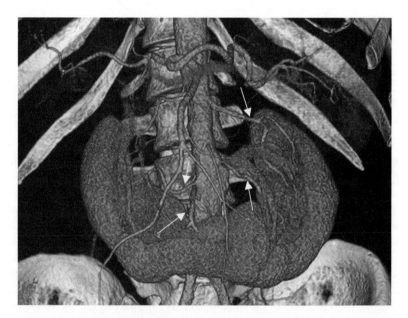

Fig. 2 3-Dimensional reconstruction of a CT image of an abdominal aortic aneurysm and coexistent horseshoe kidney. Note the multiple aberrant renal arteries (*arrows*)

third of horseshoe kidneys have renal arteries in the usual anatomic position but the remaining two thirds have either single or multiple arteries (Fig. 3). While the isthmus of a horseshoe kidney may occasionally be a fibrous band that might be amenable to division, more commonly it is composed of a thick ribbon of renal parenchyma (Fig. 4). Division of this thick parenchyma may be hazardous since the arterial distribution of the kidney is segmental with poor collateralization between the segments and the blood supply to the isthmus may be asymmetric and unpredictable arising from one side or the other.[4,5] As a result, exposure and division of the isthmus in this setting carries a risk of

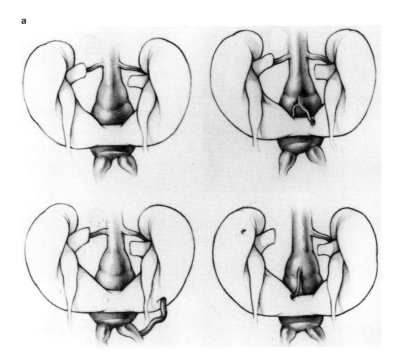

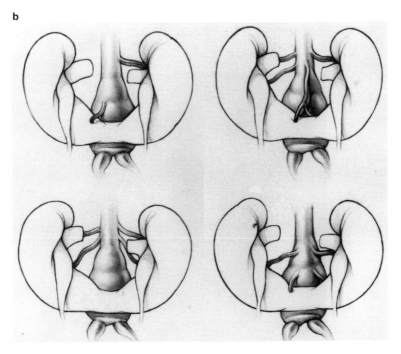

Fig. 3 Diagram of renal arterial patterns found in 19 patients with aortic aneurysms and coexistent horseshoe kidneys. (**a**) Four common patterns each found in more than one patient. (**b** and **c**) Seven uncommon patterns each found in a single patient. (Reprinted with permission from O'Hara et al.[4])

c

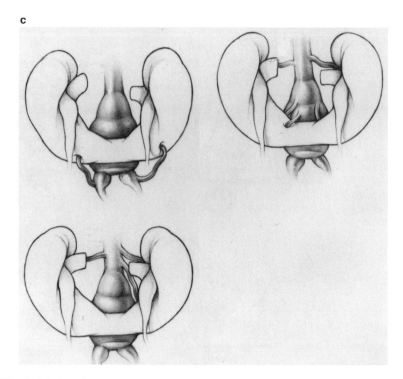

Fig. 3 (continued)

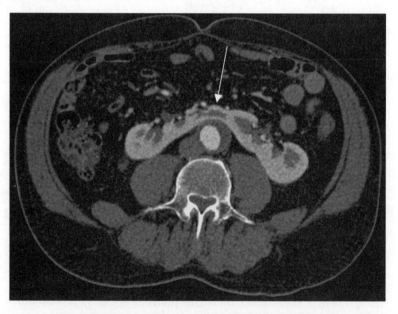

Fig. 4 CT scan demonstrating horseshoe kidney overlying a small abdominal aortic aneurysm. Note the isthmus (*arrow*) containing renal parenchyma and collecting system overlying the aorta. Division at this point would be hazardous

renal infarction, hydronephrosis, or possible urine leak or from an injury to the collecting system, a complication that may lead to subsequent graft infection, since approximately 13% of patients with horseshoe kidney are reported to have chronic urinary infection.[6]

Diagnosis and Imaging

Most would agree that it is best for the surgeon to be aware of the presence of coexistent horseshoe kidney or renal ectopia prior to the time of abdominal aortic aneurysm repair because its presence has the potential to substantially complicate the procedure whether either an open or an endovascular approach is utilized to repair the aneurysm. During an open aneurysm repair, an experienced surgeon could probably define most of the anomalous anatomy, but clearly more operative time would be required and the procedure would likely entail more potential for injury. Furthermore, it might not be possible to completely determine the arterial and collecting system anatomy with certainty or gain adequate exposure for safe aneurysm repair from the anterior, transperitoneal approach. Depending on the arterial distribution (Fig. 3) encountered, endovascular aneurysm exclusion with the current commercially available endografts may not be feasible without sacrifice of substantial renal parenchyma.

On physical examination of the abdomen, the size of an abdominal aortic aneurysm may be overestimated in the presence of a coexistent horseshoe kidney because of the presence of the renal mass overlying the aneurysm. Interestingly, ultrasonography is usually able to correctly estimate the size of the associated aneurysm but was only able to demonstrate the associated horseshoe kidney in a minority of patients. In our own series, preoperative ultrasonography was interpreted to demonstrate the horseshoe kidney in only 38% (5/13) of the patients in whom it was obtained (Fig. 5),[4] a finding also reported by others.[7] Angiography was only able to demonstrate the presence

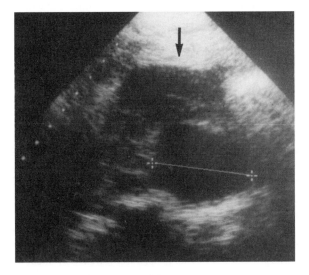

Fig. 5 Ultrasound examination of the abdominal aorta with horseshoe kidney (*arrow*) anterior to the aortic aneurysm. (Reprinted with permission from O'Hara et al.[4])

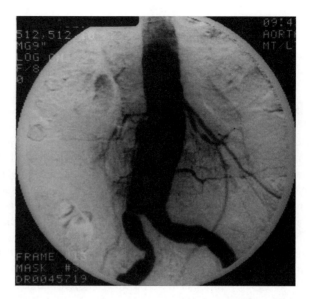

Fig. 6 Transfemoral aortogram of a patient with an abdominal aortic aneurysm and coexistent horseshoe kidney. (Reprinted with permission from O'Hara et al.[4])

of the horseshoe kidney in about two thirds of the patients in our own series, but it has been a useful tool to delineate the aberrant arterial anatomy when the presence of the renal anomaly is known (Fig. 6).[4] Currently, MRI scanning or, preferentially, CT scanning with three-dimensional image reconstruction is the most useful diagnostic imaging method for the detection of horseshoe kidney or renal ectopia and for planning an optimal treatment strategy for coexistent abdominal aortic aneurysm repair (Fig. 7). In our own experience, which was collected over a span of 31 years, horseshoe kidney was recognized preoperatively in 84% (16/19) of patients and discovered intraoperatively in the remaining 3 (16%).[4] However, in the current era, because of the liberal use of CT or MRI scanning, it would be unusual not to have the diagnosis of coexistent horseshoe kidney available preoperatively, even for urgent procedures, provided that the patient is stable enough to undergo preoperative scanning.

Therapy

Open Repair

The technical aspects of the management of anomalous renal arteries have evolved to the point that open abdominal aortic aneurysm repair in the presence of coexistent horseshoe kidney, with preservation of the renal blood supply, collecting system and renal mass, is virtually always feasible, provided that the patient is an acceptable surgical risk. Two approaches transperitoneal and left retroperitoneal are used, and each has inherent advantages. The first abdominal aortic aneurysm repair in the presence of horseshoe kidney was performed at the Mayo Clinic in 1956.[8] For this procedure, a transperitoneal approach was utilized and no arterial or venous anomalies were encountered. The aneurysm

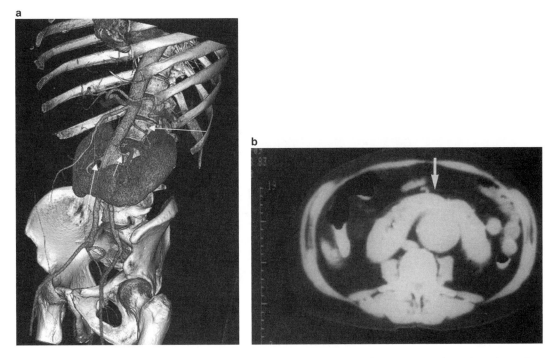

Fig. 7 (**a**) 3-Dimensional reconstruction of a CT image of an abdominal aortic aneurysm and coexistent horseshoe kidney. Note the multiple aberrant renal arteries (*arrows*). (**b**) CT scan demonstrating horseshoe kidney overlying an abdominal aortic aneurysm. Note the isthmus (*arrow*) containing renal parenchyma overlying the aorta

was replaced with an aortic homograft that was tunneled posterior to the isthmus of the horseshoe kidney. In our own experience, however, this normal pattern of renal arteries was encountered in only 26% of patients with coexistent abdominal aortic aneurysm and horseshoe kidney whereas anomalous renal arteries were encountered in the remaining 74%[4] (Fig. 3), findings also reported by other investigators.[2,6] Early in our experience, transperitoneal exposure through a midline incision was used and the aortic graft was tunneled through the aneurysm sac behind the isthmus. Often in the past, this exposure was chosen because the presence of a horseshoe kidney was not appreciated prior to abdominal aortic aneurysm repair. Perhaps the single advantage of this approach is that it offers better exposure of the distal right common iliac artery than does the left retroperitoneal approach, especially in an obese patient. Anomalous renal arteries must be reconstructed with either reimplantation or bypass but the exposure through the transperitoneal approach is sometimes less than ideal, especially if the aberrant renal arteries arise from the aorta or iliac arteries directly posterior to the horseshoe kidney (Fig. 8). Furthermore, if the length of the renal artery is inadequate to reach the graft after the aneurysm is decompressed, the renal bypass grafts required for reconstruction are often difficult to construct and to position in order to minimize the risk of kinking when performed from the transperitoneal approach.[4,5] Division of the isthmus to facilitate access to the underlying aortic aneurysm has been reported but is probably hazardous because of the risk of ischemia or injury to the anomalous collecting system.[4,5]

a

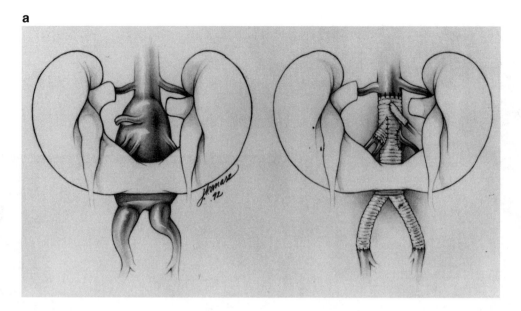

b

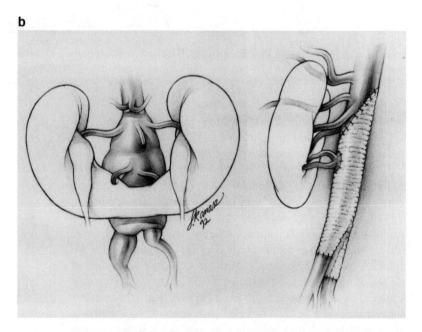

Fig. 8 Diagram of surgical exposure and reconstruction options. (**a**) Transperitoneal exposure through a midline abdominal incision with Dacron graft placed beneath renal isthmus and renal branches reconstructed by implantation or bypass grafting. (**b**) Retroperitoneal exposure through a low left thoracoabdominal incision. Dacron graft placed within the aneurysm sac and renal arterial branches reconstructed by implantation. (Reprinted with permission from O'Hara et al[4])

From a practical perspective, given the advances in preoperative imaging techniques using CT or MR scanning, the diagnosis of coexistent horseshoe kidney is rarely unsuspected prior to elective, or even emergency, abdominal aortic aneurysm repair. For these reasons we, and others, have advocated a low, left thoracoretroperitoneal approach for the repair of coexistent abdominal aortic aneurysm and horseshoe kidney (Fig. 8).[4,5,9] Ideally, the patient is placed in the left thoracoretroperitoneal position with the umbilicus centered over the break in the operating table. As near as possible, the shoulders are placed at an angle of 60° and the hips at 45° to the plane of the operating table. Positioning is aided by the use of the beanbag. The author favors an incision over the top of the ninth rib, which affords unobstructed access to the thoracic and abdominal aorta and is well tolerated in most patients. It allows the entire horseshoe kidney and collecting system to be retracted anteromedially, avoiding the renal isthmus and collecting system. The renal arteries are readily exposed through the opened aneurysm sac. Renal endarterectomy, if required, and implantation or bypass of all anomalous renal arteries as the local geometry requires are readily accomplished under direct vision through this approach. The single disadvantage of this approach may be limited access to the distal right common iliac artery, but this can usually be overcome with adequate retraction if necessary. Rarely, a counterincision superior to the right inguinal ligament or a femoro–femoral bypass graft may be required to revascularize the right leg.[4,5]

Although many reported cases of abdominal aortic aneurysm repair performed in the presence of a coexistent horseshoe or ectopic kidney have been performed without its use, some form of renal protection is probably advantageous, especially if the period of warm renal ischemia time is anticipated to be lengthy, irrespective of whether retroperitoneal or transperitoneal exposure is utilized. Depending on the local renal arterial anatomy, some authors have advocated temporary renal shunting,[10] while others have described temporary bypass construction, in situ cold perfusion, "double clamping" techniques, or even extracorporeal pump oxygenation.[11,12] It is the author's practice to infuse the renal arteries, if feasible, with a cold renal perfusate solution divided into each renal artery to extend the period of renal tolerance to ischemia during arterial reconstruction (Table 3). If practical, a total of 600 cc for the entire renal mass in the case of a single fused renal unit such as a horseshoe kidney, or the equivalent of 300 cc into each kidney in the normal situation, is infused and divided among the renal arteries present. This method seems less cumbersome and provides approximately 30–45 min of relative renal protection. It is, however, useful for the vascular surgeon to be familiar with several methods of renal protection.

Endovascular Repair

Since the first endovascular repair of an abdominal aortic aneurysm was described by Parodi in 1991,[13] it has been recognized that endovascular aneurysm repair avoids the necessity of direct dissection of the anomalous, ectopic kidney, as well as its collecting system, an advantage shared by the open, retroperitoneal approach. Furthermore, the procedure usually can be accomplished through small femoral incisions, avoiding the potential morbidity of the thoracoretroperitoneal incision in compromised patients. The principle impediment to the endovascular approach has been the anomalous renal arterial supply to the ectopic kidney, as described previously. Some have proposed endovascular repair if the arterial pattern is such that the main renal arteries can be preserved, only small accessory renal branches (<3 mm diameter) are sacrificed and preoperative renal function is normal.[14] Nevertheless, although generally well tolerated, small segmental renal infarcts were detected in 20–50% of the patients in whom renal branches were purposely covered during endografting.[1,14,15] One of four patients (25%) with endovascular exclusion of an abdominal aortic aneurysm with coexistent horseshoe kidney had a sustained postoperative 33% increase in serum creatinine levels despite normal preoperative renal function.[16] Preprocedure CT scanning and aortography were relatively insensitive in detecting small accessory renal vessels. As a consequence, more renal parenchyma may be at ischemic risk during endografting than is appreciated at the time of graft implantation. There is also the theoretical risk of type II endoleak because of the open accessory renal arteries.[14,17] However, since there is usually minimal, low-pressure, back-bleeding from renal arteries, the clinical significance of open accessory renal arteries is uncertain unless they function as outflow for a type II endoleak from a patent inferior mesenteric or lumbar artery.

It seems reasonable to consider endovascular repair for patients with coexisting abdominal aortic aneurysms and renal ectopia if they are prohibitively high risk for open aneurysm repair, have favorable renal anatomy that will put minimal renal parenchyma at ischemic risk, and have normal preoperative renal function. Most patients, however, should probably be offered open aneurysm repair.

Complications and Results

Because the coexistence of an abdominal aortic aneurysm and a horseshoe kidney or other form of renal ectopia is a relatively unusual occurrence, there exist relatively few large published series on the results of surgical treatment of the aortic aneurysm in this setting. Most published information concerning the early and late results of treatment by either open surgical or endovascular aneurysm repair consists of case reports and literature reviews. While there are no large series of endovascular abdominal aortic aneurysm repairs reported to date, the early results of the four largest series of open surgical treatment published so far are summarized in Table 4.[4,9,18,19] While the early postoperative mortality ranges from 0% to 16%, these results are undoubtedly heavily influenced by the mix of emergency and elective procedures as well as the extent of the associated patient morbidities and aneurysmal disease in the respective patient populations. It is well known that the presence of abnormal preoperative renal function is associated with increased postoperative morbidity and mortality after all forms of aortic surgery.[9,11,12,20] In our own

Table 4 Early outcomes following open repair of coexistent abdominal aortic aneurysms and horseshoe kidney or renal ectopia in recent selected series.

Abdominal aortic aneurysm and coexistent horseshoe kidney or renal ectopia				
Author	Year	Patients	Early postoperative deaths	Complications
de Virgilio et al.[18]	1995	16	0	29% (includes dialysis)
Shortell et al.[19]	1995	8	0	Dialysis 13% (1/8)
O'Hara et al.[4]	1993	19	16% (3/19)	Dialysis 16% (3/19)
Crawford et al.[9]	1988	13	15% (2/13)	Not specified

series, the presence of preoperative renal failure was the strongest indicator of a poor outcome following open aortic aneurysm repair in the presence of a coexistent horseshoe kidney.[4] Thirty-two per cent (6/19) of the patients in our own series had preoperative renal insufficiency and 3 of these (50%) required postoperative hemodialysis. Conversely, none of the 13 patients (68%) with normal preoperative renal function required postoperative hemodialysis, a difference that was statistically significant ($p = 0.02$). The early mortality rate for the entire series was 16% (3/19), 6% (1/16) for those patients not requiring postoperative dialysis, and 67% (2/3) for those patients who did require postoperative hemodialysis ($p = 0.05$).[4]

References

1. Kaplan DB, Kwon CC, Marin ML et al. Endovascular repair of abdominal aortic aneurysms in patients with congenital renal vascular anomalies. J Vasc Surg 1999; 30: 407–16.
2. Bauer SB. Anomalies of the upper urinary tract. In: Wein AJ (ed.), Campbell-Walsh Urology. 9th Ed., Philadelphia, WB Saunders Co., Chapt. 113, pp. 3269–304, 2007.
3. Park JM. Normal development of the urogenital system. In: Wein Jr AJ (ed.), Campbell-Walsh Urology. 9th Ed., Philadelphia, WB Saunders Co., Chapt. 106, pp. 3121–48, 2007.
4. O'Hara PJ, Hakaim AG, Hertzer NR, Krajewski LP, Cox GS, Beven EG. Surgical management of aortic aneurysm and coexistent horseshoe kidney: Review of 31-year experience. J Vasc Surg 1993; 17: 940–7.
5. Kasirajan K, O'Hara PJ. Renal ectopia and renal fusion in patients requiring abdominal aortic operations. In: Ernst CB, Stanley JC (eds.), Current Therapy in Vascular Surgery. St Louis (MO), Mosby, pp. 257–61, 2001.
6. Glenn JF. Analysis of 51 patients with horseshoe kidney. N Engl J Med 1959; 261: 684–7.
7. Taylor DC, Sladen JG, Maxwell T. Aortic surgery and horseshoe kidney: A challenging surgical problem. Can J Surg 1987; 30: 431–3.
8. Phelan JT, Bernatz PE, DeWeerd JH. Abdominal aortic aneurysm associated with a horseshoe kidney: Report of a case. Mayo Clin Proc 1957; 32: 77–81.
9. Crawford ES, Coselli JS, Safi HJ, Martin TD, Pool JL. The impact of renal fusion and ectopia on aortic surgery. J Vasc Surg 1988; 8(4): 375–83.
10. Schneider JR, Cronenwett JL. Temporary perfusion of a congenital pelvic kidney during abdominal aortic aneurysm repair. J Vasc Surg 1993; 17: 613.
11. Hollis HW, Rutherford RB: Abdominal aortic aneurysms associated with horseshoe or ectopic kidneys: Techniques of renal preservation. Semin Vasc Surg 1988; 1: 148.
12. Hollis HW, Jr., Rutherford RB, Crawford GJ, Cleland BP, Marx WH, Clark JR. Abdominal aortic aneurysm repair in patients with pelvic kidney. Technical considerations and literature review. [Review] [11 refs]. J Vasc Surg 1989; 9(3): 404–9.
13. Parodi JC, Palmax JC, Barone HD. Transfemoral intraluminal graft implantation for abdominal aortic aneurysms. Ann Vasc Surg 1991; 5: 491–9.
14. Ruppert V, Umscheid T, Rieger J et al. Endovascular aneurysm repair: Treatment of choice for abdominal aortic aneurysm coincident with horseshoe kidney? Three case reports and review of literature. J Vasc Surg 2004; 40: 367–70.
15. Aquino RV, Rhee RY, Muluk SC et al. Exclusion of accessory renal arteries during endovascular repair of abdominal aortic aneurysms. J Vasc Surg 2001; 34: 878–84.
16. Jackson RW, Fay DM, Wyatt MG et al. The renal impact of aortic stent-grafting in patients with a horseshoe kidney. Cardiovasc Intervent Radiol 2004; 27: 632–6.

17. Frego M, Bianchera G, Angriman I et al. Abdominal aortic aneurysm with coexistent horseshoe kidney. Surg Today 2007; 37: 626–30.

18. de Virgilio C, Gloviczki P, Cherry KJ et al. Renal artery anomalies in patients with horseshoe or ectopic kidneys: The challenge of aortic reconstruction. Cardiovasc Surg 1995; 3: 413–20.

19. Shortell CK, Welch EL, Ouriel K, Green RM, DeWesse JA. Operative management of coexistent aortic disease and horseshoe kidney. Ann Vasc Surg 1995; 9: 123–8.

20. de Virgilio C and Gloviczki P. Aortic reconstruction in patients with horseshoe or ectopic kidneys. Semin Vasc Surg 1996; 9: 245–52.

Chapter 19

Abdominal Aortic Aneurysms in Transplant Patients

Michael J. Englesbe

Abstract Physicians who manage aortic and iliac aneurysms will see increasing numbers of posttransplant patients present to the practice. Although the data is limited, there is a general agreement that aneurysm disease in transplant patients has a more aggressive course. Presumably, this is related to the long-term management of these patients on potent immunosuppressive medications. Preheart transplant patients with a history of ischemic cardiomyopathy should likely be screened for aortic aneurysms. Aortic aneurysms should be repaired in transplant patients when they are 5 cm in diameter, and iliac aneurysms should be repaired when they reach 3 cm. It is important to maintain transplant patients on their immunosuppressive medications throughout the perioperative period, though the potent immunosuppressant medication rapamycin requires special management. Patients with complicated postoperative courses should have their immunosuppression titrated accordingly, and a transplant physician should be involved in patient management. There are a few specific technical considerations for aneurysm repair in a previous heart and lung transplant recipient. If a liver transplant recipient requires an open aneurysm repair, the surgeon should be aware of the potential presence of an aortic conduit providing arterial inflow to the liver. When possible, pancreas and kidney transplant recipients should be most easily managed by an endovascular approach. If this is not possible, secondary to anatomic suitability then special consideration may be necessary to minimize the risk of postaneurysm repair organ failure.

Keywords Aortic aneurysm, Iliac aneurysm, Organ transplant, Immuno-suppression, Renal failure

Introduction

Organ transplantation is a lifesaving treatment for many patients with organ failure. As of 2004, there are over 1,50,000 people living in the United States with functioning organ transplants and over 90,000 people on the transplant

G. Upchurch and E. Criado (eds.) *Aortic Aneurysms, Contemporary Cardiology*
DOI: 10.1007/978-1-60327-204-9_19, © Humana Press, a part of
Springer Science+Business Media, LLC 2009

waiting list.[1] This population will continue to grow in size. This is due to both the improving long-term survival of transplant patients and a rate of transplantation that continues to increase by approximately 4% a year.[1] With the increasing use of donor organs that previously would have been discarded, patients who in the past had been considered too old or to sick for transplantation are now receiving lifesaving transplants.[2–4] These same older patients with increased comorbitities are at increased risk to develop aneurysms, and a consideration of their posttransplant status is necessary to optimize the care of their aneurysm disease.

Previously, the majority of patients who presented with aortic aneurysm disease were heart transplant patients. This was likely related to the close association between risk factors for ischemic heart disease and aneurysmal disease. Increasingly, liver and kidney transplants are being done on patients with risk factors for aneurysm disease. These patients represent a clinical challenge, with respect to management of their immunosuppression, management of their medical comorbidities, and the unique technical aspects of repairing aortic aneurysms in transplant patients.

In this chapter, we will discuss aortic and iliac aneurysm disease in transplant patients. We will overview the pathophysiology of aneurysm disease in the transplant patient and we will mention how it differs from nontransplant patients. The natural history of aneurysm disease in transplant patients will be discussed. Finally, the immunosuppressive and technical management of aortic and iliac aneurysms in transplant patients will be reviewed.

Pathophysiology

The pathophysiology of aneurysm disease, at both the cellular and hemodynamic level, has been detailed extensively in other sections of this volume. There is a general agreement in the literature that abdominal aortic aneurysms (AAAs) in transplant patients have a more aggressive course.[5–9] Unfortunately, this belief is based on small case series, which are inadequately powered to draw strong conclusions. There is even less data focusing on thoracic aortic aneurysm disease in transplant patients. In addition, there is minimal data addressing why aneurysm disease follows a different clinical course in transplant patients. Presumably, the immunosuppression medications that maintain the transplanted organ have an impact on the disease process. In addition, the hemodynamics of posttransplant patients may affect rates of aneurysmal expansion. In summary, even though conclusive empiric evidence is lacking, it seems prudent to give transplant patients with aneurysm disease special attention.

Overview of Immunosuppressive Medications

Immunosuppressive medications have broad ranging physiological effects, and these medications may affect the pathophysiology of aortic aneurysm disease. These medications are required in order to maintain the integrity of the transplant, primarily functioning to prevent a T-cell-mediated acute cellular rejection. There are three basic categories of immunosuppression medications that the majority of posttransplant patients take on a daily basis, including: calcineurin inhibitors, antimetabolites, and corticosteroids. In addition, patients may receive potent immunosuppression medications as induction therapy at the time of transplant or for treatment of acute cellular rejection. These medications usually include high-dose steroids and antithymocyte globulins. Another potent immunosuppressant that is being used on a more frequent basis is rapamycin. The specific immunosuppressive mechanisms of rapamycin are poorly understood, but rapamycin has been shown to be a potent smooth muscle cell inhibitor and is now commonly used as a coating on coronary stents. It is clear that rapamycin has a significant effect on the vascular wall, and has been shown to inhibit aneurysm growth in animal models.[10] Whether systemic rapamycin has a significant impact on clinical aneurysm disease remains unclear.

Transplant patients are also susceptible to another type of rejection known as antibody-mediated rejection. This form of rejection is poorly understood and these patients are at high risk for graft loss. These patients are treated aggressively with plasmapheresis, intravenous immunoglobulins, and B-cell-specific antibodies, such as rituximab. Following this aggressive treatment, these patients are profoundly immunosuppressed, and as a result, are at high risk for infectious complications. This profound degree of immunosuppression presumably also has effects on the pathophysiology of aneurysmal disease, but these remain to be characterized.

Modulation of Inflammation

The histopathological abnormality underlying thoracic aortic aneurysms is medial degeneration. This is characterized by a loss of smooth muscle cells, fragmentation and diminished numbers of elastic fibers, and increased accumulation of proteoglycans.[11] In contrast, AAAs are primarily characterized by atherosclerotic degeneration of the aortic wall. The pathophysiology of both thoracic aneurysms and AAAs involves a significant amount of cellular inflammation.[12] Presumably, immunosuppression medications will have an effect on the inflammatory process involved in aneurysm degeneration of the aortic wall. T cells and T-cell promoting cytokines, such as INF-γ, IL-2 IL-12, and IL-18, are thought to be important in the generation of an atheroma.[13] Calcineurin inhibitors inhibit IL-2 signaling and T-cell activation, while antimetabolites inhibit T-cell proliferation. Based on this mechanistic data, it is reasonable to speculate that immunosuppression medications may inhibit aneurysm degeneration. Interestingly, much of the experimental biology on aneurysm animal models have shown inhibition of aneurysm degeneration when experimental animals are placed on immunosuppressants.

These experimental findings are in contrast to clinical observations that transplant patients have a more virulent course of aneurysm disease. This observation is likely related to the fact that animal models cannot reproduce the complex milieu of the atherosclerotic lesion. Atherosclerotic disease has a more rapid progression in transplant patients. Most kidney transplant patient die with a functioning kidney transplant from complications of coronary artery disease, the most common cause of death.[14] Rapid progression of atherosclerotic disease is a multifactorial process, likely related to posttransplant hypertension, corticosteroid use, and posttransplant diabetes. Posttransplant renal insufficiency in particular is a common problem following lung, heart, and liver transplantation, and renal insufficiency is an important risk factor for atheroma generation and vascular calcification.[14,15]

In summary, immunosuppression medications likely foster the development of atherosclerotic lesions and as a result contribute to the pathophysiology of aortic aneurysm disease.

Posttransplant Hemodynamics

Posttransplant hemodynamic issues may also affect the natural history of aneurysm disease in transplant patients. While aneurysms grow at a rate of approximately 0.2–0.4 cm per year in the general population, aneurysms have been noted to grow at a rate of 1 cm per year following transplantation.[5,16,17] Similarly, the rate of growth of aneurysms accelerates in the posttransplant period in cardiac transplant patients. Cardiac transplant patients, in particular, have significant hemodynamic changes following transplantation, with significantly higher cardiac output and systemic blood pressure. Similarly, the majority of postabdominal transplant patients have hypertension following transplant, likely related to the use of calcineurin inhibitors. These hemodynamic changes following transplantation may effect the progression of vascular atherosclerosis in the aneurysm wall, accounting for increased wall stress in the aorta. Most likely, the increased rate of aneurysm expansion following transplant is a multifactorial process involving modulation of the inflammatory system, acceleration of atherosclerosis, and hemodynamic changes.

Prevalence and Screening of Aneurysmal Disease in Transplant Patients

It is speculated that the prevalence of aortic aneurysms is higher in transplant patients. Presumably, this is due to the frequent overlap of risk factors for any organ disease requiring transplant and for aortic aneurysm disease. In particular, this is true in older kidney transplant patients and patients with ischemic cardiomyopathy. More specifically, one report noted that the prevalence of aortic aneurysms was 6.2% in patients who had a heart transplant for ischemic cardiomyopathy, compared with a prevalence of 2.7% in patients who had a heart transplant for other indication. The prevalence of aortic aneurysms was only 0.4% in patients who had abdominal organ transplants.[5] In addition, other series report a prevalence of aortic aneurysms in heart transplant candidates to be between 1% and 4%.[8,18–20] As a basis for comparison, the prevalence of aortic aneurysms in men aged 65–80 in the general population ranges from 4% to 7.5%.[21,22] The fact that the prevalence seems to be the lower in patients who are being evaluated for heart transplant is likely explained by the fact that during the period when the prevalence studies of aortic aneurysm and heart transplant patients were preferred, heart transplants were not offered to older patients with ischemic cardiomyopathy. As the transplant population ages and as more heart and kidney transplant operations are done on older patients, more posttransplant patients will need treatment of their aortic aneurysms. Nonetheless, it is unclear whether there is a higher prevalence of aortic aneurysms in transplant patients.

Since the general population is not screened for aortic aneurysms, and since there is no clear data suggesting that there is a higher prevalence of aortic aneurysms in transplant patients, it is reasonable to ask whether it is appropriate to screen the transplant patient for an aortic aneurysm. Once again, the available data is inadequate to conclusively inform this decision.

As expected, one center reports that changes in screening practices increased the rate of aortic aneurysm diagnosis from 3% prior to a screening program to 5.8% once an aortic aneurysm screening program was initiated as a standard part of the preheart transplant workup.[5] When considering an AAA screening program for pretransplant patients, it is important to consider the clinical course of aneurysmal disease in transplant patients. As mentioned above, there is data noting an increased rate of aortic aneurysm expansion in the postheart transplant period. Note that the patients with previous transplants (heart, kidney, and liver) tolerate elective aortic aneurysm repair well, while transplant patients who present with rupture due particularly poorly.[5]

Which Transplant Patients Should Be Screened for Aneurysm Disease?

It is difficult to draw conclusions based on limited data. Nonetheless, considering the prevalence of risk factors for aortic aneurysms in patients with ischemic cardiomyopathy, the reported increased rate of aneurysm expansion in heart transplant patients following transplant, and the poor prognosis in transplant patients who present with rupture, it is reasonable that all patients who present for heart transplant evaluation with a history of ischemic cardiomyopathy should be screened for an AAA disease. In patients who present for evaluation for a lung transplant, pancreas transplant, or liver transplant, screening for AAA is not supported. Finally, patients being evaluated for renal transplant do not need to be screened for aortic aneurysm, unless there is a clinical suspicion on physical examination or a strong family history of aneurysm disease. In reality, patients who present for any type of transplant generally have had a comprehensive evaluation, and previous imaging studies are usually available to review and potentially diagnose an aortic aneurysm.

Clinical Management

Managing Immunosuppression in the Perioperative Period

In general, immunosuppressive medications are critical to maintain the integrity of the transplanted organ, and they should not be stopped in the perioperative period. All ambulatory immunosuppressive medications are given by mouth and these medications should just be continued. If a transplant patient is going to be in the hospital for less than 3 days, oral immunosuppressants are continued and immunosuppressant levels are not checked. If the patient has a prolonged period of taking nothing by mouth related to a postoperative ileus or other complications, then the surgeon must be concerned about whether the patient is getting adequate immunosuppression. In general, the patient should still be managed with oral medications, but the dose may need to be titrated. Intravenous immunosuppressants are labor-intensive, associated with significant complications, and thus rarely necessary. In general, major surgery and critical illness are profound immune suppressants. Rejection in the perioperative period is very uncommon. When transplant surgical patients are critically ill, immunosuppression doses are generally lowered. If an aneurysm patient has a complicated postoperative course, a practitioner experienced in transplant care should be consulted. A summary of perioperative immunosuppressant and recommendations is detailed in Table 1.

Table 1 Management of transplant immunosuppression in aneurysm patients

Immunosuppressive medication	Perioperative considerations in aneurysm patients
Calcineurin inhibitors (cyclosporin, tacrolimus)	1. Continue throughout peri-operative period. 2. Intravenous administration rarely needed. 3. Dose titration needed if complex postoperative course. 4. Acutely nephrotoxic if serum levels are too high.
Corticosteroids	1. Stress dose steroids generally not needed in perioperative period. 2. Aggressively wean if postoperative course complicated by life-threatening infection.
Antimetabolites (mycophenolic acid, azathioprine)	1. May consider stopping or reducing dose of these medications if postoperative course complicated by a life-threatening infection.
Rapamycin	1. Inhibits fibroblast function resulting in significant wound complications. 2. Consider transition to alternative medication preoperatively if open surgery is required.
Monoclonal and polyclonal antibodies	1. Avoid elective surgery in patients who have recently received these potent immunosuppressants.
Intravenous immunoglobulins	2. Avoid elective surgery in patients who were recently received this medication for management of transplant rejection.
Plasmapheresis	1. Profoundly immunosuppressive, so avoid in peri-operative period. 2. Consider post-plasmapheresis coagulopathy in the peri-operative period.

Posttransplant patients are more likely to have surgical complications. Whether this is specifically related to the immunosuppressive medications, or related to other perioperative risk factors, remains unclear. Most surgeons have observed differences in tissue integrity among patients who have been maintained on long-term steroids. Nonetheless, altering immunosuppressive regimen in the perioperative period is rarely indicated. One significant exception to this rule involves the relatively new and increasingly popular immunosuppressant, rapamycin. Rapamycin is a potent inhibitor of smooth muscle cell and fibroblast migration, and as a result, is a profound inhibitor of wound healing. In the authors experience and others, wound complications following major surgery on patients who are maintained on rapamycin approaches 100%.[23–25] Rapamycin not only affects soft tissue healing, but patients are also at increased risk of organ space complications, such as urine leak following kidney transplantation. Potential wound complications from a femoral incision associated with endovascular approaches in patients maintained on rapamycin should be expected. Strong consideration should be given to stopping rapamycin in the perioperative period for a patient who is undergoing an elective major open vascular surgical operation. Alternative immunosuppression will be needed in the perioperative period, and this should be managed by the patient's transplant physician. It is not necessary to stop rapamycin in patients who are undergoing an endovascular procedure, though wound complications will surely be more common.

When to Repair Aneurysms in Transplant Patients?

When planning an elective AAA repair in a transplant patient, careful consideration should be given to the timing of the operation. Close communication with the patient's primary transplant physician is mandatory. If a transplant patient was recently treated for severe infection or rejection, elective aortic surgery should be avoided until the patient is more stable. The limited available data seems to indicate that transplant patients have a more aggressive course of their aneurysm disease. In addition, there have been some reports of aneurysms rupturing in transplant patients at sizes that are generally considered low risk for rupture.[5] Stable transplant patients should have their aortic aneurysm repaired once it reaches 5 cm in diameter, and their iliac artery aneurysm repaired once it is 3 cm. Repair at a smaller diameter should be considered in female patients and in patients that are small in stature. Transplant patients with known aneurysms should be followed closely with serial imaging.

Aortic aneurysms are frequently diagnosed in patients undergoing an evaluation for transplantation. Careful consideration must be given regarding whether to fix the aneurysm before or after the transplant operation. In general, the risk of severe perioperative complications and death is high in patients sick enough to be considered for either lung, heart, or liver transplantation. Open aneurysm repair is generally deferred until after transplant. This decision becomes more complicated when endovascular repair of the aneurysm is considered. Patients frequently wait for months to years for their transplant. In this case, delay of repair of the aneurysm may not be appropriate. Transplant physicians need significant education regarding the risks and benefits of aneurysm repair in patients who are being considered for transplant. Since renal complications following aneurysm repair are so common, patients waiting for a kidney transplant should generally have their aneurysm repaired prior to kidney transplant.

Technical Considerations of Aneurysm Repair in Transplant Patients

Chronic renal failure is a well-recognized complication following all types of organ transplants.[15] This is thought to be related to long-term use of calcineurin inhibitors, which are the mainstay of maintenance immunosuppression for the majority of transplant recipients. The 5-year risk of chronic renal failure in nonrenal transplant recipients ranges from 7% to 21%, depending on the type of organ transplant.[15] Even patients with seemingly normal renal function will frequently have a moderate degree of renal impairment. As a result, great care should be taken to minimize intravenous contrast during the evaluation and management of their aortic aneurysm. Aggressive hydration and use of other medications to prevent nephrotoxicity following contrast injection should be used.

Heart and Lung Recipients
In patients with known heart or lung transplants, technical considerations for repair of the aneurysm are generally the same as nontransplant patients. Repair of a thoracic aneurysm in these patients will obviously be more complicated if done through an open incision. As a result, endovascular repair of thoracic aneurysms in heart and lung transplant recipients is preferred, when anatomically feasible.

Liver Recipients
Aneurysm repair in liver transplant recipients requires special technical consideration. Patients with a previous liver transplant will generally no longer have significant portal hypertension, if the portal vein is patent and the graft is functioning well. Nonetheless, they frequently may still have massive

splenomegaly, and as a result great care should be taken when doing an open aneurysm repair in a liver transplant patient. Approximately 5% of liver transplant patients will have an aortic conduit supplying inflow to the hepatic artery. This conduit is sewn either to the supraceliac (Fig. 1a) or infrarenal aorta (Fig. 1b). The location of this conduit must be considered in any liver transplant patient undergoing aneurysm repair. Luckily, liver transplant patients tend to be relatively free of adhesions throughout the abdomen with the exception of the right upper quadrant. In general, consideration of a previous liver transplant is not critical when deciding whether to approaching aneurysm through an open or endovascular approach.

Pancreas Recipients

Pancreas transplant recipients are most easily managed by an endovascular technique. The pancreas transplant is usually sewn to the right common iliac artery, though it may be sewn to the aorta or the external iliac artery. Due to the fragile nature of the pancreas parenchyma, it is generally very difficult to mobilize a pancreas transplant without jeopardizing its integrity. The pancreas is generally also sewn to its loop of small intestine. As a result, exposure of the aorta or the iliac arteries usually requires detaching the bowel anastomosis, and it can be very difficult to reconstruct.

Pancreas transplants do not provide a survival advantage to the recipient, the pancreas transplant may need to be removed if a life-threatening AAA aneurysm requires management. If endovascular stents are placed across the arterial inflow to a pancreas transplant that is still functioning, the transplant

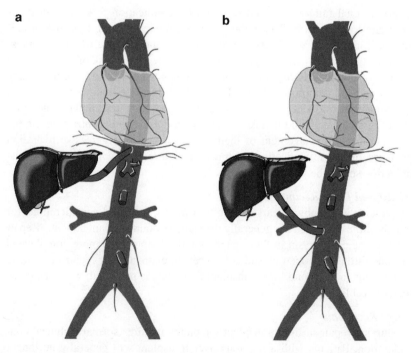

Fig. 1 The location of a supraceliac (**a**) and an infrarenal (**b**) aortic conduit to a liver transplant. The conduit is constructed when there is inadequate arterial inflow from the hepatic artery at the time of the transplant. An aortic conduit is present in approximately 5% of liver transplant patients

should be removed in the immediate postoperative period. If a pancreas is present, but is no longer functioning and does not take up contrast on CT scan or angiogram, then the transplant does not need to be removed following stent deployment across the transplant anastomotic site.

Kidney Recipients

Aneurysm disease in patients who have received a kidney transplant is a problem that is frequently encountered by vascular surgeons. This is related to improved survival following transplantation and the increased use of transplantation in patients with comorbidities that also put them at risk for AAA development.[26] In these patients, endovascular repair of the aneurysm is preferable when technically and anatomically possible. Loss of a functioning kidney transplant is associated with remarkably higher mortality for the recipient.[4] As a result, every effort should be made to maintain the function of the transplant while also adequately treating the aneurysm. This is particularly difficult in patients with iliac artery aneurysms.

Complete imaging of the aneurysm and the kidney transplant is critical, using MRI (Fig. 2a–c) and angiography. The kidney transplant is usually sewn between 3 and 10 cm from the internal and external iliac artery bifurcation.

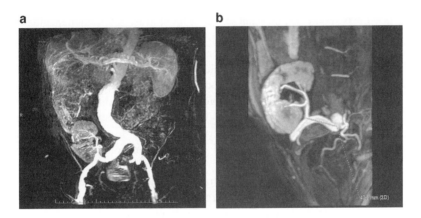

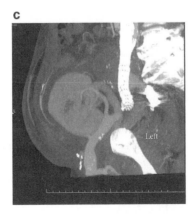

Fig. 2 Magnetic resonance imaging of renal transplant sewn to the right external iliac artery (**a**). The aneurysm terminates approximately 4 cm from the renal transplant anastomosis (**b**). Appearance following endovascular repair of the AAA and RCIA aneurysm (**c**)

Generally, the external iliac artery is spared from aneurysm degeneration. Nonetheless, efforts to adequately stent across the distal aspect of an iliac artery aneurysm may frequent jeopardize the inflow to the kidney transplant. This is particularly technically challenging when there are tortuous iliac vessels. If endovascular repair cannot be done safely without jeopardizing the kidney transplant, open repair should be preferred. If approached through the abdomen, the retroperitoneal kidney transplant will not need to be mobilized during the vascular operation. Mobilization of the kidney transplant in order to get adequate exposure for aneurysm repair is very difficult. The transplant will be densely adherent to the retroperitoneal structures, and renal parenchymal injury is common cause of significant bleeding, which can be difficult to manage.

There are several potential renal protective measures a surgeon can undertake prior to performing an open AAA repair in a patient with a kidney transplant. An axillary to femoral graft can be considered prior to the repair of an iliac aneurysm on the side of a kidney transplant. This technique ensures adequate inflow to the kidney transplant, while iliac arteries are clamped. Similarly, some authors suggest attempts at cold perfusion of the kidney transplant while arterial inflow is clamped.[7,27] Another option is the cannulation of the femoral artery and vein on the side of the kidney transplant for extracorporeal membrane oxygenation (ECMO). This technique works well, but obviously requires significant expertise and infrastructure in managing the ECMO circuit. Although all of these options may help preserve renal function, in the authors experience, they are generally unnecessary. More specifically, if a renal transplant recipient has a stable low creatinine and needs a complex aneurysm repair done in open fashion, the operation should be completed without taking these specific renal protective measures. Considering the complexity of the patients is important to remember the potential complications related to aggressive attempts to preserve the kidneys. In contrast, if a kidney transplant patient has marginal renal function, then consideration of these adjunct techniques is appropriate.

An apparent aneurysm near kidney transplant anastomotic site is most likely an anastomotic pseudoaneurysms. Surgical management of this problem frequently leads to transplant nephrectomy. Every effort should be made to manage kidney transplant pseudoaneurysm through endovascular techniques, such as coils or thrombin injection.

Summary

1. Surgeons who operate on patients with AAAs will increasingly be faced with aneurysm disease in transplant patients.
2. The pathophysiology of aneurysm disease in transplant patient is poorly understood. Limited data is available, but studies suggests a more malignant course of aneurysm disease in transplant patients.
3. Transplant patients with known aneurysms should be followed closely and perhaps AAAs should be fixed at a smaller size in transplant patients.
4. Patients undergoing heart transplant evaluation for ischemic cardiomyopathy should be screened for AAA.
5. Immunosuppressive medications should be continued throughout an uncomplicated perioperative course, with the important exception to this rule being rapamycin.

6. Posttransplant renal failure is very common in all types of transplant patients, and special attention to renal function is necessary when managing patients with AAAs.
7. Endovascular repair is preferable for the management of aortic and iliac aneurysms in kidney and pancreas transplant recipients.

References

1. Port FK, Merion RM, Finley MP, Goodrich NP, Wolfe RA. Trends in organ donation and transplantation in the United States, 1996–2005. Am J Transplant 2007;7 Suppl 1:1319–26.
2. Sung RS, Guidinger MK, Christensen LL, et al. Development and current status of ECD kidney transplantation. Clin Transpl 2005:37–55.
3. Merion RM, Pelletier SJ, Goodrich N, Englesbe MJ, Delmonico FL. Donation after cardiac death as a strategy to increase deceased donor liver availability. Ann Surg 2006;244(4):555–62.
4. Merion RM, Ashby VB, Wolfe RA, et al. Deceased-donor characteristics and the survival benefit of kidney transplantation. JAMA 2005;294(21):2726–33.
5. Englesbe MJ, Wu AH, Clowes AW, Zierler RE. The prevalence and natural history of aortic aneurysms in heart and abdominal organ transplant patients. J Vasc Surg 2003;37(1):27–31.
6. Fazel S, Lawlor DK, Forbes TL. Abdominal aortic aneurysms following orthotopic heart transplantation. Vasc Endovascular Surg 2004;38(2):149–55.
7. Favi E, Citterio F, Tondolo V, et al. Abdominal aortic aneurysm in renal transplant recipients. Transplant Proc 2005;37(6):2488–90.
8. Piotrowski JJ, McIntyre KE, Hunter GC, Sethi GK, Bernhard VM, Copeland JC. Abdominal aortic aneurysm in the patient undergoing cardiac transplantation. J Vasc Surg 1991;14(4):460–5; discussion 5–7.
9. Vantrimpont PJ, van Dalen BM, van Riemsdijk-van Overbeeke IC, Maat AP, Balk AH. Abdominal aortic aneurysms after heart transplantation. J Heart Lung Transplant 2004;23(2):171–7.
10. Lawrence DM, Singh RS, Franklin DP, Carey DJ, Elmore JR. Rapamycin suppresses experimental aortic aneurysm growth. J Vasc Surg 2004;40(2):334–8.
11. Guo DC, Papke CL, He R, Milewicz DM. Pathogenesis of thoracic and abdominal aortic aneurysms. Ann N Y Acad Sci 2006;1085:339–52.
12. Golledge J, Muller J, Daugherty A, Norman P. Abdominal aortic aneurysm: pathogenesis and implications for management. Arterioscler Thromb Vasc Biol 2006;26(12):2605–13.
13. Libby P, Theroux P. Pathophysiology of coronary artery disease. Circulation 2005;111(25):3481–8.
14. Rosas SE, Mensah K, Weinstein RB, Bellamy SL, Rader DJ. Coronary artery calcification in renal transplant recipients. Am J Transplant 2005;5(8):1942–7.
15. Ojo AO, Held PJ, Port FK, et al. Chronic renal failure after transplantation of a nonrenal organ. N Engl J Med 2003;349(10):931–40.
16. Bernstein EF, Dilley RB, Goldberger LE, Gosink BB, Leopold GR. Growth rates of small abdominal aortic aneurysms. Surgery 1976;80(6):765–73.
17. Bernstein EF, Chan EL. Abdominal aortic aneurysm in high-risk patients. Outcome of selective management based on size and expansion rate. Ann Surg 1984;200(3):255–63.
18. Reitz BA, Baumgartner WA, Oyer PE, Stinson EB. Abdominal aortic aneurysmectomy in long-term cardiac transplant survivors. Arch Surg 1977;112(9):1057–9.
19. Reichman W, Dyke C, Lee HM, Hanrahan J, Szentpetery S, Sobel M. Symptomatic abdominal aortic aneurysms in long-term survivors of cardiac transplantation. J Vasc Surg 1990;11(3):476–9.

20. Muluk SC, Steed DL, Makaroun MS, et al. Aortic aneurysm in heart transplant recipients. J Vasc Surg 1995;22(6):689–94; discussion 95–6.

21. Scott RA, Vardulaki KA, Walker NM, Day NE, Duffy SW, Ashton HA. The long-term benefits of a single scan for abdominal aortic aneurysm (AAA) at age 65. Eur J Vasc Endovasc Surg 2001;21(6):535–40.

22. Vardulaki KA, Prevost TC, Walker NM, et al. Incidence among men of asymptomatic abdominal aortic aneurysms: estimates from 500 screen detected cases. J Med Screen 1999;6(1):50–4.

23. Mehrabi A, Fonouni H, Wente M, et al. Wound complications following kidney and liver transplantation. Clin Transplant 2006;20 Suppl 17:97–110.

24. Burgos FJ, Pascual J, Quicios C, et al. Post-kidney transplant surgical complications under new immunosuppressive regimens. Transplant Proc 2006;38(8):2445–7.

25. Kuppahally S, Al-Khaldi A, Weisshaar D, et al. Wound healing complications with de novo sirolimus versus mycophenolate mofetil-based regimen in cardiac transplant recipients. Am J Transplant 2006;6(5 Pt 1):986–92.

26. Merion RM. 2006 SRTR Report on the State of Transplantation. Am J Transplant 2007;7 Suppl 1:1317–8.

27. Ierardi RP, Coll DP, Kumar A, Solomon BR, Kerstein MD, Matsumoto T. Abdominal aortic aneurysectomy after kidney transplantation: case report and review of the literature. Am Surg 1996;62(11):961–6.

Chapter 20

Inferior Vena Cava: Embryology and Anomalies

Brian Knipp, Paul Knechtges, Thomas Gest, and Thomas Wakefield

Abstract Reconstruction of the abdominal aorta and its visceral branches is one of the most common operations performed by practicing vascular surgeons. These procedures can be challenging depending on the patient anatomy and the state of the aorta. In cases of aneurysm rupture, time is of the essence; there is very little margin for error. An intimate knowledge of the anatomy of the caval venous system and its tributaries, including familiarity with developmental anomalies, is critical to safe, rapid, and precise anatomical dissection.

Keywords Venous anomalies, Preaortic/retroaortic vein, Inferior vena cava, Duplicated IVC, Vena cava anomalies

Embryology

The inferior vena cava and its tributary branches develop during the fourth to the eighth week of gestation through a complex pattern of venous development, anastomosis, and regression.[1] From caudal to cranial, the segments are referred to as the postrenal, renal, prerenal, and hepatic segments.[2–4] There are a number of documented anomalies of the inferior vena cava and its branches which can be understood more clearly based on the embryologic patterns of development. Knowledge of these developmental patterns and possible variations can prevent inadvertent and potentially life-threatening complications during aortic and retroperitoneal surgery.

The development of the inferior vena cava involves both the visceral and the parietal system. The first of the three pairs of parietal veins to develop are the posterior cardinal veins, dominant in the fourth week of gestation, which drain blood from the lower extremities in two discrete dorsal channels which, early on, do not communicate (Fig. 1a).[3] Anterior cardinal veins drain the cephalic portion of the fetus, and both pairs of veins coalesce into the sinus venosus, the site of the developing cardiac structures.[5] During the sixth week of gestation, the subcardinal veins then appear anteromedial to the posterior cardinal veins. These vessels join near the mesonephri to form a midline anastomosis, the preaortic intersubcardinal anastomosis,[6] and empty into the posterior cardinal

G. Upchurch and E. Criado (eds.) *Aortic Aneurysms, Contemporary Cardiology*
DOI: 10.1007/978-1-60327-204-9_20, © Humana Press, a part of
Springer Science+Business Media, LLC 2009

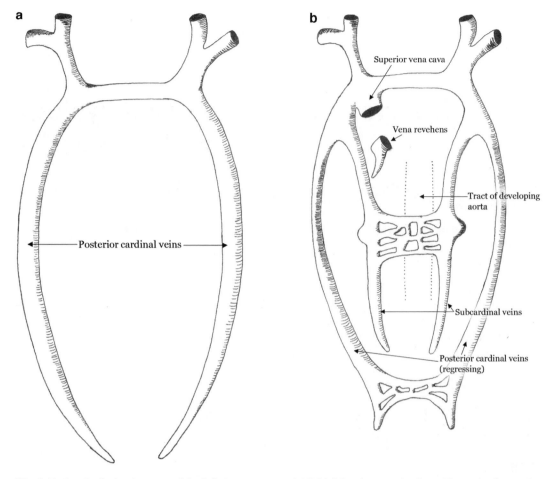

Fig. 1 Embryologic development of the inferior vena cava. (**a**) Initial development begins with a pair of posterior cardinal veins. (**b**) A second pair of veins, the subcardinal veins, arises and coalesces in the mesonephros

veins in the cranioventral aspect of the developing fetus, in proximity to the future location of the terminal arch of the azygos vein (Fig. 1b).

Concomitant with the development of the parietal venous circulation, the hepatic venous system develops from the coalescence of the vitelline veins, which drain the yolk sac and become the portal venous system. As the liver develops, the drainage of this coalescence becomes interrupted by the primitive hepatic sinusoids.[3] These sinusoids are drained by the efferent venae revehentes, which combine to form the right and left hepatic veins which then drain into the right atrium. Downward extensions from the venae revehentes anastomose with the cranial extent of the developing inferior vena cava. The posterior cardinal veins begin to form midline anastomoses and the cranial aspects begin to regress (Fig. 1b).[4,7]

A third pair of primitive parietal veins develops, known as the supracardinal veins, which are dominant in the seventh week.[5] Arising from the cranial end of the posterior cardinal veins, these vessels descend and together with subcardinal

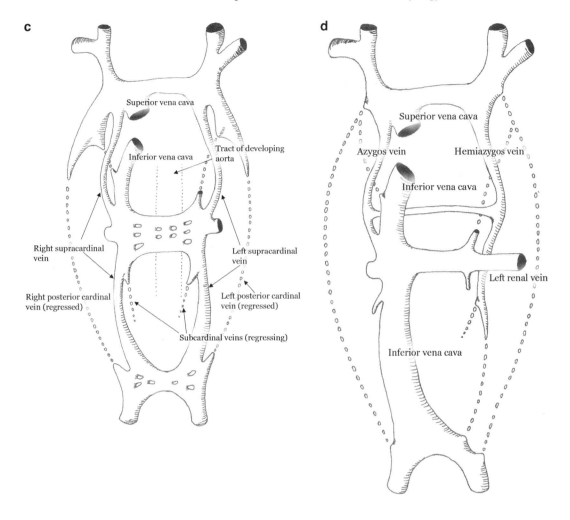

Fig. 1 (continued) (**c**) The supracardinal veins arise last, as the posterior cardinal and subcardinal veins begin to regress. (**d**) The completed vena cava. Dotted lines represent obliterated vessels

veins form a complex set of anastomoses in the mesonephric region known as the aortic collar. The usual pattern of development is regression of the intersupracardinal anastomosis, posterior to the aorta, while the intersubcardinal anastomosis anterior to the aorta persists and develops into the right and left renal veins (Fig. 1c). Errors in these regression patterns lead to renal vein anomalies, as discussed later.[8] The anastomosis of the right supracardinal and right subcardinal vein becomes the renal segment of the vena cava, and the extension of the right supracardinal vein to its anastomosis with the inferior aspect of the posterior cardinal veins becomes the postrenal segment. Beyond this anastomosis, the posterior cardinal veins contribute the iliac venous bifurcation and the common iliac veins. The superior aspects of the supracardinal veins persist as the azygos and hemiazygos systems. The subcardinal veins inferior to the aortic collar regress, as does the right subcardinal vein superior to the anastomosis to the hepatic veins. The superior portion of the left subcardinal vein persists as the left adrenal vein (Fig. 1d).

Venous Anomalies

Epidemiology of Venous Anomalies

Anomalies of the inferior vena cava and its branches occur frequently in patients with other congenital abnormalities of the cardiovascular system, but also can occur in the asymptomatic patient with no other discernable defects. While early aortic surgery often took place without the aid of preoperative computed tomography, this has become infrequent in the modern era and therefore these anomalies are more commonly diagnosed preoperatively. The landmark treatise on vena caval anomalies was published in 1925 by McClure and Butler; this report documented 14 patterns of caval variation in the feline, many of which are seen also in humans.[9] Estimates of the prevalence of these anomalies in the general population range from 0.8% to 5.8% based on radiographic studies,[2,4,10–19] 0.9% to 3.7% based on surgical series,[7,17,20–24] and 1.7%

Table 1 Review of literature series for caval anomalies.

Author	Year	Study type	N patients	Overall anomalies	Double IVC	Left IVC	RLRV	CLRV	AIVC-AC
Gladstone[6]	1929	Autopsy	876		2 (0.2%)	1 (0.1%)			
Seib[26]	1934	Autopsy	176		5 (2.8%)	1 (0.6%)	3 (1.7%)	16 (9.1%)	
Pick and Anson[27]	1940	Autopsy	202				7 (3.5%)	34 (16.8%)	
Reis and Esenther[28]	1959	Autopsy	500		11 (2.2%)	1 (0.2%)	12 (2.4%)	30 (6.0%)	
Davis and Lundberg[25]	1968	Autopsy	270	9 (3.3%)			5 (1.9%)	4 (1.5%)	
Royster et al.[23]	1974	Autopsy	159	3 (1.9%)			3 (1.9%)		
Hoeltl et al.[17]	1990	Autopsy	354	6 (1.7%)			4 (1.1%)	2 (0.6%)	
Reed et al.[13]	1982	CT scan	433				8 (1.8%)	19 (4.4%)	
Alexander et al.[14]	1982	CT scan	1200		1 (0.1%)	1 (0.1%)	1 (0.1%)	3 (0.3%)	
Mayo et al.[4]	1983	CT scan	1140		5 (0.4%)	4 (0.4%)	1 (0.1%)	1 (0.1%)	
Ueda et al.[15]	1983	CT scan	874		6 (0.7%)	9 (1.0%)			
Ueda et al.[15]	1983	CT scan	1260						1 (0.1%)
Kukubo et al.[16]	1988	CT scan	1100		12 (1.1%)	2 (0.2%)	4 (0.4%)	6 (0.5%)	
Hoeltl et al.[17]	1990	CT scan	4520	36 (0.8%)	1 (0.02%)	2 (0.04%)	29 (0.6%)	4 (0.1%)	
Matano et al.[12]	1993	CT scan	130	3 (2.3%)		2 (1.5%)	1 (0.8%)	0 (0%)	
Aljabri et al.[11]	2001	CT scan	1788	103 (5.8%)	7 (0.4%)	3 (0.2%)	57 (3.2%)	29 (1.6%)	
Karaman et al.[10]	2007	CT scan	1856				51 (2.7%)	17 (0.9%)	
Holden et al.[18]	2005	CT scan	100		1 (1.0%)		3 (3.0%)	7 (7.0%)	
Kawamoto et al.[19]	2005	CT scan	100				2 (2.0%)	9 (9.0%)	
Anderson et al.[7]	1961	Surgical	2500						15 (0.6%)
Royster et al.[23]	1974	Surgical	228	2 (0.9%)			2 (0.9%)		
Bartle et al.[21]	1987	Surgical	289	6 (2.1%)	1 (0.3%)	1 (0.3%)	4 (1.4%)	1 (0.3%)	
Hoeltl et al.[17]	1990	Surgical	215	8 (3.7%)			6 (2.8%)	2 (0.9%)	
Shindo et al.[22,a]	2000	Surgical	166	4 (2.4%)	2 (1.2%)			1 (0.6%)	
Lin et al.[20]	2004	Surgical	170				2 (1.2%)	16 (9.4%)	
Truty and Bower[24]	2007	Surgical	2427	35 (1.4%)	2 (0.1%)	3 (0.1%)	26 (1.1%)	4 (0.2%)	

Data are presented as number of patients (percentage of patients in study)

IVC inferior vena cava. *RLRV* retroaortic left renal vein, *CLRV* circumaortic left renal vein. *AIVC-AC* absent inferior vena cava with azygos continuation

[a]In this study, a preaortic confluence of the iliac veins accounted for the missing anomaly

to 3.3% based on autopsy series.[6,17,23,25–28] (see Table 1). Despite the increase in preoperative imaging, studies have demonstrated that these anomalies are often missed during preoperative workup by both the surgeon and the radiologist. These undiagnosed anomalies can lead to vascular injury and potentially life-threatening hemorrhage during aortic and retroperitoneal surgery. In a series from the Mayo Clinic, of eight patients with venous anomalies undergoing aortic reconstruction which was complicated by significant (>500 cc) blood loss, seven were undiagnosed preoperatively.[24]

Retroaortic and Circumaortic Left Renal Vein

During the sixth through the eighth week of development, the subcardinal and supracardinal veins form a central anastomotic web around the aorta, as earlier discussed. The anterior segment of the web becomes the left renal vein, while the posterior portion regresses. Failure of regression of the posterior portion leads to circumaortic left renal vein (Fig. 2), while persistence of the posterior segment and regression of the anterior segment lead to a retroaortic left renal vein (Fig. 3).[8] There are four classifications of retroaortic left renal vein. In type I, the left renal vein passes directly behind the aorta and inserts at the normal location on the IVC. Type II descends from its takeoff at the renal hilum and intersects the IVC at approximately L4/5. Types I and II tend to occur with similar frequency in the literature.[10,17] Type III is the circumaortic left renal vein, which occurs more frequently than type I or II, as discussed below. Type IV descends from the renal pelvis to insert on the left common iliac vein. There are very few case reports of this type of anomaly in the literature.[10,29]

The presence of a retroaortic left renal vein is a very dangerous clinical situation, associated with a significant risk of damage, hemorrhage, and interoperative death if the vessel is not identified and protected during aortic surgery.[29] In radiographic series, the incidence of retroaortic left renal vein

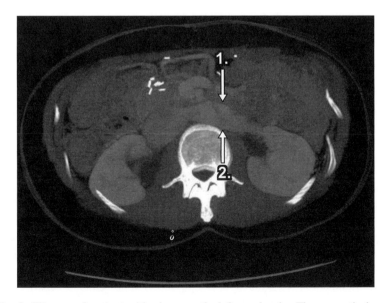

Fig. 2 CT scan of patient with circumaortic left renal vein. The preaortic branch (*arrow 1*) and the retroaortic branch (*arrow 2*) of left renal vein are seen

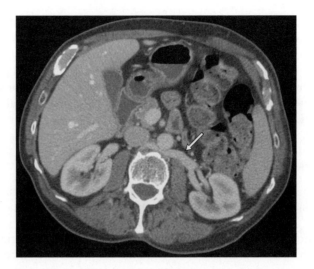

Fig. 3 CT scan of patient with retroaortic left renal vein (*arrow*)

ranges from 0.1% to 3.2%.[4,10–14,16–19] Surgical series cite rates from 0.9% to 2.8%,[17,20–21,23–24] and autopsy series cite from 1.1% to 3.5%.[17,23,25–28] In a study by Brener et al., 9 of 20 (45%) retroaortic left renal veins were injured during dissection, leading to two nephrectomies and two deaths. They concluded that the most dangerous maneuver with respect to venous injury during aortic dissection is circumferential dissection of the proximal aorta.[30] In the Mayo series, 5 of 26 cases of retroaortic left renal vein were injured (19%); only one was identified preoperatively. In this series, the diagnostic accuracy of preoperative imaging was only 19% for retroaortic left renal vein and 25% for circumaortic left renal vein. All diagnoses were made by CT scanning; ultrasound was uniformly unable to diagnose this condition. Limiting analysis to CT scanning only, the preoperative diagnostic accuracy was still only 45% for retroaortic left renal vein and 33% for circumaortic left renal vein.[24] Bartle et al. recommend a superior approach to obtain proximal control once a retroaortic left renal vein has been identified.[21]

The circumaortic left renal vein is arguably more dangerous than the retroaortic renal vein, as the presence of the preaortic branch can lead to a false sense of security if preoperative diagnosis of the anomaly is not made.[22] This anomaly is likely underreported due to the fact that surgeons do not generally look for a retroaortic left renal vein branch once the preaortic vein has been found. Nonetheless, the rate is reported to range from 0% to 9% in the radiographic literature,[4,10–14,16–19] 0.2% to 9.4% in surgical series,[17,20–22,24] and 0.6% to 16.8% in autopsy series.[17,25–28] In 15% of cases, multiple preaortic or retroaortic left renal vein branches exist. The retroaortic branch of the circumaortic left renal vein tends to run obliquely to the aorta, putting it at increased risk from clamp injury. Once the diagnosis of circumaortic left renal vein has been made, however, one branch (ideally the more diminutive) can be ligated safely. Bartle et al. recommend securing proximal control of the aorta below the level of the circumaortic left renal vein, as opposed to approaching it superiorly as recommended for the purely retroaortic left renal vein.[21]

While a retroaortic left renal vein is generally asymptomatic, they occasionally present with symptoms of venous outflow obstruction from the renal, pelvic, or gonadal vessels (Table 2). One study has documented an association between retroaortic left renal vein and varicocele. In a case control study of 277 patients, the rate of retroaortic left renal vein was 9.3% in patients with a left or bilateral varicocele compared with 2.2% of control patients.[31] The authors conclude that the retroaortic left renal vein may be part of the etiology of varicocele, and conversely the presence of varicocele in a patient undergoing aortic surgery should suggest the potential presence of a retroaortic left renal vein. Koc et al. presented case reports of two female patients with pelvic congestion syndrome and double retroaortic left renal veins, suggesting a correlation.[32] Gibo et al. documented a case of gross hematuria secondary to retroaortic left renal vein in a 13-year-old female; left renal venous hypertension was verified with pullback pressures.[33]

One rare but potential complication of a retroaortic left renal vein in a patient with an abdominal aortic aneurysm is rupture of the aneurysm into the left renal vein secondary to compression of the vein by the expanding aneurysm against the vertebral bodies leading to pressure necrosis. These patients generally do not present with high output cardiac failure or massive lower extremity edema, as do patients with aortocaval fistulae. Instead they generally present with one or more of the following: left flank pain due to stretch of Gerota's fascia from venous congestion of the kidney, hematuria, and acute renal failure which tends to resolve with prompt repair of the fistula. A physical finding of this condition is a new left flank bruit. A palpable thrill in the left renal vein noted during surgical dissection can be a diagnostic clue to the presence of this complication.

Table 2 Most common presenting symptoms of caval anomalies.

Most common symptoms
Retroaortic or circumaortic left renal vein
Asymptomatic
Varicocele
Pelvic congestion syndrome
Unexplained hematuria
Left-sided or duplicated vena cava
Asymptomatic
Lower extremity swelling
Recurrent deep venous thrombosis
Venous stasis ulceration
Absent retrohepatic vena cava with azygos continuation, absent pararenal
or infrarenal vena cava
Asymptomatic
Lower extremity swelling
Recurrent deep venous thrombosis
Venous stasis ulceration
Hemoptysis
Marsupial cava
Asymptomatic

Left-Sided Vena Cava

During normal development, the infrarenal vena cava develops from the right supracardinal vein during the seventh to eighth week of gestation. The posterior cardinal veins, which develop earlier during the fourth week, provide the outflow from the lower extremities by developing into the iliac veins. These veins form ventral and dorsal anastomoses in the midline, and then divide again as they run caudally. Once the right supracardinal vein develops, it descends and joins the iliac confluence in the dorsal location. The anterior anastomosis regresses; persistence of this anastomosis and joining of the right supracardinal vein at this point lead to preaortic iliac vein confluence, which will be discussed separately. The left supracardinal vein generally regresses, as do the posterior cardinal veins above the iliac confluence.

If the left supracardinal vein persists and the right vein regresses, this leads to a left-sided vena cava. This is generally a mirror image transposition below the renal veins; the left gonadal vein inserts on the vena cava and the right inserts on the right renal vein (Figs. 4 and 5). The vena cava crosses to the right side at approximately the level of the renal arteries, generally crossing in front of the aorta. Prevalence of this anomaly ranges from 0.04% to 1.5% in radiographic series,[4,11–12,14–17] 0.1% to 0.3% in surgical series,[21,24] and 0.1% to 0.6% in autopsy series.[6,26,28]

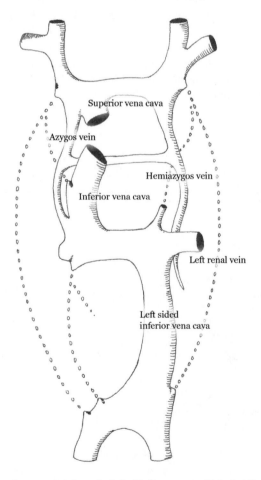

Fig. 4 Diagrammatic representation of a left-sided vena cava. Note that the caudal segment of the right supracardinal vein has regressed inappropriately and the left side has persisted

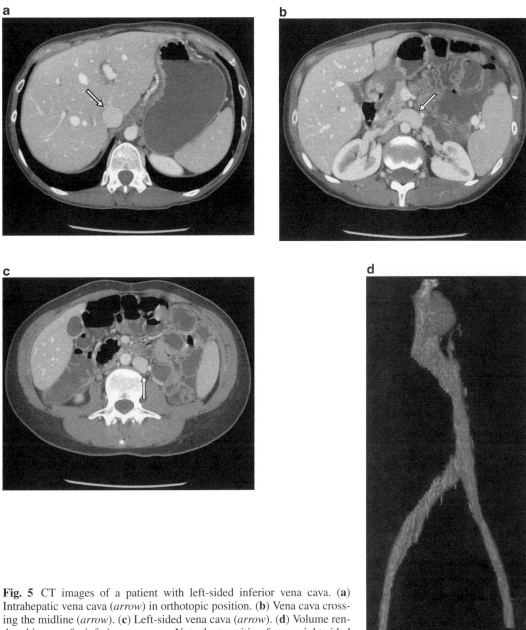

Fig. 5 CT images of a patient with left-sided inferior vena cava. (**a**) Intrahepatic vena cava (*arrow*) in orthotopic position. (**b**) Vena cava crossing the midline (*arrow*). (**c**) Left-sided vena cava (*arrow*). (**d**) Volume rendered image of a inferior vena cava. Note the transition from a right-sided structure superiorly to a left-sided structure inferiorly (*See Color Plates*)

In general, a left-sided inferior vena cava is asymptomatic, as the caliber of the vessel is equivalent to that of the cava in the orthotopic position. However, there is one case report in the literature of a left-sided IVC presenting as a right-sided May-Thurner syndrome (compression of the right iliac venous outflow tract by the overlying right iliac artery).[34]

Preoperatively, a cavagram should be obtained through a left femoral vein puncture to accurately roadmap the caval anomaly, the renal veins, and the level of crossing of the IVC to the right. Exposure options for the aorta in this case include dissection and mobilization of the IVC, division of the right renal vein, and division of the IVC.[21] However, caval division and reanastomosis are frequently associated with thrombosis. Clamping of the cava is also frequently associated with hemodynamic instability, which is generally poorly tolerated in elderly patients. Alternatively, a retroperitoneal approach to the aorta, supraceliac proximal control, or intra-aortic control with a balloon are potential strategies for managing a left-sided vena cava during aortic dissection.[24]

Duplicated Vena Cava

During embryologic development, persistence of both the right and left supracardinal veins leads to a duplicated vena cava. There are a variety of patterns to the duplicated IVC, based on the embryologic development of multiple venous channels and anastomoses between the left and right supracardinal veins (Figs. 6 and 7).[35]

The duplicated vena cava has been reported as early as 1909.[36] The prevalence of duplication of the vena cava depends on the modality used to diagnose it.

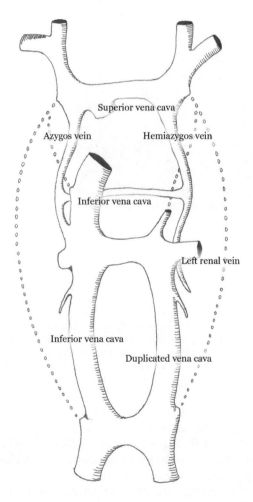

Fig. 6 Diagrammatic representation of a duplicated vena cava. In this case, there is no regression of the caudal segment of either supracardinal vein

a

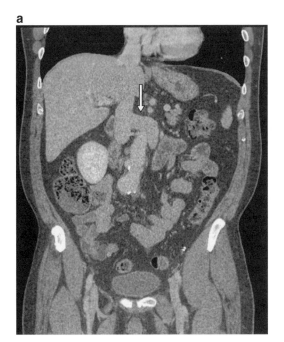

b

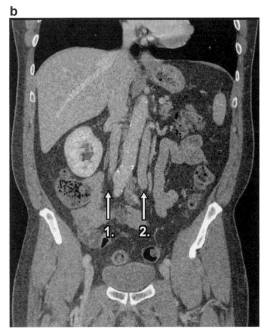

c

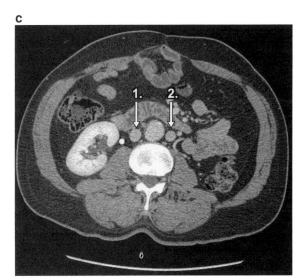

Fig. 7 CT images from a patient with a duplicated vena cava. (**a**) Coronal multiplanar reconstruction demonstrating crossover (*arrow*) of the left-sided caval structure with continuation of the right-sided cava. Right-sided cava (*arrow 1*) and left-sided cava (*arrow 2*) in coronal multiplanar reconstruction (**b**) and axial section (**c**)

Radiological series report rates from 0.02% to 1.1%,[4,11,14–17] surgical series from 0.1% to 1.2%,[21–22,24] and autopsy series from 0.2% to 2.8%.[6,26,28] There is a suggestion in the literature that this anomaly may be more prevalent in females.[35] The left-sided IVC may be diminutive and easily mistaken for a gonadal vein, in which case it is easily missed on CT scanning. Interoperatively, it can be distinguished from the gonadal vessel by tracing its caudal extent to the iliac vein which identifies it as a vena cava. Larger caliber left vena cavae can be identified preoperatively, and may cause more interoperative difficulty.

One preoperative clue that there may be a potential duplicated vena cava may be the position of the left kidney. Some authors have suggested that the left kidney being either at the level of the right kidney or lower is suggestive of duplicated vena cava, as the left IVC is thought to exert caudal traction on the developing left kidney.[35] In addition, because of the duplicate nature of the anomaly, there is often size discrepancy between the two cavae, which can lead to thrombosis of one or both vessels.[34]

For exposure, the left IVC can often be ligated as there is usually communication with the right IVC at the level of the iliacs.[1] In fact, there may be numerous retroaortic communicating branches between the two vena cavae, a situation which led to large volume blood loss and inability to perform an in situ aortobifemoral graft in a patient reported by Bartle et al.[13] Again, a preoperative cavagram should be obtained via left femoral vein puncture to assess the size of the left vena cava, its anastomoses (if any) with the right venous system, and its relation to the renal vein.

Vena Caval Interruption with Azygos Continuation

In a 1961 report, Anderson et al. documented anomalous inferior vena cava with azygos continuation (AIVC-AC) in 15 of 2500 patients with congenital heart defects, for a rate of 0.6%; these were primarily diagnosed with angiocardiography in children with cyanotic heart lesions such as cor biloculare, atrioventricular canal, anomalous connections of the pulmonary veins, double outflow right ventricle, large atrial septal defects, pulmonary stenosis or atresia, or a combination of these. Abdominal organ abnormalities such as heterotaxia, polysplenia, or asplenia are also associated with this anomaly. In patients without cardiac anomalies, this anomaly is very rare; in a series of 1055 autopsies, no cases were found.[7]

The mechanism of AIVC-AC is failure of union of the hepatic and subcardinal segments to form the prerenal IVC. Drainage therefore persists through the right supracardinal vein into the azygos system (AIVC-AC) or through the left supracardinal vein into the hemiazygos system (AIVC-HC); both routes may persist (Figs. 8 and 9).

AIVC-AC can present with hemoptysis secondary to azygos and bronchial hypertension, although it is usually asymptomatic. Lower extremity swelling, deep venous thrombosis,[37] ulceration, and other signs of venous obstructive disease have been reported. Cho et al. reported a case of an otherwise healthy 32-year-old male with no other prothrombotic risk factors who presented with a right popliteal deep venous thrombosis and extensive embolism to bilateral segmental pulmonary arteries.[38] CT scanning revealed that the patient had AIVC-AC. The patient was placed on lifelong coumadin anticoagulation.

Radiographically, AIVC is suggested by a paraspinous shadow adjoining the right hemidiaphragm on chest x-ray representing the hypertrophic azygos vein draining into the superior vena cava (Fig. 10). This can be misdiagnosed as a right paratracheal mass.

In cases of AIVC, current management recommendations for symptomatic patients include lifetime anticoagulant therapy, compression therapy, and leg elevation, as well as avoiding prolonged immobility and oral contraceptive use.[39]

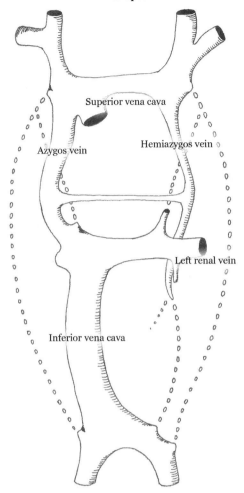

Fig. 8 Diagrammatic representation of absence of the vena cava with azygos continuation. This anomaly is due to the failure of union of the vena revehens with the prerenal segment of the cava

Marsupial Cava

If the dorsal segment of the posterior cardinal ring at the iliac venous bifurcation regresses and the anterior segment persists, this leads to a condition known as preaortic IVC/iliac confluence, also known as *marsupial cava*. This anomaly is very rare; one case (0.04%) was reported in the Mayo series.[24] It can be potentially deadly if unrecognized during dissection of the iliac arterial segments. Venous congestive symptoms are unusual in this anomaly. The critical maneuver is isolation of the right iliac artery without dissecting the preaortic confluence of the veins. If possible, either intra-arterial balloon occlusion or use of an aortic tube graft should be considered to minimize manipulation of the caval confluence.[24]

Absence of the Infrarenal Cava

Absence of the vena cava either in the prerenal segment or in its entirety with consequent collateral flow through the lumbar and azygos systems is thought to be not a true congenital condition but secondary to intrauterine thrombosis

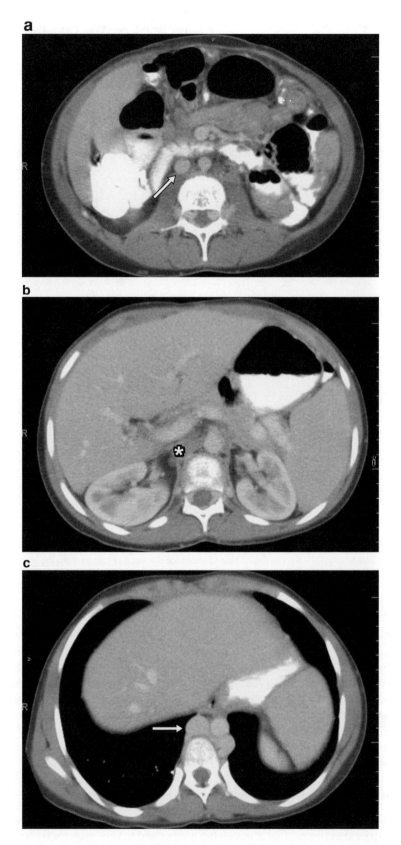

Fig. 9 CT images from a patient with absent inferior vena cava with azygos continuation. (**a**) Demonstrates orthotopic vena cava (*arrow*) below renal veins. (**b**) The vena

d

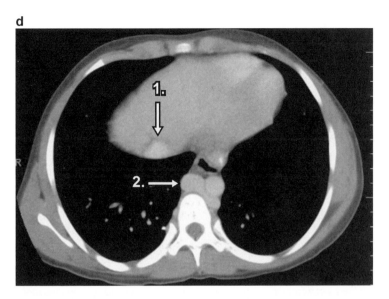

e

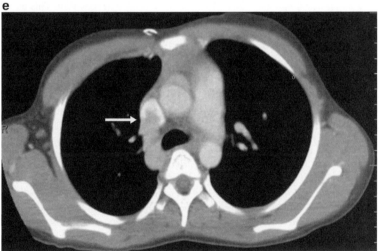

Fig. 9 (continued) cava is absent at this level (*asterisk*) and venous drainage is via retroperitoneal collaterals. (**c**) At this level, the retroperitoneal collateral venous drainage forms a confluence and drains into the azygos vein (arrow). (**d**) Venous contrast from the hepatic circulation can be seen emptying directly into the right atrium (*arrow 1*). The dilated azygos vein is again noted (*arrow 2*). (**e**) Lower extremity venous return via the azygos (minimally opacified) is seen here mixing in the superior vena cava (*arrow*)

of the vena cava. Ramanathan et al. reported a single case of absent infrarenal vena cava in a young female patient where peripartum records were available and documented caval thrombosis extending into the right renal vein. They suggest that this finding, as well as the fact that simple abnormal development of the right supracardinal vein would not explain the failure of the right postcardinal vein to persist, support the theory that this abnormality is not developmental but acquired secondary to caval thrombosis.[40]

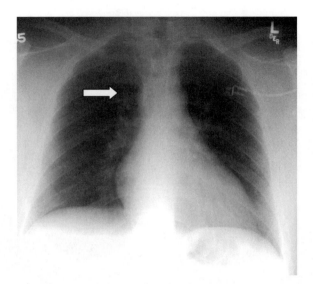

Fig. 10 Chest x-ray from a patient with anomalous IVC with azygos continuation. Note the right paratracheal structure (*arrow*) which is the dilated azygos vein. This anomaly was discovered during a laparotomy for apparent paraganglionoma

The most common presentation is an asymptomatic finding on CT scanning; the most common symptoms are due to deep venous thrombosis. Balzer et al. reported a case of a patient presenting with a retroperitoneal mass and bleeding who underwent laparotomy which demonstrated rupture of an aneurysmal collateral vein in the setting of absence of the infrarenal cava. This was managed via a PTFE interposition graft to reconstruct the cava, as well as bilateral arteriovenous fistulae. The reconstruction was patent at 4 months.[37]

Management of absence of the infrarenal inferior vena cava is similar in principle to that for other caval anomalies. For the asymptomatic patient, risk reduction is recommended. For patients with a history of venous thrombotic or thromboembolic disease, long-term or lifelong anticoagulation is appropriate. Surgical reconstruction may be attempted in life-threatening situations, as above, or in cases of recalcitrant symptoms. Shah et al. reported a case of an otherwise healthy 30-year-old male with a history of multiple deep venous thrombi, chronic venous stasis, and ulceration who was managed conservatively with aggressive compression therapy, exercise, anticoagulation, and a venous pump.[41] Similarly, Dougherty et al. report a case of an otherwise healthy 41-year-old male who presented with recurrent venous stasis ulceration and was discovered to have complete absence of the vena cava from the level of the iliac bifurcation to the right atrium; outflow was via multiple lumbar collaterals draining into an enlarged azygos system. This patient underwent PTFE bypass grafting from the right iliac vein to the azygos vein and creation of an arteriovenous fistula. This reconstruction maintained patency up to 30 months.[42]

Multiple Venous Anomalies

While the previously described anomalies of the vena cava can be problematic interoperatively when present in isolation, they can also be found in a variety of combinations. Occasionally, it is necessary to abort attempts at an intra-abdominal surgical approach and pursue other options such as extra-anatomic bypass or endovascular repair.[21]

General Principles in the Management of Vena Caval Anomalies

The most frequent nonoperative complication of caval anomalies is deep venous thrombosis of the iliac or femoral veins.[43] In a series of 97 consecutive patients diagnosed with deep venous thrombosis, 5 of 31 patients with iliac vein involvement were found to have abnormalities of the vena cava including absent renal segment and absent postrenal segment to complete absence of the entire inferior vena cava. Only one of the five patients had a hypercoagulable state identified. These patients tended to be younger than other patients in the series.[2,38] Other studies have documented that approximately 5% of young patients with deep venous thrombosis have an associated vena caval anomaly, and this rate is higher when the thrombosis is bilateral.[34,44] In a review of all case reports in the literature through 2002 of patients with deep venous thrombosis and caval anomalies, the mean age of this patient group was found to be 27 years. A total of 54% of cases were bilateral, and 69% had no identifiable hypercoagulable disorder.[45] These data suggest that young patients with no known risk factors for hypercoagulable disorders who present with iliac vein thrombosis, especially if bilateral, should be evaluated for caval anomalies.

While there are no large studies regarding the management of patients with thrombotic disease in the setting of caval anomalies, the general consensus in the limited literature on this topic seems to favor long-term (6 months to 2 years) or lifelong anticoagulation.[37–39,44–48] Conservative measures including stocking support, leg elevation, and exercise are also recommended.[48]

A final word regarding preoperative radiology for aortic surgery. Due to the prevalence of many of these venous anomalies in the general population, they are often considered clinically insignificant normal variants by radiologists. Clear communication between the surgeon and the radiologist regarding the need to evaluate for venous anomalies may provide superior surgical planning and decrease the rate of venous injury during aortic surgery.

References

1. Giordano JM, Trout HH. Anomalies of the inferior vena cava. *Journal of Vascular Surgery*. 1986:3:924–8.
2. Obemosterer A, Aschauer A, Schnedl W, Lipp RW. Anomalies of the inferior vena cava in patients with iliac vein thrombosis. *Annals of Internal Medicine*. 2002:136:37–41.
3. Chuang VP, Mena CE, Hoskins PA. Congenital anomalies of the inferior vena cava. Review of embryogenesis and presentation of a simplified classification. *British Journal of Radiology*. 1974:47;206–13.
4. Mayo J, Gray R, St. Louis E, Grosman H, McLoughlin M, Wise D. Anomalies of the inferior vena cava. *American Journal of Roentgenology*. 1983:140;339–45.
5. Mathews R, Smith PA, Fishman EK, Marshall FF. Anomalies of the inferior vena cava and renal veins: embryologic and surgical considerations. *Urology*. 1999:53;873–80.
6. Gladstone RJ. Development of the inferior vena cava in light of recent research, with especial reference to certain abnormalities, and current descriptions of the ascending lumbar and azygos veins. *Journal of Anatomy*. 1929:64;70–93.
7. Anderson RC, Adams P, Burke B. Anomalous inferior vena cava with azygos continuation (infrahepatic interruption of the inferior vena cava). *Journal of Pediatrics*. 1961:59;370–83.

8. Macchi V, Parenti A, De Caro R. Pivotal role of the sub-supracardinal anastomosis in the development and course of the left renal vein. *Clinical Anatomy*. 2003:16;358–61.

9. McClure CFW, Butler EG. The development of the inferior vena cava in man. *American Journal of Anatomy*. 1925:35;331–83.

10. Karaman B, Koplay M, Ozturk E, Basekim CC, Ogul H, Mutlu H, Kizilkaya E, Kantarci M. Retroaortic left renal vein: multidetector computed tomography angiography findings and its clinical importance. *Acta Radiologica*. 2007:48;355–60.

11. Aljabri B, MacDonald PS, Satin R, Stein LS, Obrand DI, Steinmetz OK. Incidence of major venous and renal anomalies relevant to aortoiliac surgery as demonstrated by computed tomography. *Annals of Vascular Surgery*. 2001:15;615–8.

12. Matano R, Gennaro M, Mohan C, Ascer E. Association of intra-abdominal pathologies and vascular anomalies with infrarenal aortic aneurysm: a computed tomographic study. *Cardiovascular Surgery*. 1993:1;27–9.

13. Reed MD, Friedman AC, Nealy P. Anomalies of the left renal vein: analysis of 433 CT scans. *Journal of Computer Assisted Tomography*. 1982:6;1124–6.

14. Alexander ES, Clark RA, Gross BH, Colley DP. CT of congenital anomalies of the inferior vena cava. *Computerized Radiology*. 1982:6;219–26.

15. Ueda J, Hara K, Kobayashi Y, Ohue S, Uchida H. Anomaly of the inferior vena cava observed by CT. *Computerized Radiology*. 1983:7;145–54.

16. Kukubo T, Oyama K, Ohtomo K, Yashiro N, Itai Y, Iio M, Masuyama S. CT of anomalies of the inferior vena cava and left renal vein. *Nippon Acta Radiologica*. 1988:48;10–16.

17. Hoeltl W, Hruby W, Aharinejad S. Renal vein anatomy and its implication for retroperitoneal surgery. *Journal of Urology*. 1990:143;1108–14.

18. Holden A, Smith A, Dukes P, Pilmore H, Yasutomi M. Assessment of 100 live potential renal donors for laparoscopic nephrectomy with multi-detector row helical CT. *Radiology*. 2005:237;973–80.

19. Kawamoto S, Lawler LP, Fishman EK. Evaluation of the renal venous system on late arterial and venous phase images with MDCT angiography in potential living laparoscopic renal donors. *American Journal of Roentgenology*. 2005:184;539–45.

20. Lin CH, Steinberg AP, Ramani AP, Abreu SC, Desai MM, Kaouk J, Goldfarb DA, Gill IS. Laparoscopic live donor nephrectomy in the presence of circumaortic or retroaortic left renal vein. *Journal of Urology*. 2004:171;44–6.

21. Bartle EJ, Pearce WH, Sun JH, Rutherford RB. Infrarenal venous anomalies and aortic surgery: avoiding vascular injury. *Journal of Vascular Surgery*. 1987:6;590–3.

22. Shindo S, Kubota K, Kojima A, Iyori K, Ishimoto T, Kobayashi M, Kamiya K, Tada Y. Anomalies of the inferior vena cava and left renal vein: risks in aortic surgery. *Annals of Vascular Surgery*. 2000:14;393–6.

23. Royster TS, Lacey L, Marks RA. Abdominal aortic surgery and left renal vein. *American Journal of Surgery*. 1974:127;552–4.

24. Truty MJ, Bower TC. Congenital anomalies of the inferior vena cava and left renal vein: implications during open abdominal aortic aneurysm reconstruction. *Annals of Vascular Surgery*. 2007:21:186–97.

25. Davis CJ, Lundberg GD. Retroaortic left renal vein. A relatively frequent anomaly. *American Journal of Clinical Pathology*. 1968:40;700–3.

26. Seib G. The azygos system of veins in American whites and American negroes, including observations on the inferior caval venous system. *American Journal of Physiology and Anthropology*. 1934:19;39–163.

27. Pick JW, Anson BJ. The renal vascular pedicle. An anatomical study of 430 body-halves. *Journal of Urology*. 1940:44;411–34.

28. Reis RH, Esenther G. Variations in the pattern of renal vessels and their relation to the type of posterior vena cava in man. *American Journal of Anatomy*. 1959:104;295–318.

29. Turgut HB, Bircan MK, Hatipoglu ES, Dogruyol S. Congenital anomalies of left renal vein and its clinical importance. *Clinical Anatomy*. 1996:9;133–5.

30. Brener BJ, Darling RC, Frederick PL, Linton RR. Major venous anomalies complicating abdominal aortic surgery. *Archives of Surgery*. 1974:108:159–65.

31. Karazincir S, Balci A, Gorur S, Sumbas S, Kiper AN. Incidence of the retroaortic left renal vein in patients with varicocele. *Journal of Ultrasound in Medicine*. 2007:26;601–4.

32. Koc Z, Ulusan S, Tokmak N, Oguzkurt L, Yildirim T. Double retroaortic left renal veins as a possible cause of pelvic congestion syndrome: imaging findings in two patients. *British Journal of Radiology*. 2006:79;e152–5.

33. Gibo M, Onitsuka H. Retroaortic left renal vein with renal vein hypertension causing hematuria. *Clinical Imaging*. 1998:22;422–4.

34. Burke RM, Rayan SS, Kasirajan K, Chaikof EL, Milner R. Unusual case of right-sided May-Thurner syndrome and review of its management. *Vascular*. 2006:14;47–50.

35. Lewis SJ. Observations on a double inferior vena cava: a case report with a literature review. *Clinical Anatomy*. 1992:5;227–33.

36. Pattern C. Persistence of the embryonic arrangement of the post-renal part of the cardinal veins. *Anatomischer Anzeiger*. 1909:34;189–91.

37. Balzer KM, Pillny M, Luther B, Grabitz K, Sandmann W. Spontaneous rupture of collateral venous aneurysm in a patient with agenesis of the inferior vena cava: A case report. *Journal of Vascular Surgery*. 2002:36:1053–7.

38. Cho BC, Choi HJ, Kang SM, Chang J, Lee SM, Yang DG, Hong YK, Lee DH, Lee Yong Won, Kim SK. Congenital absence of inferior vena cava as a rare cause of pulmonary thromboembolism. *Yonsei Medical Journal*. 2004:45:947–51.

39. Gil RJ, Perez AM, Arias JB, Pascual FB, Romero SR. Agenesis of the inferior vena cava associated with lower extremities and pelvic venous thrombosis. *Journal of Vascular Surgery*. 2006:44:1114–6.

40. Ramanathan T, Hughes MD, Kumar RM, Vivekanand SG, Grover A. Perinatal inferior vena cava thrombosis and absence of the infrarenal inferior vena cava. *Journal of Vascular Surgery*. 2001:33:1097–9.

41. Shah NL, Shanley CJ, Prince MR, Wakefield TW. Deep venous thrombosis complicating a congenital absence of the inferior vena cava. *Surgery*. 1996:120:891–6.

42. Dougherty MJ, Calligaro KD, DeLaurentis DA. Congenitally absent inferior vena cava presenting in adulthood with venous stasis and ulceration: a surgically treated case. *Journal of Vascular Surgery*. 1996:23:141–6.

43. Artico M, Lorenzini D, Mancini P, Gobbi P, Carloia S, David V. Radiological evidence of anatomical variation of the inferior vena cava: report of two cases. *Surgical and Radiologic Anatomy*. 2004:26:153–6.

44. Ruggeri M, Tosetto A, Castaman G, Rodeghiero F. Congenital absence of the inferior vena cava: a rare risk factor for idiopathic deep vein thrombosis. *Lancet*. 2001:357:441.

45. Yun SS, Kim JI, Kim KH, Sung GY, Lee DS, Kim JS, Moon IS, Lim KW, Koh YB. Deep venous thrombosis caused by congenital absence of inferior vena cava, combined with hyperhomocysteinemia. *Annals of Vascular Surgery*. 2004:18;124–9.

46. Saito H, Sano N, Kaneda I, Arakawa M, Ishida S, Takahashi S, Sakamoto K. Multisegmental anomaly of the inferior vena cava with thrombosis of the left inferior vena cava. *Cardiovascular and Interventional Radiology*. 1995:18;410–3.

47. Chee YL, Culligan DJ, Watson HG. Inferior vena cava malformation as a risk factor for deep venous thrombosis in the young. *British Journal of Haematology*. 2001:114:878–80.

48. Sakellaris G, Tilemis S, Papakonstantinou O, Bitsori M, Tsetis D, Charissis G. Deep venous thrombosis in a child associated with an abnormal inferior vena cava. *Acta Paediatrica*. 2005:94:242–4.

Chapter 21

Aortocaval Fistula

Tamara N. Fitzgerald, Bart E. Muhs, and Alan Dardik

Abstract A fistula between the inferior vena cava and aorta is a rare finding, occurring in 0.2–1.3% of abdominal aortic aneurysms (AAA). The incidence is 1% in asymptomatic and 3–4% in symptomatic aneurysms. Most fistulas occur as a complication of AAA, but 5–10% can occur because of mycotic aneurysms. Ehlers-Danlos and Marfan's syndromes or Takayasu's arteritis can also cause fistulas. Rarely low-velocity penetrating trauma, such as a stab wound, can result in an aortocaval fistula. However, the majority of penetrating injuries to the aorta result in either death or hemodynamic instability necessitating surgical exploration, such that a fistula does not have the opportunity to form. Nevertheless, congestive heart failure in a young patient with a history of trauma should alert the physician to a possible aortocaval fistula.

Keywords Aortocaval fistula, Aortic Disease, Aortic Aneurysm, Congestive Heart Failure

Presentation

The simultaneous presentation of abdominal aortic aneurysms (AAA) and congestive heart failure (CHF) usually represents unrelated processes. Therefore, the CHF should be treated prior to AAA repair. However, the persistence of CHF despite treatment suggests a fistula or some other ominous finding.

Patients may complain of back or abdominal pain. On physical examination, there may be a pulsatile abdominal mass, 75% will have an audible continuous bruit and 25% a palpable thrill. In a study performed at the Mayo clinic, 94% of patients with aortocaval fistulas were symptomatic at presentation, but only 17% had a triad of pain, pulsatile mass, and abdominal bruit.[1]

CHF associated with aortocaval fistula is one of a hyperdynamic, high output state. Therefore, patients may present with tachycardia, hypertension, decreased diastolic blood pressure, cardiac dilation with an associated murmur, jugular venous distension, hepatomegaly, swollen legs, or venous stasis disease. There have also been reports of saphenous vein bruit.[2] Previously undiagnosed congenital abnormalities such as patent foramen ovale, or central malignancies, may contribute to circulatory overload and heart failure. Renal

G. Upchurch and E. Criado (eds.) *Aortic Aneurysms, Contemporary Cardiology*
DOI: 10.1007/978-1-60327-204-9_21, © Humana Press, a part of
Springer Science+Business Media, LLC 2009

failure is often present. Rarely patients may present with lower gastrointestinal bleeding in cases with visceral ischemia or hematuria if venous engorgement of the bladder is present. Lower extremity claudication may also be present.

Diagnosis

The initial test to confirm the presence of an AAA is usually an ultrasound, but this is not the best imaging option. Occasionally a fistula may be discovered with color flow on the duplex ultrasound, but this is rare, and preoperative planning is not routinely performed with ultrasound. In the past, aortocaval fistulas were more often discovered unexpectedly in the operating room, during the course of open repair of an aneurysm.

Aortography is the gold standard for diagnosis, but now, more commonly, computed tomography (CT) and magnetic resonance (MR) angiograms are used to assess AAA and associated fistula. CT is more commonly used, especially as patients routinely receive CT to determine endovascular repair (EVAR) candidacy. This leads to increased preoperative detection of fistulas. Early filling of the inferior vena cava (IVC) after intra-aortic contrast injection is indicative of a fistula (Fig. 1). MR angiography can demonstrate this finding as well, but is less commonly used.

Treatment

The natural history of an aortocaval fistula is progressive CHF leading to death. Therefore, the fistula and associated AAA should be immediately repaired. However, even with successful surgical repair, there is an associated 22–51% mortality largely due to blood loss, cardiac decompensation, and pulmonary embolus. Survival rates are generally higher for elective repairs and lower for emergency repairs of ruptured AAA or elective repairs of AAA in which the fistula was not preoperatively diagnosed. Today, with proper preoperative angiographic study, it is increasingly rare for a fistula to go undiagnosed and encountered unexpectedly during open aneurysm repair.

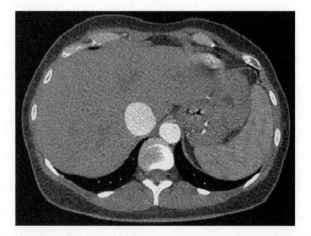

Fig. 1 Arterial phase computed tomography (*CT*) demonstrating an aortocaval fistula. In addition to contrast in the aorta, contrast is also simultaneously present in the inferior vena cava (*IVC*)

Preoperatively, all patients with suspected aortocaval fistula should receive a transesophageal echocardiogram to evaluate cardiac performance and hemodynamics as well as to demonstrate alternative sites of, or potential additional, fistulas, including those due to a previously undiagnosed patent foramen ovale. The central venous pressure is usually elevated and patients may have varying degrees of renal failure. Therefore, in patients with severe symptoms requiring therapy, a pulmonary artery catheter should be used to evaluate left-to-right shunt or high output cardiac failure, and it can also be used to guide fluid management. In most cases, renal function will return to normal after a successful repair.

The hemodynamic consequences of AAA-IVC fistula repair should be anticipated intraoperatively. Both the cardiac output and the mixed venous oxygen content should fall to normal values. Continued fall in cardiac output to low values likely reflects low filling pressures that will be responsive to fluids. Mild acidosis may be present after repair as well.

Operative Repair

Traditional open repair is performed either from the transperitoneal or from the retroperitoneal approach, depending on aneurysm configuration and surgeon preference. Although successful operation is expected with proper preoperative diagnosis and planning, complications include bleeding, infection, hemodynamic instability, impotence, colon ischemia, cardiac failure, prolonged ventilator dependence, stroke, air embolism, pulmonary embolism, acute limb ischemia, and death.

Repair should proceed in standard fashion including dissection, vessel control, and heparinization. Acute fistulas are easily entered, whereas chronic fistulas can be encased in fibrous tissue or an inflammatory mass. Chronic fistulas may also have thinned, large arteries and bulging veins, adding to the difficulty of vascular isolation. Patients must be adequately prepped so that major bleeding can be controlled. For high abdominal fistulas, the chest should be prepped. The fistula and IVC do not need to be isolated or dissected individually. After aneurysm exclusion and opening of the sac, back bleeding from the fistula is characteristically quite large. Sponge sticks may be used to compress the IVC (Fig. 2). Venous control may also be achieved by intermittent clamping of the artery, but Fogarty and Foley catheters may also be used. Control of the IVC may diminish venous return to the heart, and should be performed cautiously. Massive venous bleeding upon opening the aneurysm sac should alert the surgeon to an undiagnosed fistula, but can be generally easily controlled (Fig. 2).

Once control of the aorta has been achieved, repair of the fistula should be performed from within the aneurysm sac. Care should be taken not to manipulate the aneurysm as clot may be dislodged into the fistula and lead to a pulmonary embolus. The vein should be repaired first, usually by primary closure, but Teflon pledgets may be helpful. Next, the aortic aneurysm should be repaired with a standard aortic graft.

Rarely, aortocaval fistula is a complication of aortitis. If the surgical field is contaminated due to severe aortic infection, routine principles of vascular surgery are followed and the septic tissue should be debrided. The fistula is oversewn, the artery closed proximally and distally, and extra-anatomic arterial bypass performed. Once the abdomen is closed, a subcutaneous bypass can be placed in a clean surgical field to allow adequate perfusion of the legs.

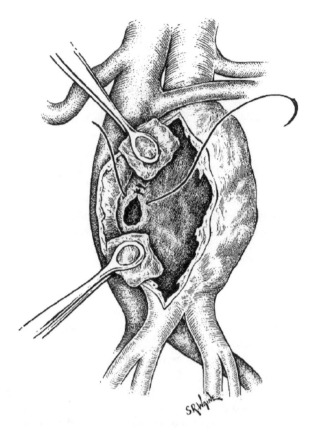

Fig. 2 Technique for controlling bleeding from an aortocaval fistula and fistula repair via an intra-aortic suture closure. From Dardik et al[3]

Alternatively, a prosthetic graft can be placed into the contaminated field after the aorta has been debrided and thoroughly irrigated with saline or antibiotic solution. An antibiotic coated graft can be used, if available. Once the graft has been placed, an omental pedicle should be used to cover the graft.

Endovascular Repair

As preoperative diagnosis of fistulas with CT becomes more common, endovascular stent-graft repair becomes an important consideration. Given the relatively high operative mortality and morbidity of open repair, the EVAR option offers the potential benefits of decreased blood loss, virtually no chance for air embolus, decreased hospital stay, and a more rapid return to normal activities. Once anatomical suitability has been determined, typically by the presence of adequate proximal and distal sealing zones, then EVAR may be an acceptable approach for repair of an aneurysm with an IVC fistula.

The immediate efficacy of EVAR has been demonstrated in an animal model,[4] but as with all aortic stent grafts, careful follow-up must be maintained to evaluate endoleaks.[5-7] Endoleaks can cause fistulas to reoccur. However, isolated non-aneurysmal aortocaval fistulas represent a different disease process than AAA. The purpose of treatment in AAA is to prevent rupture, whereas in aortocaval fistula, the primary measurement of success is restoration of normal physiology via the treatment of a large arteriovenous shunt. This has implications for follow-up. Traditional follow-up of EVAR has included contrast CT on a yearly basis to evaluate the presence of endoleak. This usually exposes patients to substantial radiation and nephrotoxic contrast. In EVAR for AAA, the purpose of surveillance is to eliminate any endoleak that presents a risk for rupture. Conversely, in aortocaval fistulas, a small, hemodynamically insignificant endoleak likely needs no treatment at all. It has been proposed that nonaneurysmal, aortocaval fistula treated via EVAR can be followed adequately by yearly IVC duplex scanning. If elevated arterial velocities are not encountered, then the radiation and contrast of a CT can be eliminated. Abnormal duplex examinations should prompt a contrast CT or MR angiogram for additional delineation.

There have been reports of aortocaval fistula treatment with coil embolization, with coils placed into the midfistula tract.[8] This method is likely suitable only for very small fistulas with long fistula tracks. Large, short fistulas are high-flow phenomena. Endovascular coils placed in these high-flow communications carry a high risk of coil embolization to the lungs. Future endovascular solutions may involve occlusion devices, similar to the Amplatzer septal occluder or the Helix occluder device (W.L. Gore) used to treat intracardiac septal defects with large shunts.

The endovascular treatment of aortocaval fistulas lacks long-term data to evaluate the outcome of this treatment modality. Most case reports have only 1-year follow-up,[7,9] and randomized, controlled trials or multicenter studies are unlikely to ever occur given the rarity of this condition. Nevertheless, endovascular options appear promising and deserve additional study.

Aortocaval fistula repair is associated with a 50% mortality. In the presence of persistent renal failure, the results are dismal. Aortocaval fistulas should be repaired as soon as possible after diagnosis in order to minimize end-organ damage from sustained high cardiac output. EVAR is a new approach to repair an aortocaval fistulas and the associated aortic aneurysm, and will be considered more often as CT is used preoperatively to identify aortocaval fistulas. However, long-term data must be obtained to determine the durability of this technique.

References

1. Davis, P.M., P. Gloviczki, and K.J. Cherry, Aorto-caval and ilio-iliac ateriovenous fistulae: Rare and challenging problems. Am J Surg, 1998. 176:115.
2. Phillips, A.W., A. Chaudhuri, and F.J. Meyer, Bilateral long saphenous bruits: A marker of aortocaval fistula. Eur J Vasc Endovasc Surg, 2006. 32:529–531.
3. Dardik, H., I. Dardik, M.G. Strom, L. Attai, N. Carnevale, and F.J. Veith, Intravenous rupture of arteriosclerotic aneurysms of the abdominal aorta. Surgery, 1976. 80: 647–651.
4. Boudghene, F., et al., Aortocaval fistulae: A percutaneous model and treatment with stent grafts in sheep. Circulation, 1996. 94:108–112.
5. Maeda, H., et al., Surgery for ruptured abdominal aortic aneurysm with an aortocaval and iliac vein fistula. Surg Today, 2007. 37:445–448.
6. Pathak, S., et al., Endovascular repair of a recurrent aortocaval fistula and anastamotic false aneurysm. Brit J Radiol, 2006. 79:e62–e63.
7. Vetrhus, M., et al., Endovascular repair of abdominal aortic aneurysms with aortocaval fistula. Eur J Vasc Endovasc Surg, 2005. 30:640–643.
8. Kashyap, V.S., et al., Aortocaval fistula. J Am Coll Surg, 2006. 203(5):780.
9. Waldrop, J.L., Jr., B.W.t. Dart, and D.E. Barker, Endovascular stent graft treatment of a traumatic aortocaval fistula. Ann Vasc Surg, 2005. 19:562–565.

Chapter 22

Acute Limb Ischemia After Abdominal Aortic Aneurysm Repair

Paul J. Riesenman and William A. Marston

Abstract Acute limb ischemia is a potential complication of open surgical and endovascular repair of abdominal aortic aneurysms. This complication may present in the early postoperative period or late in follow-up and may be related to technical, patient, and/or graft-related factors. For endovascular aneurysm repair, device-specific factors have been associated with endograft limb occlusion and consequential limb ischemia.

Keywords Limb occlusion, limb ischemia

Introduction

Both open surgical and endovascular aneurysm repair (EVAR) are effective forms of treatment for infrarenal abdominal aortic aneurysms (AAAs).[1] Acute limb ischemia may potentially complicate either treatment modality[2] and may add considerable morbidity to the patient's outcome. Arterial occlusion may be detected intraprocedurally during either form of intervention or it may present in the postoperative period. Postoperatively, patients with arterial occlusion may develop classical clinical symptoms of acute limb ischemia. The severity of these symptoms depends on the degree and level of arterial occlusion, and this may threaten the viability of the affected lower extremity. Once identified and if clinically indicated, an operative or endovascular intervention must be initiated to minimize the potential for tissue loss. Several technical or patient-related factors may place the patient at risk for this complication. Additionally, graft or endograft-related factors may result in graft/endograft limb occlusion, and this complication must be appropriately addressed in order to reestablish and maintain perfusion to the affected lower extremity. While well-known factors such as distal arterial stenosis or occlusion enhance the risk for limb occlusion following open surgery or EVAR, other endograft-specific factors unique to EVAR should be considered in order to minimize or address this potential complication.

G. Upchurch and E. Criado (eds.) *Aortic Aneurysms, Contemporary Cardiology*
DOI: 10.1007/978-1-60327-204-9_22, © Humana Press, a part of
Springer Science+Business Media, LLC 2009

Open Surgery

The etiology of acute limb ischemia following open surgical reconstruction of an AAA is primarily related to the time of presentation. Acute ischemic events in the early postoperative period usually are related to intraoperative technical problems, whereas patients who present with acute limb ischemia during follow-up will most likely have graft-limb occlusion due to inadequate outflow from progressive atherosclerotic disease of their distal arterial vessels. In either situation, the potential for a proximal embolic source is a possibility and should be evaluated if clinically indicated.

Early/Postoperative Limb Ischemia

Early postoperative acute limb ischemia following open AAA repair has an incidence of 1.7–3%.[2–4] This complication is one of the most common indications for an additional intervention following the initial surgical procedure.[3] Many of the causes of acute limb ischemia in this setting may be directly attributed to the operative procedure including embolization, arterial injury, and graft-related complications.

Embolization of atheroembolic debris or intramural thrombus mobilized during operative exposure and vessel clamping may result in distal arterial occlusion and acute ischemic changes in the lower extremities immediately following open AAA repair. Additionally, embolic material may gain access to the distal vasculature if a thorough intraluminal irrigation is not performed prior to completion of the distal anastomosis. The size of these particles will often be small, and the clinical relevance of these microemboli is variable as ischemic changes are often transient and do not result tissue loss, although patients with advanced peripheral arterial disease may be more vulnerable in this setting.

The femoral vessels in patients with aneurismal disease are typically calcified to a varying degree, and many patients also have significant intraluminal obstruction leading to challenges in access and closure of these vessels. Technical issues that may lead to thrombosis and limb ischemia include clamp trauma, raising an intimal flap, and narrowing of the vessel lumen at the time of closure.

A careful consideration of placement of the surgical graft can minimize potential graft-related complications which may manifest as acute limb ischemia. Avoidance of heavily calcified areas of the common femoral artery by use of the proximal superficial femoral artery (SFA) or profunda femoral artery (PFA) is a useful alternative. We commonly perform anastomoses to the distal common femoral artery with profundaplasty to optimize outflow, particularly in patients with occluded SFAs. In heavily calcified arteries, consideration should be given to the use of intraluminal balloon occlusion of the inflow from the iliac artery to avoid the use of clamps that may crush the artery leading to potential embolization or intimal flaps. Patients presenting with occlusion of the SFA and severe PFA disease should undergo concomitant procedures to reopen either the SFA or the PFA to provide adequate graft limb outflow and reduce the risk of early limb thrombosis.

Kinks or external compression of the prosthesis by surrounding structures may impede outflow leading to obstruction and/or thrombosis. Care should be taken to avoid external compression of the graft during reapproximation of the aortic wall and periaortic tissues. If the aortic wall or periaortic tissues cannot adequately cover the graft from adjacent bowel without constriction, an omental flap can be utilized; however, the aortic wall is usually not limiting as this is redundant in aneurysmal disease. Redundant length in the graft limbs should also be minimized as this may be a potential source of graft kinking.

The assessment of the limbs immediately after aneurysm repair is a critical component of the procedure. After reperfusion of the femoral vessels, arteries should be interrogated with a Doppler or duplex scanner for evidence of adequate flow. Distal pulses and/or Doppler signals should also be confirmed and the limb must be examined carefully to ensure that adequate perfusion is present. The optimal time to correct lower extremity perfusion problems is prior to leaving the operating room in order to minimize the potential for irreversible tissue loss. If any questions concerning the adequacy of lower extremity perfusion are raised, immediate evaluation with duplex ultrasound scanning or arteriography should be performed. The choice of these methods depends on availability and patient related factors. We favor duplex scanning in patients with contraindications to contrast administration and in cases where the question concerning perfusion arises after closure of the incisions has been completed. Otherwise, we favor intraoperative angiography as long as this is rapidly available in the operative suite. Based on the results of the diagnostic study, correction of the perfusion problem is immediately performed. Consideration should be given to four compartment fasciotomy based on the duration and extent of limb ischemia prior to reperfusion.

Late Limb Ischemia

Late acute limb ischemic events following open AAA repair are most likely a consequence of progressive occlusive processes in the distal arterial vessels. Distal atherosclerotic disease and intimal hyperplasia at the distal anastomotic sites may make the graft limbs prone to thrombosis as outflow is impeded.

The incidence of late graft-limb occlusion has been reported to range from 0.1% to 5.3% in long-term durability studies through variable follow-up.[5–8] Biancari et al. reported on 208 operative survivors of elective and emergent AAA repair with a mean follow-up of 8 years.[5] Eleven patients (5.3%) developed graft limb occlusion during follow-up, with four of these cases attributed to distal occlusive processes. Adam et al. reported on 957 patients treated for nonruptured AAAs over a mean follow-up of 41 months.[6] Eleven cases (1.1%) of limb occlusion necessitating a secondary intervention were reported, with only one of these occurring during the patient's initial hospitalization for their AAA repair. In a review of 1047 cases performed at the Cleveland Clinic by Hertzer et al., only one case (0.1%) of late limb occlusion was identified during a mean follow-up of 57 months.[7] Additionally, Hallet et al. reported on 307 patients treated at the Mayo clinic and found a 2% ($n = 6$) incidence of graft thrombosis with the majority of these cases occurring at more than 30 days.[8] Both of these later studies were strengthened by their efforts to establish long-term follow-up.

Late graft limb occlusion can potentially be minimized by clinically monitoring patients for symptoms of peripheral arterial disease. Routine graft scanning with duplex ultrasound is not warranted given the low incidence of late problems, so further evaluation is only recommended when symptoms develop at follow-up. Areas of stenosis at the anastomotic sites or distal arterial vessels may require operative or endovascular intervention to ensure adequate distal runoff from the graft limbs.

Endovascular Aneurysm Repair

As with open surgery, acute limb ischemia following EVAR is a recognized complication of this form of intervention, and has been reported to occur in 1.3–6.8% of patients.[4,9] Although limb ischemia is largely attributed to endograft limb occlusion, similar etiologies as those describe for open repair may be the cause of this complication following EVAR.[9] The potential risk of endograft limb occlusion has been associated with endograft design-specific factors, as well as technical considerations at the time of EVAR (Fig. 1).

Endograft Limb Occlusion

Endograft limb occlusion has been reported to be a common complication necessitating intervention following EVAR.[10] This complication tends to be detected intraoperatively or in the early postoperative period, with approximately half of reported cases occurring within approximately 30 days.[11,12] Early studies reporting high rates of endograft limb occlusion involved endografts with an unsupported configuration.[13–15] Additionally, some anatomic characteristics and procedure-related risk factors have been associated with this complication (Fig. 2).

Anatomic Considerations

Proper preoperative evaluation and consideration of the patient's vascular anatomy are essential for minimizing the potential of endograft limb occlusion. Patients with clinical symptoms or physical examination findings concerning for peripheral arterial disease should undergo further evaluation as distal arterial outflow stenoses or occlusions are risk factors for graft occlusion. Although the iliac arterial system is routinely interrogated for luminal diameter

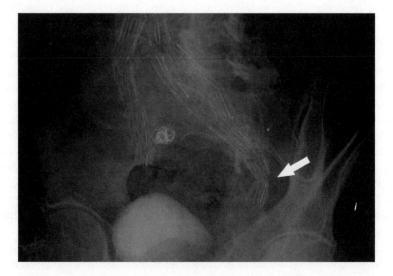

Fig. 1 Abdominal radiograph in a patient presenting with acute onset claudication 3 months after endovascular repair of an abdominal aortic aneurysm with extensive bilateral iliac involvement necessitating endograft limb deployment in the external iliac artery. A kink is appreciated in the distal endograft limb (*arrow*)

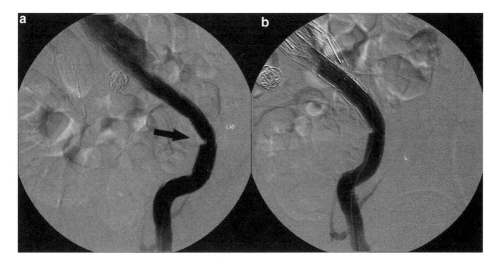

Fig. 2 (**a**) Arteriogram of a left endograft iliac limb following catheter-directed thrombolysis for acute limb thrombosis. A distal kink and luminal filling defect is observed in the distal endograft limb (*arrow*). (**b**) Completion arteriogram following placement of a 12 × 60 mm Luminexx stent (C.R. Bard, Inc., Murray Hill, NJ) and balloon angioplasty

and tortuosity in order to assess delivery sheath accommodation, these characteristics also affect the patency of endograft limbs. As opposed to open repair, where the surgeon has the advantage of constructing an unimpeded course for the graft limbs, endograft limbs must conform to the tortuosity, tapering, and intraluminal compressive forces of the iliac arteries.

Several anatomic characteristics of the aortoiliac system have been associated with endograft limb occlusion. At the aortic bifurcation, risk factors associated with limb occlusion include angulation of the iliac origin in relation to the course of the iliac artery, abrupt luminal transition from the aorta to the iliac system, and extrinsic compression from thrombus within the aneurysm or from the contralateral endograft limb.[15] A limiting aortic diameter at this level may potentially be overcome through the use of a kissing endovascular balloon technique during limb deployment, or use of an aortomonoiliac endograft design. Tortuosity and regions of stenosis secondary to atherosclerotic disease encountered throughout the course of the iliac system may also contribute to endograft limb occlusion as these may result in limb kinks and extrinsic compression. Additionally, extension of the endograft limb into the external iliac artery has also been associated with endograft limb occlusion.[11,16] Although this association may be a consequence of the smaller arterial diameters encountered in the external iliac artery, it has been suggested that the loss of hypogastric artery outflow may contribute to endograft limb occlusion in this setting.[16]

Although angiographic evaluation may reveal an optimal technical result at the conclusion of the initial endovascular procedure, endograft limb patency remains at risk due to conformational changes in the endograft as it adapts to aneurysmal remodeling over time. Reductions in aneurysm sac length have been associated with endograft buckling and kinking.[17] Additional observations have noted that late endograft kinking may be more likely, and present earlier, when the arterial vessels are more tortuous at the time of EVAR.[18]

Device-Specific Considerations and Outcomes

General conclusions about the anticipated frequency endograft limb occlusion are difficult to make, given the variability in endograft design. Several single-institution studies describing the frequency of endograft limb occlusion have been reported with this complication occurring in 0.6–45.6% of all patients who have undergone EVAR[9,11–16,18–22] (Table 1). Conclusions from these studies are difficult to make, given different definitions of limb complications (kinking, stenosis, occlusion, and/or thrombosis), variable follow-up,

Table 1 Studies reporting endograft limb complications following EVAR.

Study	Year	Patients	Limbs at risk	Endograft(s)	Limb complications[a] (%) Patients	Limbs	Follow-up (months)
Umscheid et al.[18]	1999	264	528		14.0	7.8	
		124	248	Vanguard			
		81	162	Stentor			
		41	82	Talent			
		18	36	AneuRx			
Tillich et al.[19]	1999	33	66	Vanguard	9.1	4.5	8.8
Baum et al.[20]	2000	89	149		14.6	12.1	10.6
		74	122	Talent	6.8	4.9	
		15	27	Ancure	53.0	44.0	
Amesur et al.[13]	2000	68	130	Ancure	45.6	36.2	
Carpenter et al.[15]	2001	173	310			7.7	9.7
		111	189	Talent		3.7	
		31	59	Ancure		28.8	
		25	50	AneuRx		0.0	
		4	8	Lifepath		0.0	
		2	4	Zenith		0.0	
Krajcer et al.[21]	2002	40	80	Ancure	15.0	8.8	
Parent et al.[14]	2002	67	125	Ancure	23.8	11.2	15.9
Carroccio et al.[16]	2002	351	702		7.4	3.7	20
		255	510	Talent	7.8	3.9	
		35	70	AneuRx	2.8	1.4	
		25	50	Excluder	0.0	0.0	
		18	36	Vanguard	22.2	11.1	
		10	20	Teramed	0.0	0.0	
		8	16	Ancure	12.5	6.3	
Erzurum et al.[11]	2004	823			2.7		
		373	746	Zenith	2.4	1.2	
		230	460	AneuRx	2.6	1.3	
		68	136	Ancure	10.3	5.1	
		61		Other	0.0		
		39	78	Talent	5.1	2.6	
		30	60	Excluder	0.0	0.0	
		22	44	Quantum	4.5	2.3	
Maldonado et al.[9]	2004	311			4.8		22.5
		238		Ancure	5.9		
		30		Excluder	0.0		
		28		AneuRx	3.6		
		15		Zenith	0.0		
Sivamurthy et al.[12]	2006	248	486	Zenith	5.2	2.7	24.0
Hiramoto et al.[22]	2007	325	650	Zenith	0.6	0.3	27.5

[a] Kinking, stenosis, occlusion, and/or thrombosis

inclusion or exclusion of adjunctive limb procedures at the time of EVAR, and inclusion of multiple endograft designs. It is more instructive to look at each device design and its associated incidence of limb thrombosis, including some devices no longer in the market to consider design issues related to this complication.

The Ancure endograft (Guidant, Menlo Park, CA) was the first commercially manufactured device to be placed into clinical trials in the United States and is no longer available on a commercial basis. This device was constructed as an unsupported bifurcated or aortomonoiliac configured endograft. This unsupported design was initially employed due to its smaller size, conformability, and ability to traverse tortuous iliac anatomy at the time of deployment. The lack of structural support made it prone to external compression, as well as developing folds in the graft material secondary to size mismatch between graft and vessel. High rates of endograft limb occlusion led to the practice of reinforcing these limbs with intravascular stents as both an intraoperative therapeutic[15] and a prophylactic measure.[23]

Amesur et al. reported on a series of patients treated with the Ancure device and noted that 47 of 130 limbs treated (36%) required reinforcement with stents due to luminal compromise at the time of deployment or during follow-up.[13] They noted that none of the patients who underwent limb reinforcement with adjunctive limb stenting experienced endograft limb occlusion through a mean follow-up of 14 months.

Parent et al. reported an overall incidence of endograft limb stenosis or occlusion of 23% in 67 patients using the Ancure endograft.[14] Nine patients (13%) underwent endograft limb stenting for abnormalities noted upon completion angiography, and none developed endograft limb complications during a mean follow-up of 15.9 months. The remaining 58 patients had normal appearing endograft limbs at the conclusion of EVAR and did not undergo adjunctive stenting. Seven (12%) of these patients developed limb stenosis or occlusion during follow-up; three of which presented with acute lower extremity ischemia necessitating operative intervention.

In a study including 823 patients treated with either the Ancure device or one of several supported endograft designs, Erzurum et al. reported a median time to limb occlusion of 34.9 days. They found that endograft configuration was significantly associated with endograft limb occlusion with this complication occurring in 5.1% of Ancure limbs and 0–2.6% of supported endograft limbs.[11]

Carroccio et al. reported an endograft limb occlusion rate of 3.7% in 702 at-risk limbs during a mean follow-up of 20 months.[16] Half of the cases of limb occlusion occurred within 30 days of surgery, and 69% required an intervention to reestablish blood flow to the affected extremity. No association between endograft limb occlusion and any of the six commercially manufactured devices was demonstrated, although the cohort was dominated by the Talent (Medtronic, Santa Rosa, CA) device (73% of at-risk limbs).

Although adjunctive stenting for unsupported endograft limbs appears to be beneficial in preventing limb occlusion, this practice may also be beneficial when utilizing endograft limbs with a supported configuration. Sivamurthy et al. compared patients who underwent adjunctive primary stenting of endograft limbs at the time of EVAR with the Zenith AAA endovascular graft (Cook, Inc., Bloomington, IN).[12] Indications for adjunctive stenting were endograft limb angulation, compression, and kinking. After a mean follow-up of 2 years, no cases of limb occlusion occurred in 85 at-risk stented limbs, while occlusion was observed in 3.6% (13 of 361) of unstented limbs. Approximately half the cases of obstruction occurred within 30 days of EVAR and 73% occurred at ≤6 months. This higher rate of occlusion in unstented endograft limbs occurred despite more favorable vascular anatomy and more favorable initial EVAR results.

Interventions for Endograft Limb Occlusion

Following endograft limb occlusion, the severity of the patient's symptoms may necessitate an emergent intervention to restore and maintain limb patency to the affected vascular territory. A less invasive endovascular intervention would be preferable and is often technically successful. Endovascular options depend on the etiology of the occlusion and include angioplasty, stenting, AngioJet thrombectomy, and thrombolysis. Krajcer et al. reported on six patients with symptomatic thrombosis, all of whom underwent successfully treatment with AngioJet thrombectomy (Possis Medical, Minneapolis, MN).[21] Erzurum et al. reported on 25 patients treated endovascularly ($n = 12$) and with extra-anatomic bypass ($n = 13$) for endograft limb occlusion.[11] Nine (75%) of the initial endovascular approaches were successful at resolving the occlusion and none of these patients experienced recurrent endograft limb occlusion.

When the patient's extremity is acutely threatened secondary to endograft limb occlusion and an endovascular revision is technically unsuccessful or prohibitive, extra-anatomic bypass is indicated. When a femoral–femoral bypass is to be performed, care should be taken to evaluate the contralateral endograft limb supplying the donor vessel, as contralateral endograft limb obstruction has been responsible for extra-anatomic bypass failure in this setting.[11]

Other Causes of Limb Ischemia Fowllowing EVAR

Although lower extremity ischemia following EVAR is largely attributed to endograft limb occlusion, cases of atheroembolization necessitating intervention have been reported [9,24] Operative dissection and obtaining vascular control of the femoral or iliac vessels may release atheroembolic debris. Additionally, wire and sheath manipulation may further disrupt atherosclerotic plaques or intraaneurysmal material. The evaluation for distal occlusion and need for intervention should be similar to that described for open surgical repair.

In addition to disruption of atheroembolic debris, wire and sheath manipulation has been reported to result in arterial access vessel injury in 4.8–8% of patients undergoing EVAR.[4,25] This iatrogenic trauma may result in rupture, dissection, or pseudoaneurysms which may give rise to thromboembolic processes and vessel occlusion. Care should be taken to assess the iliofemoral anatomy at the time of evaluation for EVAR candidacy. Patients with access vessels that are found to be tortuous and severely atherosclerotic may be better served with a more proximal level of arterial access. At the conclusion of each EVAR procedure, device limb and iliac vessel anatomy should be evaluated to identify any luminal irregularity for consideration for treatment in order to avoid potential limb occlusion.

Conclusion

Acute limb ischemia is a recognized complication of both open surgical repair of AAAs and EVAR. Early acute limb ischemic events following open repair are most commonly due to technical factors of the repair, while late events are often secondary to progressive atherosclerotic disease. Acute limb ischemia following EVAR has mainly been associated with endograft limb occlusion and this complication tends to be present in the early postoperative period. Early reports of high rates of limb ischemia following EVAR were associated with the use of unsupported endografts limbs which were inherently prone to occlusion. Adjunctive stenting of unsupported limbs greatly reduced the incidence of this complication and the present use of supported endograft limbs has been associated with a lower incidence of endograft limb obstruction.

References

1. EVAR trial participants. Endovascular aneurysm repair versus open repair in patients with abdominal aortic aneurysm (EVAR trial 1): randomised controlled trial. Lancet 2005;365(9478):2179–86.
2. Cao P, Verzini F, Parlani G, et al. Clinical effect of abdominal aortic aneurysm endografting: 7-year concurrent comparison with open repair. J Vasc Surg 2004; 40(5):841–8.
3. Sayers RD, Thompson MM, Nasim A, Healey P, Taub N, Bell PR. Surgical management of 671 abdominal aortic aneurysms: a 13 year review from a single centre. Eur J Vasc Endovasc Surg 1997;13(3):322–7.
4. Drury D, Michaels JA, Jones L, Ayiku L. Systematic review of recent evidence for the safety and efficacy of elective endovascular repair in the management of infrarenal abdominal aortic aneurysm. Br J Surg 2005;92(8):937–46.
5. Biancari F, Ylonen K, Anttila V, et al. Durability of open repair of infrarenal abdominal aortic aneurysm: a 15-year follow-up study. J Vasc Surg 2002;35(1):87–93.
6. Adam DJ, Fitridge RA, Raptis S. Late reintervention for aortic graft-related events and new aortoiliac disease after open abdominal aortic aneurysm repair in an Australian population. J Vasc Surg 2006;43(4):701–5; discussion 5–6.
7. Hertzer NR, Mascha EJ, Karafa MT, O'Hara PJ, Krajewski LP, Beven EG. Open infrarenal abdominal aortic aneurysm repair: the Cleveland Clinic experience from 1989 to 1998. J Vasc Surg 2002;35(6):1145–54.
8. Hallett JW, Jr., Marshall DM, Petterson TM, et al. Graft-related complications after abdominal aortic aneurysm repair: reassurance from a 36-year population-based experience. J Vasc Surg 1997;25(2):277–84; discussion 85–6.
9. Maldonado TS, Rockman CB, Riles E, et al. Ischemic complications after endovascular abdominal aortic aneurysm repair. J Vasc Surg 2004;40(4):703–9; discussion 9–10.
10. Elkouri S, Gloviczki P, McKusick MA, et al. Perioperative complications and early outcome after endovascular and open surgical repair of abdominal aortic aneurysms. J Vasc Surg 2004;39(3):497–505.
11. Erzurum VZ, Sampram ES, Sarac TP, et al. Initial management and outcome of aortic endograft limb occlusion. J Vasc Surg 2004;40(3):419–23.
12. Sivamurthy N, Schneider DB, Reilly LM, Rapp JH, Skovobogatyy H, Chuter TA. Adjunctive primary stenting of Zenith endograft limbs during endovascular abdominal aortic aneurysm repair: implications for limb patency. J Vasc Surg 2006;43(4):662–70.
13. Amesur NB, Zajko AB, Orons PD, Makaroun MS. Endovascular treatment of iliac limb stenoses or occlusions in 31 patients treated with the ancure endograft. J Vasc Interv Radiol 2000;11(4):421–8.

14. Parent FN, 3rd, Godziachvili V, Meier GH, 3rd, et al . Endograft limb occlusion and stenosis after ANCURE endovascular abdominal aneurysm repair. J Vasc Surg 2002;35(4):686–90.

15. Carpenter JP, Neschis DG, Fairman RM, et al . Failure of endovascular abdominal aortic aneurysm graft limbs. J Vasc Surg 2001;33(2):296–302; discussion 302–3.

16. Carroccio A, Faries PL, Morrissey NJ, et al . Predicting iliac limb occlusions after bifurcated aortic stent grafting: anatomic and device-related causes. J Vasc Surg 2002;36(4):679–84.

17. Harris P, Brennan J, Martin J, et al . Longitudinal aneurysm shrinkage following endovascular aortic aneurysm repair: a source of intermediate and late complications. J Endovasc Surg 1999;6(1):11–6.

18. Umscheid T, Stelter WJ. Time-related alterations in shape, position, and structure of self-expanding, modular aortic stent-grafts: a 4-year single-center follow-up. J Endovasc Surg 1999;6(1):17–32.

19. Tillich M, Hausegger KA, Tiesenhausen K, Tauss J, Groell R, Szolar DH. Helical CT angiography of stent-grafts in abdominal aortic aneurysms: morphologic changes and complications. Radiographics 1999;19(6):1573–83.

20. Baum RA, Shetty SK, Carpenter JP, et al . Limb kinking in supported and unsupported abdominal aortic stent-grafts. J Vasc Interv Radiol 2000;11(9):1165–71.

21. Krajcer Z, Gilbert JH, Dougherty K, Mortazavi A, Strickman N. Successful treatment of aortic endograft thrombosis with rheolytic thrombectomy. J Endovasc Ther 2002;9(6):756–64.

22. Hiramoto JS, Reilly LM, Schneider DB, Sivamurthy N, Rapp JH, Chuter TA. Long-term outcome and reintervention after endovascular abdominal aortic aneurysm repair using the Zenith stent graft. J Vasc Surg 2007;45(3):461–5; discussion 5–6.

23. Aburahma AF, Stone PA, Bates MC, Khan TN, Prigozen JM, Welch CA. Endovascular repair of abdominal aortic aneurysms using 3 commercially available devices: midterm results. J Endovasc Ther 2004;11(6):641–8.

24. Aljabri B, Obrand DI, Montreuil B, MacKenzie KS, Steinmetz OK. Early vascular complications after endovascular repair of aortoiliac aneurysms. Annals of vascular surgery 2001;15(6):608–14.

25. May J, White GH, Yu W, et al . Concurrent comparison of endoluminal versus open repair in the treatment of abdominal aortic aneurysms: analysis of 303 patients by life table method. J Vasc Surg 1998;27(2):213–20; discussion 20–1.

Chapter 23

Mesenteric Ischemia Following Abdominal Aortic Aneurysm Repair

Kerianne H. Quanstrum and Gilbert R. Upchurch, Jr.

Abstract Intestinal infarction following abdominal aortic aneurysm (AAA) repair is lethal. Prevention is the key to combating this complication. It has been shown that heightened vigilance to avert, detect, and intervene early on intestinal ischemia in the setting of AAA repair can decrease the incidence and mortality of this frequently lethal disease.

Keywords Mesenteric ischemia, Intestinal ischemia incidence, Mesenteric arterial anatomy.

Definition

The term intestinal ischemia refers to a spectrum of disease. The common endoscopic grading system includes: grade I ischemia, which affects the mucosa and may lead to sloughing, grade II ischemia, which penetrates the muscularis layer, and grade III or transmural ischemia, which includes gross bowel infarction.

Incidence

Fortunately, intestinal ischemia is not a common problem following elective (i.e., nonruptured) open AAA repair. The literature sites an incidence of 1–2% in this setting. If subclinical ischemia evident only on endoscopy is included, the rate increases to 4.5%, as demonstrated in a study by Bast et al. in which 100 patients underwent routine colonoscopy following open AAA repair.[1]

Those patients who undergo open repair of ruptured AAAs are at highest risk for intestinal ischemia, with a variable incidence of 3–30%. When Bast et al. assessed this subset of patients, 17.6% were found to demonstrate some degree of ischemia on routine postoperative colonoscopy.[1]

Data on intestinal ischemia following elective endovascular AAA repair have only begun to emerge, but initial studies report rates of clinically evident

G. Upchurch and E. Criado (eds.) *Aortic Aneurysms, Contemporary Cardiology*
DOI: 10.1007/978-1-60327-204-9_23, © Humana Press, a part of
Springer Science + Business Media, LLC 2009

colon ischemia similar to those seen with open repair, ranging from 1.3% to 2.9%.[2-4] In one study that examined both small and large bowel ischemia following elective endovascular AAA repair, incidence of small bowel ischemia was somewhat higher than that seen in open repair, 0.8% compared to 0.2–0.6%, and was attributed to microembolization of aneurysm plaque.[2]

As is the case with open ruptured repair, endovascular repair of ruptured AAA results in higher rates of intestinal ischemia compared to the elective setting. In a study by Champagne et al. in which patients with ruptured AAA underwent routine postoperative endoscopy following endovascular repair, 23% showed evidence of ischemia, including 8% who required operation.[5] Further, this study corroborated the hypothesis that atheroembolization is a major contributor to intestinal ischemia in endovascular ruptured AAA repair, as pathology specimens from all three of the patients requiring operation revealed atheroemboli underlying the areas of necrotic bowel.

Mesenteric Arterial Anatomy

Prior to discussing the causes of intestinal ischemia following AAA repair, a review of mesenteric arterial anatomy is in order. The mesenteric arterial system involves extensive collateralization (Fig. 1), such that chronic intestinal ischemia rarely occurs unless at least two of the three main mesenteric arteries are compromised. The celiac and the superior mesenteric artery (SMA) exchange collaterals via the pancreaticoduodenal arteries (Fig. 2). The SMA and the inferior mesenteric artery (IMA) collateralize via the marginal artery of Drummond, which joins the left branch of the SMA's middle colic artery to the ascending branch of the IMA's left colic artery (Figs. 3 and 4). In addition, the meandering mesenteric artery, also known as the central anastomotic artery, provides a route of direct anastomosis between the trunks of the SMA and IMA (Figs. 5 and 6). The IMA also collateralizes with the iliac system via the capillary network in the rectal wall, through which the IMA's superior hemorrhoidal artery exchanges with the middle and inferior hemorrhoidal branches of the internal iliac, or hypogastric, arteries (Figs. 1, 3, and 4). Finally, the internal iliac arteries themselves receive collaterals from the external iliac, lumbar, and femoral arteries.

Etiology

The causes of intestinal ischemia in the setting of AAA repair are several, and can be divided into anatomic, embolic and mechanical, and physiological entities (Table 1).

Anatomic

Given the collateral flow within the mesenteric arterial system, ligation or exclusion of the IMA, as often performed during AAA repair, should not, on its own, compromise intestinal blood flow in the setting of otherwise nondiseased vessels. A patient with an AAA, however – a disease whose risk factors include increased age, smoking, coronary artery disease, high cholesterol, etc. – often has coexistent atherosclerotic disease. In the setting of atherosclerosis of all three main mesenteric vessels, for example, ligation of the IMA – or

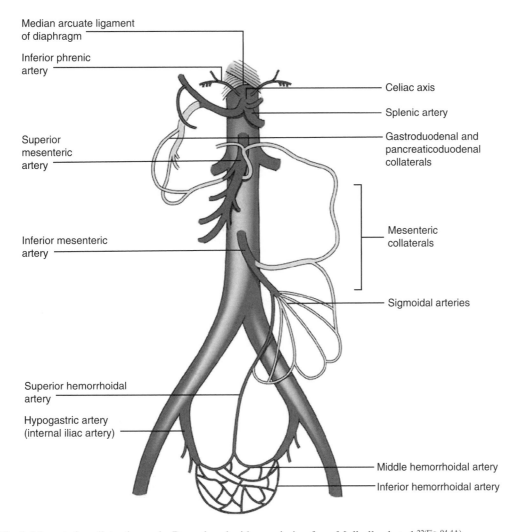

Fig. 1 Mesenteric collateral vessels. Reproduced with permission from Mulholland et al.[22(Fig. 94.4A)]

exclusion of the IMA, as necessarily occurs during endovascular AAA repair – could be the critical event that precipitates overt bowel ischemia. In the setting of celiac stenosis, in which SMA is the main source of blood flow to the stomach and duodenum via the pancreaticoduodenal collaterals, ligation or exclusion of the IMA, leaving the SMA as the primary source of blood supply to the entire gastrointestinal tract, could similarly prove disastrous. In the setting of SMA stenosis, on the other hand, the role of the internal iliac arteries as collateral flow to the left colon gains importance if IMA is ligated. As it is not infrequent, particularly during endovascular repair of AAA, that one, and occasionally both, of the internal iliac arteries must be sacrificed, the patient may be at risk for bowel ischemia if conscious steps are not taken to maintain flow to the left colon. Finally, in the setting of atherosclerosis of the IMA, the left colon will be receiving most of its blood supply from other sources, including collaterals from the SMA or internal iliac arteries. Ligation, then, at

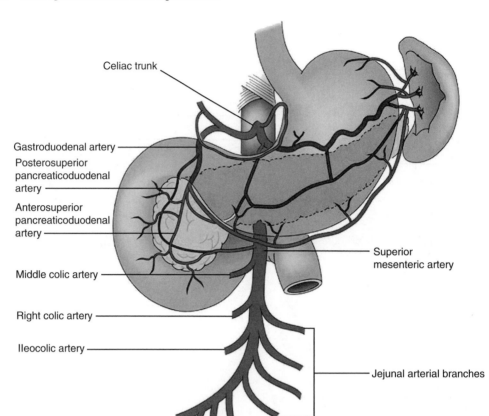

Celiac trunk

Gastroduodenal artery

Posterosuperior
pancreaticoduodenal
artery

Anterosuperior
pancreaticoduodenal
artery

Middle colic artery

Right colic artery

Ileocolic artery

Superior
mesenteric artery

Jejunal arterial branches

Ileal arterial branches

Fig. 2 Distribution of the celiac artery and superior mesenteric artery (*SMA*). Reproduced with permission from Mulholland et al.[22](Fig. 94.1)

the root of the IMA should not affect that supply to any great extent, provided that the collateral sources are left intact.

Embolic and Mechanical

Embolization of atherosclerotic plaque or thrombos during aortic clamping in open AAA repair, or during intraluminal stent manipulation in endovascular repair, is another factor likely to be at work in the event of intestinal ischemia. As mentioned earlier, based on histological review of the pathology specimens of patients who underwent operation for necrotic bowel, this mechanism is strongly suggested to be a contributor to bowel ischemia in the setting of endovascular AAA repair. Undue compression of mesenteric vessels by retractors during open AAA repair has also been hypothesized to contribute to bowel ischemia. Finally, in the setting of AAA rupture, when intestinal ischemia is most common, it is thought that the resulting retroperitoneal hematoma compresses the mesenteric vessels to compromise flow.

Physiologic

Particularly in the setting of atherosclerotic disease affecting the mesenteric arteries, physiological factors alone, including intra- or perioperative hypotension,

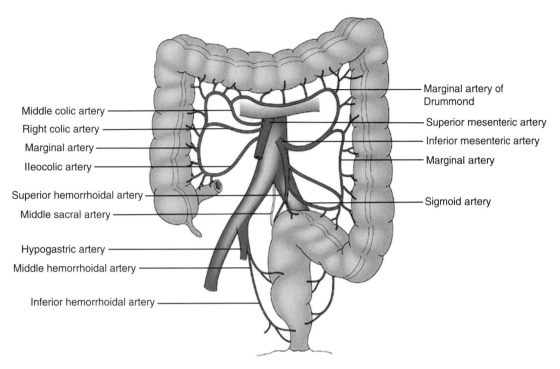

Fig. 3 Distribution of the superior mesenteric artery (*SMA*) and inferior mesenteric artery (*IMA*). Reproduced with permission from Mulholland et al.[22](Fig. 94.2)

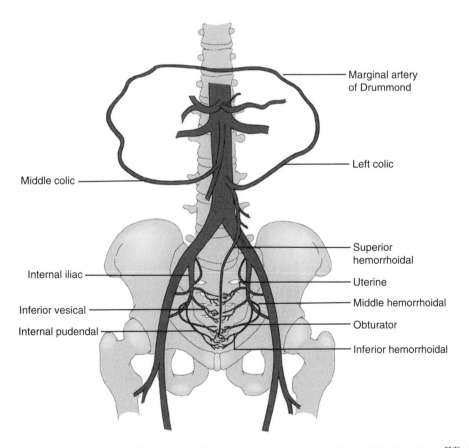

Fig. 4 Marginal artery of Drummond. Reproduced with permission from Mulholland et al.[22](Fig. 95.3)

Fig. 5 Selective inferior mesenteric artery (*IMA*) angiography demonstrates the marginal artery of Drummond (*single arrow, image right*) and the larger meandering mesenteric artery, or central anastomotic artery (*paired arrows, image left*). Reproduced with permission from Mulholland et al.[22(Fig. 94.3)]

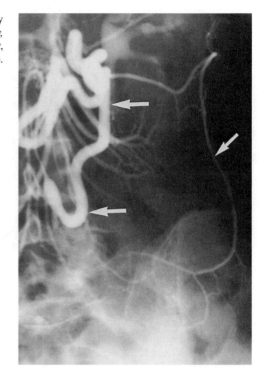

Fig. 6 Angiography demonstrates an enlarged inferior mesenteric artery (*IMA*) (*black arrow*) and meandering mesenteric artery (*white arrow*) in the setting of celiac and superior mesenteric artery (*SMA*) occlusion. Reproduced with permission from Mulholland et al.[22(Fig. 94.16B)]

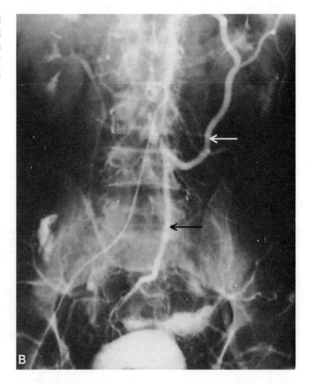

Table 1 Causes of mesenteric ischemia during AAA repair.

Anatomic	Embolic and Mechanical	Physiologic
Preexisting atherosclerosis of one or more mesenteric vessels	Embolization of atherosclerotic plaque: during aortic clamping in open repair or during intraluminal stent manipulation in endovascular repair Compression of mesenteric vessels by retractors during open repair Compression of mesenteric vessels by retroperitoneal hematoma in the setting of AAA rupture	Hypotension, hypovolemia, low cardiac output, use of pressors, e.g., leading to poor visceral perfusion

hypovolemia, or use of pressors, might be sufficient to precipitate intestinal ischemia. Piotrowski et al. published findings suggesting that preoperative shock was the most important risk factor for colon ischemia following open repair of ruptured AAA, while large intraoperative blood loss was also predictive.[6] In contrast, a study by Meissner et al. found no correlation between intestinal ischemia following ruptured AAA repair and either perioperative shock or volume administration, but documented that low perioperative cardiac output and use of alpha-adrenergic pressors were predictive.[7] While reports in the literature are conflicting as to which physiological mechanism is most predictive of bowel ischemia, it is intuitive that each can contribute.

Diagnosis and Management

Diagnosis

For purposes of intraoperative detection of inadequate intestinal perfusion during AAA repair, several methods have been proposed. Other than in cases of gross ischemia or infarction, visual inspection of the bowel is generally inadequate to recognize malperfusion. Management of the IMA appears critical. Relatively simple adjuncts to determine the safety of IMA ligation versus the need for implantation into the aortic graft include Doppler ultrasound of the relevant mesenteric vessels,[8] endoluminal pulse oximetry of the bowel wall,[9] or laser Doppler monitoring of serosal blood flow[10,11] following IMA occlusion. Each of these methods has demonstrated good sensitivity in small, nonrandomized studies, but none has been universally adopted. Intravenous fluorescein injection followed by Wood's lamp examination of the bowel wall,[12] intraperitoneal xenon injection followed by gastrointestinal-activity monitoring,[13] and measurement of intraluminal pH[14] are other methods that have been proposed. None of these methods is universally accessible due to the need for specialized equipment, however, and none has been rigorously validated in the literature.

The classic presenting sign of intestinal ischemia following AAA repair is bloody diarrhea. Classic symptoms such as abdominal pain out of proportion to physical examination may be masked by the use of epidural anesthesia or intravenous narcotics; while fever, leukocytosis, lactic acidosis, or general sepsis are less specific signs whose significance may be confounded by the physiological changes associated with the operation itself. Regardless, postoperative diarrhea, whether bloody or not, is uncommon following AAA repair, when ileus would be the more expected scenario, and thus should lead to consideration of sigmoidoscopy. Similarly, any suspicion of intestinal ischemia on the part of the surgeon, whether because of clinical presentation or the mere presence of risk factors for the event, should prompt endoscopic examination. Liberal use of endoscopy has been suggested to avoid the catastrophic event of intestinal infarction. In the setting of ruptured AAA repair, in fact, when intestinal ischemia is most frequent, several authors have promoted routine postoperative endoscopy in the first 24–48 h. following surgery. Vascular surgeons at Case Medical Center instituted routine colonoscopy following open ruptured AAA repair, with resultant improved mortality rates for ischemic colitis that they attributed to earlier diagnosis and treatment.[15] In a second study, these authors instituted the same mandate for *endovascular* repair of ruptured AAA.[5] While an effect on mortality was not documented due to the lack of a comparison group, it is notable that among the patients in the study found to have any degree of intestinal ischemia, not a single death occurred during 30-day follow-up. The effects on outcome of routine endoscopy after ruptured AAA repair await more rigorous examination to determine whether this strategy should become common practice. Of note, flexible sigmoidoscopy, as opposed to full colonoscopy, is usually sufficient to diagnose intestinal ischemia, as the rectosigmoid colon is involved in 95% of cases in which intestinal ischemia occurs.[16]

Management

Management of intestinal ischemia varies with endoscopic findings (Table 2). Mucosal ischemia alone (i.e., grade I), associated with a near-zero mortality rate, generally warrants only supportive management, including optimization of fluid status, bowel rest, empirical antibiotics, serial abdominal examinations, and repeat endoscopy to confirm resolution or evaluate for progression that may warrant more aggressive management. With more advanced ischemia that penetrates the muscularis propria (grade II), recovery also commonly occurs with conservative management alone. In this case, however, patients are at risk of developing strictures as the bowel wall heals, and thus they should undergo contrast enema once the acute phase of ischemia has resolved. Finally, transmural involvement of the bowel (grade III) requires urgent laparotomy. Even in the setting of prompt operation, mortality can run as high as 90%, generally due to sepsis and multisystem organ failure.

Table 2 Management of intestinal ischemia.

Grade I	Grade II	Grade III
Supportive: Optimization of fluid status, bowel rest, empirical antibiotics, serial abdominal examinations, consideration of followup endoscopy	Supportive management, including lower threshold for follow-up endoscopy; contrast enema to evaluate for intestinal strictures after the acute phase of ischemia has resolved	Urgent exploratory laparotomy

Recommendations

Preoperative Planning

Preoperative assessment of the patency and dominance of the celiac, SMA, IMA, and internal iliac arteries is essential prior to AAA repair. First and foremost, a complete history and physical examination should be obtained to detect any history of symptoms suggesting mesenteric ischemia, such as postprandial pain, unintentional weight loss, or food fear. In most cases, CT angiography is adequate to assess the characteristics and measurements of the aortic aneurysm and its relationship to visceral and renal arteries, as well as the patency of the visceral vessels themselves. Compromise of any one or combination of the mesenteric arteries may require a more creative operative plan, varying from IMA implantation into the aortic graft, to internal iliac artery bypass, to a more complex reconstruction involving the celiac or SMA.

Treatment of the IMA

A study from Massachusetts General Hospital sited ligation of a patent IMA as the most common factor found to be present, at a rate of 75%, in patients who developed colon ischemia following open abdominal aortic surgery.[17] Implantation of the IMA into the aortic graft, therefore, has been heralded to prevent, or at least to lessen the risk of, intestinal ischemia. The efficacy of this practice has not strictly been borne out in the literature, however. Senekowitsch et al. performed a study in which patients were prospectively, randomly assigned to undergo IMA ligation or implantation.[18] There was no statistically significant difference in rates of ischemic colitis as diagnosed by routine postoperative colonoscopy and biopsy sampling. There was a nonstatistically significant trend favoring IMA implantation, however, with relative risk for ischemic colitis as low as 0.55, $p = 0.203$. Of note, in the final analysis, the study was found to be underpowered. Further, nonrandom implantation of the IMA, as dictated by surgeon judgment, is likely to have a *clinically* significant effect on the risk of developing ischemic colitis for a given patient. To answer this question definitively would require taking patients in whom it was judged by the surgeon that IMA implantation would be beneficial, and randomizing *those* patients to undergo implantation versus ligation. Of course, such a study would be unethical and impossible. We recommend, therefore, implantation of the IMA in those patients in whom it is judged to be feasible and beneficial. In some cases, the benefit – indeed, the necessity – will be obvious, such as in the patient with SMA stenosis and a large IMA supplying the majority of their intestinal blood flow (Fig. 6). For purposes of assessing benefit in more subtle cases, measurement of IMA stump pressure has been proposed, with a pressure of at least 40 mmHg thought to be sufficient to allow for safe ligation.[19] In practice, however, simple visual inspection of IMA backflow is usually employed. When the IMA must be ligated without implantation, we recommend the standard practice of ligating at the wall of the aorta in order to avoid interruption of any proximal collateral vessels.

Treatment of the Internal Iliac Arteries

It has been promulgated that maintaining patency of one or both internal iliac arteries lessens the risk of bowel compromise. Maintaining perfusion to one internal iliac artery, in fact, is often considered the standard of care in open AAA repair. Two case series, however, have demonstrated that unilateral or bilateral internal iliac artery interruption can be performed during either endovascular or open AAA repair without inducing buttock necrosis or colon ischemia requiring operation.[20,21] This can be performed provided that (1) the internal iliac arteries are interrupted as proximally as possible, ideally at their origin, in order to maintain distal collateral flow from the external iliac and femoral arteries; (2) distal embolization is avoided; and (3) ligation, when bilateral, is performed in a staged fashion. Unfortunately, neither of these case series involved a control group. The surgical tenet remains, therefore, that perfusion to one internal iliac artery should be maintained wherever possible. If ligation of both internal iliacs is necessary, this may be done without undue increase in rates of intestinal ischemia provided that the three mentioned criteria are met.

Conclusion

Intestinal infarction following AAA repair is lethal, but largely preventable in the elective setting. Vigilance on the part of the surgeon is essential. Attention to the possibility of intestinal ischemia, and due diligence in preoperative planning, procedural execution, and postoperative monitoring so as to avert its development or allow for timely intervention, respectively, can decrease the incidence and mortality of this otherwise deadly complication.

References

1. Bast TJ, van der Biezen JJ, Scherpenisse J, Eikelboom BC: Ischaemic disease of the colon and rectum after surgery for abdominal aortic aneurysm: A prospective study of the incidence and risk factors. Eur J Vasc Surg 4:253–57, 1990.
2. Zhang WW, Kulaylat MN, Anain PM, Dosluoglu HH, Harris LM, Cherr GS, Dayton MT, Dryjski ML: Embolization as cause of bowel ischemia after endovascular abdominal aortic aneurysm repair. J Vasc Surg 40:867–72, 2004.
3. Maldonado TS, Rockman CB, Riles E, Douglas D, Adelman MA, Jacobowitz GR, Gagne PJ, Nalbandian MN, Cayne NS, Lamparello PJ, Salzberg SS, Riles TS: Ischemic complications after endovascular abdominal aortic aneurysm repair. J Vasc Surg 40:703–10, 2004.
4. Dadian N, Ohki T, Veith FJ, Edelman M, Mehta M, Lipsitz EC, Suggs WD, Wain RA: Overt colon ischemia after endovascular aneurysm repair: The importance of microembolization as an etiology. J Vasc Surg 34:986–96, 2001.
5. Champagne BJ, Lee EC, Valerian B, Mulhotra N, Mehta M: Incidence of colonic ischemia after repair of ruptured abdominal aortic aneurysm with endograft. J Am Coll Surg 204:597–602, 2007.
6. Piotrowski JJ, Ripepi AJ, Yuhas JP, Alexander JJ, Brandt CP: Colonic ischemia: The Achilles heel of ruptured aortic aneurysm repair. Am Surg 62:557–60, 1996.
7. Meissner MH, Johansen KH: Colon infarction after ruptured abdominal aortic aneurysm. Arch Surg 126:979–85, 1992.
8. Hobson RW, 2nd, Wright CB, Rich NM, Collins GJ, Jr: Assessment of colonic ischemia during aortic surgery by Doppler ultrasound. J Surg Res 20:231–35, 1976.
9. Yilmaz EN, Vahl AC, van Rij G, et al: Endoluminal pulse oximetry of the sigmoid colon and the monitoring of the colonic circulation. Cardiovasc Surg 7:704–9, 1999.
10. Krohg-Sorensen K, Kvernebo K: Laser Doppler flowmetry in evaluation of colonic blood flow during aortic reconstruction. Eur J Vasc Surg 3:37–41, 1989.

11. Sakakibara Y, Jikuya T, Saito EM, et al: Does laser Doppler flowmetry aid the prevention of ischemic colitis in abdominal aortic aneurysm surgery? Thorac Cardiovasc Surg 45:32–34, 1997.

12. Bergman RT, Gloviczki P, Welch TJ, et al: The role of intravenous fluorescein in the detection of colon ischemia during aortic reconstruction. Ann Vasc Surg 6:74–79, 1992.

13. Gharagozloo F, Bulkley GB, Zuidema GD, O'Mara CS, Alderson PO. The use of intraperitoneal xenon for early diagnosis of acute mesenteric ischemia. Surgery. 1984 Apr;95(4):404–11.

14. Fiddian-Green RG, Amelin PM, Hermann JB, et al: Prediction of the development of sigmoid ischemia on the day of aortic operations: Indirect measurements of intramural pH in the colon. Arch Surg 121:654–60, 1986.

15. Champagne BJ, Darling RC, 3rd, Daneshmand M, Kreienberg PB, Lee EC, Mehta M, Roddy SP, Chang BB, Paty PSK, Ozsvath KJ, Shah DM: Outcome of aggressive surveillance colonoscopy in ruptured abdominal aortic aneurysm. J Vasc Surg 39:792–96, 2004.

16. Bjorck M, Bergqvist D, Troeng T: Incidence and clinical presentation of bowel ischaemia after aortoiliac surgery--2930 operations from a population-based registry in Sweden. Eur J Vasc Endovasc Surg 12:139–44, 1996.

17. Brewster DC, Franklin DP, Cambria RP, Darling RC, Moncure AC, Lamuraglia GM, Stone WM, Abbott WM: Intestinal ischemia complicating abdominal aortic surgery. Surg 109:447–54, 1991.

18. Senekowitsch C, Assadian A, Assadian O, Hartleb H, Ptakovsky, H, Hagmuller GW: Replanting the inferior mesentery artery during infrarenal aortic aneurysm repair: Influence on postoperative colon ischemia. J Vasc Surg 43:689–94, 2006.

19. Ernst CB, Hagihara PF, Daugherty ME, GriffenJr. WO: Inferior mesenteric artery stump pressure: A reliable index for safe IMA ligation during abdominal aortic aneurysmectomy. Ann Surg 187:641–46, 1978.

20. Mehta M, Veith FJ, Ohki T, Cynamon J, Goldstein K, Suggs WD, Wain RA, Chang DW, Griedman SG, Scher LA, Lipsitz EC: Unilateral and bilateral hypogastric artery interruption during aortoiliac aneurysm repair in 154 patients: A relatively innocuous procedure. J Vasc Surg 33:S27–32, 2001.

21. Mehta M, Veith FJ, Darling RC, 3rd, Roddy ST, Ohki T, Lipsitz EC, Paty PS, Kreienberg PB, Ozsvath KJ, Chang BB, Shah DM: Effects of bilateral hypogastric artery interruption during endovascular and open aortoiliac aneurysm repair. J Vasc Surg 40:698–702, 2004.

22. Mulholland MW, et al; Greenfield's Surgery: Scientific Principles & Practice. 4th ed. Philadelphia, PA: Lippincott Williams & Wilkins, 2006. http://thegreenfieldsolution.com

Chapter 24

Operative Therapy for the Descending and Thoracoabdominal Aorta

Himanshu J. Patel, Gilbert R. Upchurch, Jr., and G.Michael Deeb

Abstract Aortic aneurysms are the 13th leading cause of mortality in the United States. Thoracoabdominal aortic aneurysms (TAAAs), defined as straddling the diaphragm and extending anywhere between the left subclavian artery down to the aortic bifurcation, remain a less common entity compared to the more frequently presenting aneurysms involving the ascending or infrarenal aorta. In 1986, E. Stanley Crawford popularized a classification scheme for TAAA based on their extent, a surrogate for the risk of postoperative neurological deficit. This system essentially classifies the extent of aneurysm as primarily involving the thoracic aorta with varying degrees of extension into the abdominal aorta (types I and II), and contrasts them to those primarily involving the abdominal aorta with varying degrees of extension into the thoracic aorta (types III and IV). The natural history of aortic aneurysms remains that of inexorable expansion and rupture. Classic early studies on the natural history of untreated TAAA demonstrated a 2-year mortality of 76%, predominantly from aortic rupture. The strongest determinant of the risk for rupture is greatest for those aneurysms with diameters larger than 5 cm. However, other determinants of rupture include advanced age, a history of hypertension, tobacco use, or chronic obstructive pulmonary disease. Aneurysms presenting with preexisting dissection, or those that are larger, typically have higher growth rates and represent a higher risk for rupture. This chapter will discuss the indications for intervention, as well as operative approaches, both open and hybrid.

Keywords Thoracoabdominal aorta, Open operative TAAA repair, Hybrid TAAA repair

Preoperative Evaluation for Patients with Thoracoabdominal Aortic Aneurysm

Despite advances in perioperative care, thoracoabdominal aortic aneurysm (TAAA) repair remains among the most formidable of operative procedures with reported rates of mortality varying from 4%to 20%.[1-4] In addition, the

G. Upchurch and E. Criado (eds.) *Aortic Aneurysms, Contemporary Cardiology*
DOI: 10.1007/978-1-60327-204-9_24, © Humana Press, a part of
Springer Science+Business Media, LLC 2009

frequent presence of comorbid conditions including coronary artery disease, chronic obstructive pulmonary disease, renal failure, and peripheral vascular disease increases risk for major postoperative morbidity. The typical age of presentation also reaches the sixth decade of life, and can often result in a delayed functional recovery. It is in this setting that the aortic surgeon must conduct the preoperative evaluation to be certain that the outcome is optimal.

The aneurysm extent is typically evaluated with computed tomography (CT) angiography. The images are in thin 1–2 mm slices, and are obtained during peak opacification of the aorta to give the best visualization of the offending pathology, the location of critical intercostal vessels, and to determine whether branch vessel obstruction is present (Table 1). Although previously universally utilized as part of the preoperative evaluation, conventional aortography is rarely used and does not give the same detailed information obtained by CT scanning. Although other modalities may be used, including magnetic resonance imaging and echocardiography, these do not give the same detail as CT scanning.

Assessment of comorbid conditions is paramount in deciding whether the patient is able to withstand the physiological insult imposed by this operative procedure. We evaluate cardiac status in everyone for elective open repair with coronary angiography and transesophageal echocardiography. If obstructive coronary lesions are present, they are all treated with either percutaneous intervention or coronary artery bypass grafting, and TAAA repair is then performed at a later stage (usually 4–6 weeks later). If major valvular pathology is identified, this is also addressed at that time. Those patients with severely impaired ejection fraction (i.e., <35%) are often not considered for open repair. Pulmonary function is assessed by standard evaluation and those patients with FEV1 or DLCO < 60% all referred for preoperative evaluation and optimization. If patients are actively smoking, we will not operate in the elective setting until they have been free from tobacco use for at least 6 weeks. Normal renal function is important not only for risk stratification but also for potential optimization to minimize perioperative complications. Assessment of coexisting peripheral arterial disease is assisted by obtaining carotid duplex scanning and baseline ankle brachial indices. Finally, hepatic function is assessed; cirrhosis remains a relative contraindication for open operation.

In the event that open TAAA repair is contraindicated secondary to comorbid conditions, an evaluation for a hybrid endovascular approach is entertained. In this option, a thoracotomy is avoided. If the aneurysm extends into the visceral or pararenal aortic segments, a debranching procedure is indicated whereby the respective involved vessel is bypassed and then the TAAA excluded with a stent graft to include coverage of the bypassed vessel(s). By avoiding the thoracotomy, and limiting the incision to an abdominal approach only, the morbidity is theoretically decreased. Although long-term results of

Table 1 Thoracoabdominal aortic aneurysm classification.

Type	Extent of pathology
I	Distal to left subclavian artery to above renal arteries
II	Distal to left subclavian artery to aortic bifurcation
III	From sixth intercostal space to infrarenal aorta
IV	From aortic diaphragm to infrarenal aorta (total abdominal aorta)

this approach are not well characterized, early data are encouraging. Note that the debranching procedure itself is not altogether benign and has been associated with significant morbidity in some series.[5,6]

The preoperative workup for hybrid TAAA repairs is similar to that seen for open TAAA repair. We typically obtain adenosine nuclear medicine stress tests and selectively catheterize only those with abnormal results. Although the remaining preoperative testing is similar, it is primarily performed to risk stratify the patient and present him/her with an estimate of procedural morbidity. If the procedure is totally endovascular (i.e., no debranching procedure needed, or thoracic endovascular aneurysm repair (TEVAR)), we and others have performed this procedure in patients considered a prohibitive risk for open repair with good early and late results.[7,8] In contrast to medical therapy, previous work suggests that this approach may reduce the risk for early mortality even in this frequently elderly and debilitated group.[9] For those patients needing a debranching procedure, a more selective approach is taken since this additional operation requires laparotomy with its attendant morbidity.[6]

Operative Techniques for Repair of TAAA

Open Operative TAAA Repair

Open TAAA repair is approached via a left thoracoabdominal incision. If the aneurysm is confined to the descending thoracic aorta, an abdominal extension is not made. We typically extend our abdominal incision in the left paramedian line and stay in the retroperitoneal plane. All type I, II, and III TAAA repairs are done with spinal drains to minimize the risk for spinal cord ischemia. In addition, the use of extracorporeal perfusion is standard in all TAAAs. We will often use full cardiopulmonary bypass with deep hypothermic circulatory arrest for all TAAA repairs done for acute type B dissections or for those with isolated type I TAAA (as a spinal protective adjunct). Otherwise, left heart bypass with an oxygenator is used for all others.

The sequence of the operative repair for a type II TAAA is described as follows and the final result is illustrated in Fig. 1. Briefly, the proximal anastomosis is constructed first. We use a sequential clamping technique to maximize perfusion times to all viscera and the spinal cord. We attempt to reimplant lower (T8–T11) intercostal vessels in all patients unless they are thrombosed, or the adjacent aorta is heavily calcified. The diaphragm is left intact to minimize postoperative pulmonary complications. The visceral and renal vessels are then sequentially bypassed using the prefabricated side branches on the main Dacron aortic graft. In this manner, flow is maintained to the viscera throughout construction of the anastomosis. In addition, the avoidance of reimplanting the visceral vessels as a patch eliminates all aneurysmal aortic tissue and the risk of formation of visceral patch aneurysms. When renal arterial bypasses are constructed, 10 mg of furosemide is administered prior to renal artery clamping and administer a cold (4°C) renal preservation solution containing heparin and mannitol directly into the ostium. Finally, the distal aortic anastomosis is constructed, and the patient then weaned from extracorporeal support.

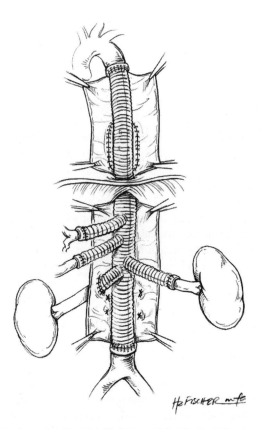

Fig. 1 A completed repair of a type II thoracoabdominal aortic aneurysm. Note the reimplantation of the lower sets of intercostal vessels, as well as individual bypasses to the visceral and renal vessels

Hybrid TAAA Repair

For those patients undergoing a purely endovascular procedure (i.e., typically pathology confined to the descending aorta), the access vessel is made ready for isolation. The delivery of the endograft is typically via a transfemoral approach, but iliac exposure is needed in approximately 15–20% (predominantly women, smaller men, or those with significant external iliac atherosclerosis). We use lumbar drains for spinal cord protection for all those patients requiring long segment (>20 cm) coverage or those who have prior infrarenal AAA repairs. The endograft is then delivered to the intended aortic segment via the isolated access vessel, and the vessel is then repaired following completion aortography.

If a debranching procedure is needed for coverage into the visceral and pararenal segments, this is performed first, and endografting is then subsequently performed after allowing for 4–6 weeks of recovery. Abdominal debranching is often performed by basing the inflow of the branch vessels on the iliac artery or occasionally the terminal infrarenal aorta. Bypasses are constructed with 7- or 8-mm Dacron or Goretex grafts and are typically an end-to-end bypass graft to the branch vessel. Endografting is then performed as described above.

In lieu of abdominal debranching, a totally endovascular approach may be undertaken at select centers who have access to custom fabricated fenestrated and branched endografts.[10] These endografts are designed specifically for the patient's individual anatomy and allow for cannulation and endografting into the branch vessels via the main aortic endograft to perform a totally endovascular TAAA. Early results are encouraging.

Postoperative Management

Recovery from repair of a TAAA requires a stay of 2–4 days in the intensive care unit for open procedures, and 1–2 days following TEVAR. During this time, permissive hypertension is maintained to improve spinal cord perfusion, and the spinal fluid is drained to maintain intrathecal pressures < 10 mmHg. Following this period, attention is paid to ambulation, resumption of enteral nutrition when bowel function returns, and aggressive pulmonary toilet. There is a phenomenon of delayed paraplegia that can occur at any time after an operation, but usually occurs within the first week. It has often been associated with hemodynamic instability, and thus we attempt to maintain permissive hypertension (systolic blood pressure 120–140 mmHg) throughout the hospitalization.[11]

Outcomes following open TAAA repair have been analyzed in multiple series. Essentially, the risk for mortality varies from 4% to 18%.[1-3] A recent analysis of the Nationwide Inpatient Sample administrative database, however, suggested a nationwide mortality estimate exceeding 20%.[4] At the University of Michigan, we have reported a mortality rate of 3% in the elective setting.[12] Other risks include those of renal failure (temporary or permanent) of 10% and a risk for spinal cord ischemia of 5–12%. In contrast, the risks of purely endovascular TAAA repair are lower, with reported rates of mortality of 1–5% and of paraplegia of 1–5%.[5-10]

Conclusion

In summary, repair of TAAAs remains a daunting task. Over the last 40 years, changes in operative and perioperative care as well as newer minimally invasive options are improving outcomes to ameliorate the risks of dissection or rupture and aneurysm-related mortality.

References

1. Crawford ES, Crawford JL, Safi HJ, et al. Thoracoabdominal aortic aneurysms: preoperative and intraoperative factors determining immediate and long term results of operations in 605 patients. J. Vasc. Surg. 1986; 3: 389–404.
2. Svensson LG, Hess KR, Coselli JS, et al. Influence of segmental arteries, extent and atriofemoral bypass on postoperative paraplegia after thoracoabdominal aortic operations. J. Vasc. Surg. 1994; 20: 255–62.
3. Coselli JS, LeMaire SA, Conklin ND, et al . Morbidity and mortality after extent II thoracoabdominal aortic aneurysm repair. Ann. Thorac. Surg. 2002; 73: 1107–15.
4. Cowan JA, Jr., Dimick JB, Henke PK et al. Surgical treatment of intact thoracoabdominal aortic aneurysms in the United States: hospital and surgeon volume-related outcomes. J. Vasc. Surg. 2003; 37: 1169–74.

5. Fulton JJ, Farber MA, Marston WA, et al. Endovascular stent graft repair of para-renal and type IV thoracoabdominal aortic aneurysms with adjunctive visceral reconstruction. J. Vasc. Surg. 2005; 41: 191–8.

6. Chiesa R, Tshomba Y, Melissano G, et al. Hybrid approach to thoracoabdominal aortic aneurysms in patients with prior aortic surgery. J. Vasc. Surg. 2007; 45: 1128–35.

7. Patel HJ, Williams DM, Upchurch GR, Shillingford MS, Dasika NL, Proctor MC, Deeb GM. Long term results from a 12 year experience with endovascular therapy for thoracic aortic disease. Ann. Thorac. Surg. 2006; 82: 2147–53.

8. Greenberg RK, O'Neill S, Walker E, et al. Endovascular repair of thoracic aortic lesions with the Zenith TX1 and TX2 thoracic endografts: intermediate-term results. J. Vasc. Surg. 2005; 41: 589–96.

9. Patel HJ, Shillingford MS, Williams DM, et al. Survival benefit of endovascular descending thoracic aortic repair for the high risk patient. Ann. Thorac. Surg. 2007; 83: 1628–34.

10. Roselli EE, Greenberg RK, Pfaff K, Francis C, Svensson LG, Lytle BW. Endovascular treatment of thoracoabdominal aortic aneurysms. J. Thorac. Cardiovasc. Surg. 2007; 133: 1474–82.

11. Wong DR, Coselli JS, Amerman K, et al . Delayed spinal deficits after thoracoab-dominal aortic aneurysm repair. Ann. Thorac. Surg. 2007; 83: 1345–55.

12. Upchurch GR, Jr., Patel HJ, Rectenwald JE, et al. Open repair of thoracoabdominal aortic aneurysms: when and how. *In* Pearce WH, Matsumura JS, Yao JST (eds.), Vascular Surgery in the Endovascular Era. Greenwood Academic. Evanston IL. 2008: pp. 146–155.

Chapter 25

Endovascular Repair of Thoracic Aortic Aneurysms

Timothy A. M. Chuter

Abstract Endovascular repair is particularly appealing in cases of thoracic aortic aneurysm because the surgical alternative requires thoracotomy and aortic cross-clamp, resulting in pulmonary dysfunction, cardiac strain, downstream ischemia, and reperfusion injury. Moreover, localized aneurysms of the thoracic aorta are relatively easy to treat by endovascular means, using simple aortoaortic stent-grafts; hence, the endovascular thoracic aortic aneurysm repair was rapidly adopted in the early 1990s.[1] Yet this area of endovascular technology remains something of a work in progress. Thoracic aortic stent-grafts still fail to meet many of the requirements of long-term success because the affected segment is long, wide, curved, far from the femoral arteries, and close to the origins of visceral or cerebral branches. There remain many obstacles to be overcome before endovascular repair can be considered safe, durable, and effective for the majority of thoracic aortic aneurysms. Some problems affect repair in any part of the thoracic aorta, while some are segment-specific; some problems are amenable to refinements of operative technique, while others must wait for fundamental advances in stent-graft technology.

Keywords Endovascular, Thoracic aortic aneurysm, Stent-graft

Arterial Access

Even in its healthy state, the descending thoracic aorta is wider and longer than the infrarenal abdominal aorta, and thoracic aortic stent-grafts have to be wider and longer than abdominal aortic stent-grafts. The additional width is a particular problem in women and patients with common femoral or external iliac stenosis, because wider stent-grafts need wider delivery systems. If the delivery system is too large to traverse the external iliac artery, one needs an alternative route of access, to the common iliac artery, or even the aorta. Although direct puncture has been described, most surgeons prefer to create a conduit to the central arterial circulation, which may be surgical or endovascular, simultaneous or staged.

G. Upchurch and E. Criado (eds.) *Aortic Aneurysms, Contemporary Cardiology*
DOI: 10.1007/978-1-60327-204-9_25, © Humana Press, a part of
Springer Science+Business Media, LLC 2009

An endovascular conduit consists of a covered stent, or stents, within the external or common iliac artery, which permits aggressive balloon-induced dilatation to the point of arterial rupture. This technique works well when the arterial narrowing spares the proximal external iliac artery. Otherwise, there is a risk that the covered stent will either occlude the internal iliac artery or fail to prevent bleeding from rupture of the proximal external iliac artery.

The simplest form of conduit is a conventional surgical graft with one end sutured to the margins of a common iliac arteriotomy.[2] An encircling loop of cloth tape compresses the conduit around the delivery system or sheath, providing hemostasis. Better still, the wall of the conduit is punctured and the sheath is inserted over a wire, as though the conduit were a native artery. A tight fit between the margins of the hole and the wall of the sheath is usually sufficient hemostasis. On occasion, a small incision at the puncture site may be needed to permit large bore sheath insertion. In theory, a blind-ended conduit can be left in an accessible location under the skin as the first part of a staged procedure. The second stage then starts with thrombectomy of the graft. A more satisfactory alternative involves attaching the proximal end of the graft to the transected end of the common iliac artery and the distal end to the side of the external iliac artery, creating a bypass with antegrade flow through the femoral artery to the limb and retrograde flow up the native external iliac artery to the internal iliac territory.[3] This graft need not be exposed during the second stage of the operation. Instead, access to the conduit can be obtained through the femoral artery.

Aortic Tortuosity

An aneurysm of the descending thoracic aorta often lengthens as it dilates, raising the distal aortic arch and creating a transverse segment of redundant aorta just above the diaphragm. The resultant angles impede stent-graft insertion and compromise both stent-graft sealing and attachment.

The aortic arch and diaphragmatic hiatus tend to fix the aorta in position, preventing the straightening that would otherwise accompany the insertion of a smoothly tapered delivery system over a stiff guidewire. Under these circumstances, the delivery system has to flex without kinking. The simplest way to make a sheath kink resistant is to thicken its wall, but this remedy is limited by the size of the access arteries. The incorporation of a spiral wire, or ribbon, into the wall of the sheath has the same effect without the added bulk, and most sheath-based delivery systems incorporate this approach. This design appears to achieve the two primary goals: atraumatic insertion and unrestricted sheath withdrawal. Indeed, the TX2 Superflex delivery system (Cook Medical, Bloomington, IN) (Fig. 1) will deploy even when tied in a knot. The TAG stent-graft (WL Gore, Flagstaff, AZ) employs a different approach. The sheath is too short to reach the level of the diaphragm. Instead of a sheath, the stent-graft has a corset of PTFE fabric with a lacing of a PTFE thread. The corset opens when the thread is removed. In rare cases, the tip of the corset may fail to open. Under these circumstances, a high pressure balloon has been used to rupture the thread.

A very stiff guidewire, such as the Lunderquist (Cook Medical, Bloomington, IN), helps the delivery system follow an atraumatic path through the aorta to

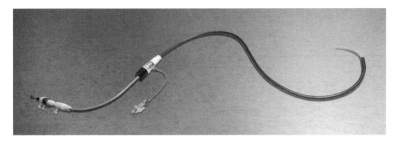

Fig. 1 Photograph of the Superflex delivery system (TX2, Cook Medical, Inc., Bloomington, IN), showing its characteristic flexibility (*See Color Plates*)

its implantation site. When "ultrastiff" is not stiff enough, additional support can be provided by applying traction to the ends of a through and through brachiofemoral wire. In such cases, a catheter or sheath helps cover the brachiocephalic portion of the wire and minimize the risk of arterial injury.

A short, angulated proximal implantation site is the single most common cause of primary technical failure. Unless the end of the stent-graft and the wall of the nondilated segment of aorta share the same longitudinal axis, blood leaks between them into the aneurysm (type I endoleak). The proximal end of the stent-graft has to assume the orientation of the implantation site (neck), while the rest of the stent-graft assumes the orientation of the aneurysm. The greater the angle, the more the stent-graft has to bend. A long neck will usually generate the necessary torque. A short neck, on the other hand, is less able to impose coaxial orientation on the stent-graft. At the very least, the lower lip of the stent-graft tends to lift from the inner curvature of an angulated distal aortic arch. There are two possible remedies: increase the effective length of the neck or uncouple the mechanical linkage between the proximal end of the stent-graft and the body of the stent-graft.

The most direct way to lengthen the neck is to cover the arteries that originate from the distal aortic arch. This used to be standard practice for several reasons: the subclavian artery is richly supplied with collaterals, asymptomatic subclavian artery occlusion is a common incidental finding, and subclavian coverage at the time of endovascular aneursysm repair rarely produces serious complications.[4] However, recent studies have shown subclavian occlusion to be associated with neurological complications, such as stroke and paraplegia.[5,6] The current consensus favors subclavian artery preservation, even in the absence of left vertebral artery dominance or left internal mammary artery (LIMA) coronary bypass.[7] For one thing, the subclavian artery is a source of collateral flow to the spine, and subclavian preservation lowers the risk of paraplegia. When the proximal end of a thoracic aortic aneurysm approaches the level of the subclavian orifice, the alternatives for subclavian preservation include: carotid-subclavian bypass (mandatory in the presence of a LIMA grafts), subclavian-carotid transposition, subclavian stenting, stent-graft fenestration, or stent-graft branching (see *The Aortic Arch* section below).

Mechanical uncoupling of the proximal stent-graft from the rest (flexibility) depends on the potential for a change in the relative lengths of the inner and outer aspects of the bend. The problem is that the stents are designed to change their diameter, not their length. Changes in length occur between stents (Fig. 2). Long stents, small gaps between stents, and wide stents all reduce the flexibility

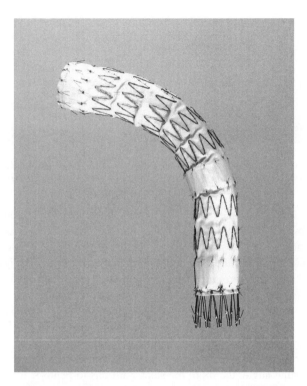

Fig. 2 Photograph of the TX2 stent-graft, showing the barbed proximal and distal stents, and demonstrating narrowing of the gaps between stents on the inner curvature of a bend. (*See Color Plates*)

of the stent-graft. Stent-grafts, such as the TAG, that appear flexible in their compressed state usually become more rigid when they open. In general, the stent-graft with the greatest potential for flexibility is the one with the shortest stents. In the Inoue stent-graft,[8,9] for example, the "stents" consist of nothing more than a series of wire rings. Similar design elements are seen in the most flexible of abdominal aortic stents, but thoracic aortic versions are not yet commercially available. This degree of flexibility comes at a price; the longitudinal dimensions of such a stent-graft cannot be entirely stable. The incorporation of a longitudinal spine helps, but only if the spine lies along the outer curve of the bend, otherwise it will buckle and eventually break.

The addition of an uncovered stent to the proximal end of the stent-graft improves attachment and orientation. The uncovered stents of the Talent[10] (Medtronic, Santa Rosa, CA) or Pythagorus (Lombard Medicals, FL) increase the influence of neck orientation on proximal stent-graft orientation without occluding flow to the great vessels of the arch. The wide loops of current generations of uncovered stents may be relatively atraumatic, but a steady stream of case reports describing stent-induced aortic rupture suggests otherwise.

The length and tortuosity of the thoracic aorta contribute to the incidence of stent-graft migration and component separation. Bends in the stent-graft generate destabilizing forces that increase with the square of graft diameter, while a wide gap between the proximal and distal implantation sites provides room for stent-graft migration. Most of the hemodynamic force on a stent-graft is generated by pressure, not flow, and these forces are just as likely to produce upward migration of the distal end of the stent-graft as distal migration of the proximal end.[11] Hence, the importance of distal stent-graft fixation and adequate intercomponent overlap. Some stent-grafts have barb-mediated fixation between the prosthesis (Fig. 2) and the arteries of the implantation site, but intercomponent connections rely on a combination of friction and stiffness.

Stent-Graft Sizing

The range of stent-graft dimensions varies (Table 1), as does the recommended degree of oversizing. The TAG is particularly intolerant of excessive oversizing, which may cause the stent-graft to fold in on itself, causing endoleak and aortic occlusion. When this happens at the time of deployment, the stent-graft can be forced to assume a circular profile using a large Palmaz stent. When this occurs later, in an unmonitored setting, the results may be fatal. In cases of widely disparate proximal and distal implantation site diameters, a series of overlapping grafts, each larger than the one before, helps avoid excessive oversizing of any individual component.

In general, the longer the inter-component, the better the overlap. The overlap zone provides for continued contact in the event of slippage, friction to resist slippage, and stiffness to resist bending. A multiple component approach also has the advantage of allowing independent control over the positions of the proximal and distal ends, with precise intraoperative adjustment of the overall conduit length through a variation in the length of the overlap.

Multiplanar angulation of the aorta greatly complicates the preoperative measurement of aortic length. Some form of multiplanar reconstruction helps, but the prediction of graft lie is more art than science. The graft may follow the center line, the inner curve, or the outer curve. Again, a multicomponent approach provides some latitude for error by allowing intraoperative adjustment of overlap length.

Table 1 Thoracic aortic stent-grafts.

TAA stent-graft	Diameter range (mm)	Lengths (mm)	Delivery sheath ID	Fixation	Stent material	Graft material
Cook Zenith TX2	22–42	108–216	20 Fr (22–34 mm) 22 Fr (36–42 mm)	Barbs	Stainless steel	Woven polyester
Gore TAG	26–45	100, 150, 200	20 Fr (26 and 28 mm) 22 Fr (31 and 34 mm) 24 Fr (37–46 mm)	Friction	Nitinol	ePTFE
Medtronic Talent	26–44	112–116	22 Fr (26–32 mm) 24 Fr (34–40 mm) 25 Fr (42–46 mm)	Bare stent	Nitinol	Woven polyester
Medtronic Valiant	26–46	112–227	22 Fr (26–32 mm) 24 Fr (34–40 mm) 25 Fr (42–46 mm)	Optional Bare stent	Nitinol	Woven polyester
Endomed	30–42	140, 160, 180, 240	22 Fr (30–36 mm)	Optional	Nitinol	ePTFE
Endofit			24 Fr (38–42 mm)	Bare stent	Nitinol	Woven polyester
Bolton Relay	22–46	103–200	19 Fr (22–32 mm) 20 Fr (34–36 mm) 21 Fr (38–40 mm) 22 Fr (42–44 mm) 23 Fr (46 mm)	Bare stent	Nitinol	Woven polyester

Neurological Complications

Endovascular thoracic aneurysm repair may be complicated by stroke or paraplegia.[5,6,12–14] In most cases of stroke, the presumed etiology is embolism of thrombus or atheroma. Risk factors include prolonged operation, which is probably a surrogate for repeated proximal aortic instrumentation, and atherosclerosis of the ascending aorta and arch, which is more prevalent in older patients. In most cases of paraplegia, the presumed etiology is the occlusion of flow to the anterior spinal artery through segmental branches of the aorta. Risk factors include intraoperative hypotension, extensive aortic coverage (especially below T8), concurrent AAA repair (especially open surgical repair), occlusion of the left subclavian artery, and occlusion of the internal iliac arteries. One should probably take measures to maintain prograde flow through the left subclavian artery in any patient with other risk factors for paraplegia. High-risk patients should also be considered for perioperative spinal drainage and preoperative reductions in antihypertensive medication.[15] The goal is to raise spinal perfusion pressure while short-lived perioperative effects resolve and collateral flow increases. Unfortunately, these interventions rest on several unknowns, such as the pharmacology and physiology of spinal blood flow regulation, and the time course of collateral development. We do know that the segmental arteries are connected by an extensive collateral network. High-resolution computed tomography angiogram shows no change in the number of patent segmental arteries before and after stent-graft implantation.[15]

The Aortic Arch

The branches of the aortic arch are accessible in the root of the neck, and there is no reason why the techniques used for branch preservation (branching, debranching, and fenestration) have to be mutually exclusive. They can be mixed and matched in a wide variety of combinations. Every additional bypass graft is one less branch on the stent-graft and vice versa. The branches of the aortic arch are readily accessible in the posterior triangle of the neck, and surgical bypass between them is a low-morbidity procedure with a good record of durable success.[16–18] In contrast, the construction of a multiply branched or fenestrated stent-graft requires precise placement of a large prosthesis within a wide, curved, mobile segment of the aorta, followed by repeated instrumentation of the brachiocephalic arteries, the aortic arch, and the ascending aorta. Opportunities for failure abound[19] and embolism is an ever present risk. The least risk strategy minimizes the complexity of the endovascular part of the operation by perfusing covered branches through bypass grafts between arteries in the neck, so long asthere is at least one patent source of inflow. If secure hemostatic stent-graft implantation requires innominate artery coverage, the situation changes. Under these circumstances, the only reliable source of inflow is the ascending aorta. A mini-sternotomy for aortic exposure may be a low-morbidity procedure, but the aortic anastomosis is not without risk. The placement of a side-biting clamp on a diseased ascending aorta might liberate a shower of emboli, causing a stroke, or tear the intima, causing type A aortic dissection.

Aortic exposure and clamping can be avoided by maintaining innominate artery flow through a single branch on the stent-graft, and limit the surgical part of the operation to a series of bypass grafts within the neck.[20] There are two distinct approaches for the creation of a single-branch modular stent-graft, depending on the route of insertion,[21] transcervical or transfemoral. Both have to satisfy the same primary requirement for success: any interruption of blood flow through the carotids to the brain has to be very brief. To date, most experience with modular stent-grafts within the aortic arch has been based on Zenith (Cook Medical, Bloomington, IN) designs, but, by the time this chapter is published, a branched TAG device will likely have been used clinically.

Our preference is for transcervical insertion through the right carotid, right subclavian, left subclavian, or innominate arteries.[20] The bifurcated stent-graft has a long thin limb and a short wide limb. The trunk of the stent-graft is implanted in the ascending thoracic aorta, the long thin limb extends to the innominate or left subclavian artery, and the short wide limb lies inside the proximal aortic arch where it serves as the proximal implantation site for an extension to the descending thoracic aorta. This route of insertion has the advantage of ensuring prompt deployment of the cerebral branch at the time of primary stent-graft insertion. Uninterrupted cerebral blood flow is also ensured by the presence of a carotid–carotid bypass. During stent-graft insertion, blood flows between the carotid arteries from left to right, and after stent-graft insertion, blood flows from right to left. The other advantages of this approach stem from the short, straight line of insertion which aids in stent-graft positioning and orientation.

The transfemoral route is longer and more tortuous. The delivery system has to bend, transmit torque, and deploy despite its greater length. More important, it has to have a mechanism for partial stent-graft deployment, so that blood can flow around the stent-graft to the brain in the interval between sheath withdrawal and deployment of the cerebral branches. Indwelling catheters and wires may help provide a secure means of access to the primary stent-graft for cerebral branch insertion, although these mechanisms are made more cumbersome by acute angles between the long axis of the attachment site and the line of stent-graft insertion.

When the aneurysm is confined to the inner curvature of the aorta, the proximal end of the aortic stent-graft can be advanced into a more proximal location while preserving an open route for flow to adjacent arch vessels through stents, or covered stents.[22]

The Thoracoabdominal Aorta

Strictly speaking, the visceral aorta lies within the abdomen, not the thorax. However, many aneurysms of the thorax extend into the abdomen and many aneurysms of the abdomen extend into the chest, so the management of thoracoabdominal aortic aneurysm (TAAA) is not entirely beyond the scope of this chapter.

The visceral arteries are less accessible that the branches of the aortic arch and the visceral bypasses required for surgical debranching of the thoracoabdominal aorta represent a significant source of morbidity in hybrid operations. The results of hybrid repair have generally been disappointing. It appears that patients who are too unhealthy to tolerate conventional TAAA repair are too unhealthy to tolerate visceral bypass.[23–26]

Branched stent-grafts offer an entirely endovascular alternative.[3,15,27,28] Early results suggest that the avoidance of a large abdominal operation contributes to the relatively low complication rates of branched stent-graft insertion. However, the primary morbidity of this approach does not stem from the stress of the insertion procedure, but from the body's response to the presence of a thoracoabdominal stent-graft. TAAA patients appear to be prone to an exaggerated form of generalized inflammatory response. Although leukocytosis, thrombocytopenia, anorexia, and fever are common findings after any form of endovascular aneurysm repair, the response is particularly marked after TAAA repair, probably because the stent-grafts are so much larger.[29,30] These patients are also at risk for spinal cord ischemia, especially during periods of relative hypotension. Although permanent symptoms can be prevented through a combination of spinal drainage and permissive hypertension, patients may remain at-risk of paraplegia for an unknown period after operation.

The technical aspects of branched stent-graft insertion lie beyond the scope of this chapter. Suffice it to say that the combination of a cuffed primary stent-graft and self-expanding covered stents appears to be easier to plan, easier to insert, and more durable than the combination of a fenestrated primary stent-graft and balloon-expanded covered stents. The cuffed technique appears to be safe, effective, durable, and versatile. Relatively few patients are excluded for lack of suitable anatomic substrate, and many centers around the world now have both the skills and the facilities to insert devices of this type. The main barriers to an expanded role for branched stent-grafts in the management of TAAA are regulatory and financial. The main areas for further research relate to the biology of the postimplantation syndrome.

Conclusion

Endovascular repair of TAA has come a long way in the last decade. The endovascular approach to TAA repair is generally believed to have much lower morbidity and mortality rates than the open surgical approach.[10,31,32] Nevertheless, the aneurysmal thoracic aorta can be a challenging endovascular environment, and many cases of TAA remain beyond the reach of current endovascular technology. Areas for advancement are easy enough to identify. The manufacturers' to-do list needs to include greater flexibility, higher expansion ratio, and predictable long-term durability. The endovascular surgeon's wish list might also include a safe, versatile, durable method of branched stent-graft assembly, a way to predict paraplegia risk, and a better understanding of postimplantation biology.

References

1. Mitchell RS, Dake MD, Sembra CP, Fogarty TJ, Zarins CK, Liddel RP, Miller DC. Endovascular stent-graft repair of thoracic aortic aneurysms. J Thorac Cardiovasc Surg 1996;111:1054–62.
2. Criado FJ. Iliac arterial conduits for endovascular access: technical considerations. J Endovasc Ther 2007;14:347–51.
3. Chuter TA, Reilly LM. Endovascular treatment of thoracoabdominal aortic aneurysms. J Cardiovasc Surg 2006;47:619–28.

4. Gorich J, Asquan Y, Seifarth H, et al. Initial experience with interntional stent-graft coverage of the subclavian artery during endovascuclar thoracic aortic repairs. J Endovasc Ther 2002;9 Suppl 2:II39–43.

5. Sullivan TM, Sundt TM, 3rd. Complications of thoracic aortic endografts: spinal cord ischemia and stroke. J Vasc Surg 2006;43 Suppl A:85A–8A.

6. Khoynezhad A, Donayre CE, Bui H, Kopchok GE, Walot I, White RA. Risk factors of neurologic deficit after thoracic aortic endografting. Ann Thorac Surg 2007;83:882–9.

7. Peterson BG, Eskandari MK, Gleason TG, Morasch MD. Utility of left subclavian artery revascularization in association with endoluminal repair of acute and chronic thoracic aortic pathology. J Vasc Surg 2006;43:433–9.

8. Inoue K, Iwase T, Sato M, Yoshida Y, Ueno K, Tamaki S, et al. Transluminal endovascular branched graft placement for a pseudoaneurysm: reconstruction of the descending thoracic aorta including the celiac axis. J Thorac Cardiovasc Surg 1997;114–61.

9. Saito N, Kimura T, Odashiro K, Toma M, Nobuyoshi M, Ueno K, et al. Feasibility of the Inoue single-branched stent-graft implantation for thoracic aortic aneurysm or dissection involving the left subclavian artery: short-to-medium-term results in 17 patients. J Vasc Surg 2005;41:206–12.

10. Fattouri R, Nienaber CA, Rousseau H, et al. Results of endovascular repair of the thoracic aorta with the Talent Thoracic stent-graft: the Talent Thoracic Resrospective Registry. J Thorac Cardiovasc Surg 2006;132:332–9.

11. Howell BA, Kim T, Cheer A, Dwyer H, Saloner D, Chuter TA. Computational fluid dynamics within bifurcated abdominal aortic stent-grafts. J Endovasc Ther 2007;14:138–43.

12. Weigang E, Hartert M, Siegenthaler MP, et al. Perioperative management to improve neurologic outcome in thoracic or thoracoabdominal aortic stent-grafting. Ann Thorac Surg 2006;82:1679.

13. Cheung AT, Pochettino A, McGarvey ML, et al. Strategies to manage paraplegia risk after endovascular stent repair of descending thoracic aortic aneurysms. Ann Thorac Surg 2005;80:1280–1289.

14. Morales JP, Taylor PR, Bell PE, Chan YC, Sabharwal T, Carrell TWG, Reidy JF. Neurological complications following endoluminal repair of thoracic aortic disease. Cardiovasc Intervent Radiol 2007;30:833–9.

15. Chuter TA, Rapp JH, Hiramoto JS, Schneider DB, Howell B, Reilly LM. Endovascular treatment of thoracoabdominal aortic aneurysms. J Vasc Surg 2007 [Epub ahead of print].

16. Criado FJ, Clard NS, Barnatan MF. Stent graft repair in the aortic arch and descending thoracic aorta: a 4-year experience. J Vasc Surg 2002;36:1121–8.

17. Czerny M, Gottard R, Zimpfer D, et al. Mid-term results of supraaortic transpositions for extended endovasccular repair of aortic arch pathologies. Eur J Cardiovasc Surg 2007;31:623–7.

18. Bergeron P, Mangialardi N, Costa P, et al. Great vessel management for endovascular exclusion of aortic arch aneurysms and dissections. Eur J Vasc Endovasc Surg 2006;32:38–45.

19. Chuter TA, Buck DG, Schneider DB, Reilly LM, Messina LM. Development of a branched stent-graft for endovascular repair of aortic arch aneurysms. J Endovasc Ther 2003;10:940–5.

20. Chuter TA, Schneider DB, Reilly LM, Lobo EP, Messina LM. Modular branched stent graft for endovascular repair of aortic arch aneurysm and dissection. J Vasc Surg 2003;38(4):859–63.

21. Verhoeven EL. Endovascular reconstruction of aortic arch by modified bifurcated stent graft for Stanford type A dissection. Asian J Surg 2007;30:296–7.

22. Hiramoto JS, Schneider DB, Reilly LM, Chuter TA. A double-barrel stent-graft for endovascular repair of the aortic arch. J Endovasc Ther 2006;13(1):72–6.

23. Quinones-Baldrich WJ, Panetta TF, Vescera CL, Kashyap VS. Repair of type IV thoracoabdominal aortic aneurysm with a combined endovascular and surgical approach. J Vasc Surg 1999;30:555–60.

24. Resch TA, Greenberg R, Lyden SP, Clair DG, Krajewski L, Kashyap VS, et al. Combined staged procedures for the treatment of thoracoabdominal aneurysms. J Endovasc Ther 2006;13:481–489.

25. Black SA, Wolfe JHN, Clark M, Harmady M, Cheshire NJW, Jenkins MP. Complex thoracoabdominal aortic aneurysms: Endovascular exclusion with visceral revascularization. J Vasc Surg 2006;43:1081–9.

26. Zhou W, Reardon M, Peden EK, Lin PH, Lumsden AB. Hybrid approach to complex thoracic aortic aneurysms in high-risk patients: Surgical challenges and clinical outcomes. J Vasc Surg 2006;13:5–10.

27. Verhoeven EL, Tielliu IF, Muhs BE, et al. Fenestrated and branched stent-grafting: a 5-years experience. Acta Chir Belg 2006;106(3):317–22.

28. Greenberg RK, West K, Pfaff K, Foster J, Skender D, Haulon S, et al. Beyond the aortic bifurcation: Branched endovascular grafts for thoracoabdominal and aortoiliac aneurysms. J Vasc Surg 2006;43:879–86.

29. Galle C, De Maertelaer V, Motte S, et al. Early inflammatory response after elective abdominal aortic aneurysm repair: A comparison between endovascular procedure and conventional surgery. J Vasc Surg 2000;32:234–46.

30. Cross KS, Bouchier-Hayes D, Leahy AL. Consumptive coagulopathy following endovascular stent repair of abdominal aortic aneurysm. Eur J Vasc Endovasc Surg 2000;19:94–95.

31. Stone DH, Brewster DC, Kwolek CJ, et al . Stent-graft versus open-surgical repair of the thoracic aorta: mid-term results. J Vasc Surg 2006;44:1188–97.

32. Bavaria JE, Appoo JJ, Makaroun MS, et al. Gore TAG Investigators. Endovascular stent grafting versus open surgical repair of descending thoracic aortic aneurysms in low-risk patients: a multicenter comparative trial. J Thorac Cardiovasc Surg 2007;133:369–77.

Chapter 26

Evaluation and Treatment of Isolated Common Iliac Artery Aneurysms

Guillermo A. Escobar and Enrique Criado

Abstract Iliac artery aneurysms are found unilateral or bilaterally with equal frequency and are more common in older males; the majority of these cases are associated to abdominal aortic aneurysms (AAAs). The pathogenesis of iliac artery aneurysms is similar to that of AAA, and most are diagnosed incidentally in asymptomatic patients. The natural history of iliac artery aneurysms is to progressively enlarge and rupture. Untreated, small (<3 cm) isolated iliac artery aneurysms are estimated to grow at a rate of about 0.5–1.1 mm/year, but may expand at a faster pace (over 2.6 mm/year) when larger than 3 cm. The risk of rupture of iliac artery aneurysm can approach 75% when they reach 5 cm in diameter. Open repair offers the greatest assurance of a lasting repair and is ideal in patients that are at low risk and/or young, although the short-term morbidity may be greater. Patients who are at high risk for open repair, technically difficult to access (obese or reoperations), and/or relatively older are best served with an endoluminal approach.

Keywords Isolated iliac artery aneurysms, Pathogenesis of IAA, IAA expansion/progression, Diagnostic evaluation of IAA, IAA repair, Endoluminal IAA

Epidemiology

The majority of iliac artery aneurysms are associated to abdominal aortic aneurysms (AAAs), whereas isolated iliac artery aneurysms are unusual. Common and external iliac arteries greater than 1.8 cm in diameter and hypogastric arteries greater that 0.8 cm are considered iliac aneurysms.[1] The exact incidence of isolated iliac artery aneurysms is not known, but approximately 10% of AAAs will have a coexisting iliac artery aneurysm most often involving the common iliac artery.[2–4] In 1921, Luke found only one iliac artery aneurysm in an autopsy series of over 12,000 bodies. In a larger and more recent autopsy series by Brunkwell, iliac artery aneurysms were twice as common. Therefore, the incidence of these aneurysms is thought to be between 1 in 6,000 to 1 in 12,000 of the autopsy population.[5,6]

G. Upchurch and E. Criado (eds.) *Aortic Aneurysms, Contemporary Cardiology*
DOI: 10.1007/978-1-60327-204-9_26, © Humana Press, a part of
Springer Science+Business Media, LLC 2009

Iliac artery aneurysms are found unilateral or bilateral with equal freuency and are more common in older males. The pathogenesis of iliac artery aneurysms is similar to that of AAA, and most are diagnosed incidentally in asymptomatic patients.[2,7] Iliac artery aneurysm are thought to be mostly degenerative, but they may also be secondary to trauma, infection, inflammatory, or autoimmune diseases, like in Kawasaki syndrome, Takayasu's arteritis, Hughes-Stovin syndrome, or Behçet's disease. Poststenotic iliac artery dilatations secondary to occlusive disease may also acquire aneurysmal dimensions. Genetic disorders affecting vessel wall, particularly Ehlers-Danlos syndrome type IV and Marfan syndrome, can have isolated iliac artery aneurysms.[1,2,8,9] Anastomotic pseudoaneurysms of the iliac arteries are not uncommon and appear at the site of the anastomosis with prosthetic grafts after aortoiliac reconstruction.

Natural History and Risk of Rupture

The natural history of iliac artery aneurysms is to progressively enlarge and rupture. Untreated, small (<3 cm) isolated iliac artery aneurysms are estimated to grow at a rate of about 0.5–1.1 mm/year, but may expand at a faster pace (over 2.6 mm/year) when larger than 3 cm.[10] The risk of rupture of iliac artery aneurysm can approach 75% when they reach 5 cm in diameter.[10,11] Elective repair generally offers a good operative outcome with a low morbidity and mortality. On the other hand, ruptured iliac artery aneurysms carry a high mortality rate similar to that of ruptured AAA (~40%).[2,7,11] Atherosclerotic internal iliac artery aneurysms are though to present with rupture 40% of the time and have an overall mortality of 31%.[7,12] The highest risk of iliac aneurysm rupture is in patients with connective tissue diseases such as Ehlers-Danlos syndrome type IV (Sack-Barabas syndrome). In addition, operative or endovascular repair of these aneurysm can be very challenging due to their fragility and often require multiple interventions during their hospitalization.[13,14]

Diagnostic Evaluation

At the time of diagnosis, almost half of iliac artery aneurysms are asymptomatic. Internal iliac artery aneurysms, on the other hand, tend to be larger at the time of diagnosis and are therefore more often associated with clinical manifestations such as pelvic pain, ureteral obstruction with ipsilateral hydronephrosis, rectal discomfort, arterioenteric fistulae with hematochezia, and aneurysm rupture. Common and external iliac artery aneurysms are mostly asymptomatic but may present with pain, claudication, palpable pulsatile masses, distal embolization, fistulization into the iliac veins, and spontaneous rupture. Iliac artery aneurysms occasionally present with lower limb swelling or deep vein thrombosis secondary to direct compression of the iliac and pelvic veins.[2,8,12,15] However, physical examination of patients with iliac aneurysms may reveal a pulsatile mass or bruit in the lower abdomen or abnormal pulsation during a rectal examination.

Ultrasonography, computed tomography angiography (CTA), digital subtraction angiography, and MRI are all utilized in the diagnosis of iliac aneurysms.

Ultrasound is the screening test of choice, but is often hampered by the presence of bowel gas and/or severe obesity which may make imaging of the pelvic vessels difficult, if not impossible. Nevertheless, when ultrasound is technically feasible, it has been found to be rather accurate in sizing iliac aneurysms compared to CTA.[10] Computerized tomography with contrast enhancement is perhaps the optimal imaging modality for evaluating iliac aneurysms, and certainly the test of choice in preparation for surgical or endovascular repair (Fig. 1). There is an exponential growth in the technology of this imaging modality. Angiography is in general inadequate to size iliac aneurysms because of the presence of mural thrombus, but may be helpful in some cases to delineate the arterial anatomy in patients with very tortuous vessels.

Repair of Iliac Artery Aneurysms

Iliac artery aneurysms noted at the time of repair of an AAA should be repaired simultaneously if they are >2.5 cm in diameter to prevent aneurysmal growth if left untreated.[10,16,17] Isolated iliac artery aneurysms without an associated aortic aneurysm should be repaired when they reach 3–3.5 cm in diameter or if they become symptomatic.[10] Symptoms are an important indication as most iliac aneurysms that rupture are preceded by pain.[10,11]

The first recorded surgical treatment of an iliac artery aneurysm was in 1827 by Valentine Mott. It consisted in the successful blind ligation of the common iliac artery in an awake patient.[18] While much experience has been accumulated with the open surgical repair of iliac aneurysms, there is a paucity of long-term data on endoluminal approaches. For this reason, open repair offers

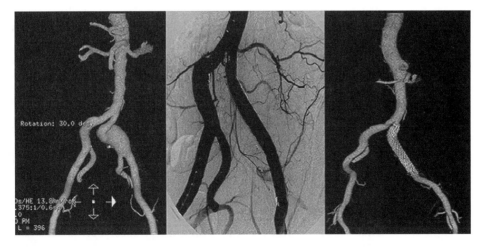

Fig. 1 Computed tomography angiography (*CTA*) of the aortoiliac segment (*left*). Digital subtraction angiography during deployment of an iliac endograft with exclusion of the left hypogastric artery after placement of a vascular occlusion plug in the proximal left hypogastric artery (*center*). Postoperative *CTA* demonstration exclusion of the aneurysm without endoleak and patency of the iliac segment (*right*)

the greatest assurance of a lasting repair and is ideal in patients who are at low risk and/or young although the short-term morbidity may be greater.

Patients who are at high risk for open repair, technically difficult to access (obese or reoperations), and/or relatively older are best served with an endoluminal approach. Technical considerations that may exclude patients from endoluminal therapy include lack of adequate vascular access and absence of landing zones in the arterial segments proximal or distal to the aneurysm. In addition, extreme tortuosity or angulation of the iliac anatomy may also preclude endoluminal intervention.

Finally, special consideration must be taken for patients with Ehlers-Danlos syndrome type IV (Sack-Barabas syndrome) who may require both open and endoluminal approaches due to the high risk of rupture and reintervention.[13,14]

Surgical Repair

The midline transperitoneal approach is best suited for the surgical repair of bilateral iliac aneurysms. Bilateral common iliac arteries are best treated with a bifurcated graft from the distal infrarenal aorta to the distal, nonaneurysmal vessel. Care must be taken to identify and spare the ureters and iliac veins, especially in cases of inflammatory aneurysms or reexplorations. Preoperative placement of ureteral stents may be helpful in identifying and preventing ureteral injury.

Unilateral aneurysms are ideally repaired via an ipsilateral extraperitoneal approach and are replaced with a prosthetic graft. The aneurysm can usually be replaced with an end-to-end anastomosis from the proximal normal iliac to the external iliac or common femoral arteries. If the aneurysm includes the origin of the hypogastric artery, then the latter is ligated as proximally as possible as long as the contralateral one is widely patent. Unilateral ligation of the hypogastric artery often results in ipsilateral gluteal claudication or less commonly in ischemic colitis, impotence, or gluteal muscle necrosis (also a concern during endoluminal exclusion or embolization of this vessel). In younger, physically, and sexually active patients, revascularization of the hypogastric artery is advisable (if technically feasible) to prevent the above-mentioned complications.

Endoluminal Repair

Experience with endoluminal treatment of iliac artery aneurysms is rapidly expanding and may eventually become the standard of care. Until then, patients without anatomical contraindication and significant operative risk are ideal candidates because it offers a less invasive approach, lower periprocedural morbidity, and faster recovery.[19] Complications cited for endograft exclusion of iliac artery aneurysms include endograft thrombosis, migration of the graft, and continued aneurysm expansion; all of which may require subsequent operative repair.[20–22] Significant advances in the technology of endoluminal devices, industry standardization of the grafts, adaptation of bifurcated aortic grafts for small necks (<1.5 cm), greater experience with the devices, and improved selection criteria have made endoluminal therapy more appealing in the management of iliac artery aneurysms.

References

1. Johnston KW, Rutherford RB, Tilson MD, Shah DM, Hollier L, Stanley JC. Suggested standards for reporting on arterial aneurysms. Subcommittee on Reporting Standards for Arterial Aneurysms, Ad Hoc Committee on Reporting Standards, Society for Vascular Surgery and North American Chapter, International Society for Cardiovascular Surgery. *J Vasc Surg*. Mar 1991;13(3):452–458.

2. Krupski WC, Selzman CH, Floridia R, Strecker PK, Nehler MR, Whitehill TA. Contemporary management of isolated iliac aneurysms. *J Vasc Surg*. Jul 1998;28(1):1–11; discussion 11–13.

3. Gliedman ML, Ayers WB, Vestal BL. Aneurysms of the abdominal aorta and its branches: a study of untreated patients. *Ann Surg*. Aug 1957;146(2):207–214.

4. Spittell PC, Ehrsam JE, Anderson L, Seward JB. Screening for abdominal aortic aneurysm during transthoracic echocardiography in a hypertensive patient population. *J Am Soc Echocardiogr*. Sep 1997;10(7):722–727.

5. Luke B, Rea K. Studies of aneurysm. *J Am Med Assoc*. 1921;72:935–936.

6. Brunkwall J, Hauksson H, Bengtsson H, Bergqvist D, Takolander R, Bergentz SE. Solitary aneurysms of the iliac arterial system: an estimate of their frequency of occurrence. *J Vasc Surg*. Oct 1989;10(4):381–384.

7. Richardson JW, Greenfield LJ. Natural history and management of iliac aneurysms. *J Vasc Surg*. Aug 1988;8(2):165–171.

8. Markowitz AM, Norman JC. Aneurysms of the iliac artery. *Ann Surg*. Nov 1961;154:777–787.

9. Kalko Y, Basaran M, Aydin U, Kafa U, Basaranoglu G, Yasar T. The surgical treatment of arterial aneurysms in Behcet disease: a report of 16 patients. *J Vasc Surg*. Oct 2005;42(4):673–677.

10. Santilli SM, Wernsing SE, Lee ES. Expansion rates and outcomes for iliac artery aneurysms. *J Vasc Surg*. Jan 2000;31(1 Pt 1):114–121.

11. Lowry SF, Kraft RO. Isolated aneurysms of the iliac artery. *Arch Surg*. Nov 1978;113(11):1289–1293.

12. Dix FP, Titi M, Al-Khaffaf H. The isolated internal iliac artery aneurysm – a review. *Eur J Vasc Endovasc Surg*. Aug 2005;30(2):119–129.

13. Pepin M, Schwarze U, Superti-Furga A, Byers PH. Clinical and genetic features of Ehlers-Danlos syndrome type IV, the vascular type. *N Engl J Med*. Mar 2000;342(10):673–680.

14. Oderich GS, Panneton JM, Bower TC, et al The spectrum, management and clinical outcome of Ehlers-Danlos syndrome type IV: a 30-year experience. *J Vasc Surg*. Jul 2005;42(1):98–106.

15. Bollinger A . The death of Thomas Mann: consequence of erroneous angiologic diagnosis? *Wien Med Wochenschr*. 1999;149(2–4):30–32.

16. Sala F, Hassen-Khodja R, Branchereau P, et al. Outcome of common iliac arteries after aortoaortic graft placement during elective repair of infrarenal abdominal aortic aneurysms. *J Vasc Surg*. Nov 2002;36(5):982–987.

17. Hassen-Khodja R, Feugier P, Favre JP, Nevelsteen A, Ferreira J. Outcome of common iliac arteries after straight aortic tube-graft placement during elective repair of infrarenal abdominal aortic aneurysms. *J Vasc Surg*. Nov 2006;44(5):943–948.

18. Mott V. Successful ligature of the common iliac artery. *Am J Med Sci*. 1827;1:156.

19. Criado E, Marston WA, Ligush J, Mauro MA, Keagy BA. Endovascular repair of peripheral aneurysms, pseudoaneurysms, and arteriovenous fistulas. *Ann Vasc Surg*. May 1997;11(3):256–263.

20. Sahgal A, Veith FJ, Lipsitz E, et al. Diameter changes in isolated iliac artery aneurysms 1 to 6 years after endovascular graft repair. *J Vasc Surg*. Feb 2001;33(2):289–284; discussion 294–285.

21. Boules TN, Selzer F, Stanziale SF, et al. Endovascular management of isolated iliac artery aneurysms. *J Vasc Surg*. Jul 2006;44(1):29–37.

22. Henry M, Amor M, Henry I, et al. Percutaneous endovascular treatment of peripheral aneurysms. *J Cardiovasc Surg (Torino)*. Dec 2000;41(6):871–883.

Chapter 27

Diagnosis, Evaluation, and Management of Isolated Hypogastric Artery Aneurysms

Gautam Agarwal and Enrique Criado

Abstract Isolated hypogastric artery aneurysms are extremely rare. A series of 12,000 autopsies reported in 1921 noted only 1 hypogastric aneurysm among 320 aneurysms identified. McLaren reported the first successful ligation of a hypogastric aneurysm in 1913. Since then, fewer than 100 cases of isolated hypogastric aneurysm have been reported in the English literature. Hypogastric aneurysms are often large and associated with significant morbidity and mortality secondary to compression of adjacent structures or rupture into the pelvis. They are technically challenging to repair due to their location deep in the pelvis and difficulty in gaining distal control of the hypogastric artery and its branches.

Keywords Hypogastric artery aneurysms, Diagnosis of Hypogastric artery aneurysms

Diagnosis

Most hypogastric aneurysms are asymptomatic due to their deep pelvic location. The majority of them are detected incidentally on imaging studies. They can also present as a pelvic mass. Compression of adjacent structures can cause neurological symptoms (radicular pain, weakness, numbness), urologic symptoms (pain, urgency, frequency, hematuria, ureteral obstruction), gastrointestinal symptoms (abdominal pain, tenesmus), or venous obstruction. Patients may present with rupture into the rectum, sigmoid, ureter, bladder, or most commonly, into the peritoneal cavity or retroperitoneum.[1–7]

Despite their deep location, it has been reported that up to 70% of iliac aneurysms are palpable on rectal, vaginal, or abdominal examination.[7] Ultrasonography, computed tomography, and magnetic resonance imaging have been all used for detecting internal iliac aneurysms. Computed tomography scan is the most favored diagnostic modality. Angiography is helpful in planning elective operations and revascularization when needed.

G. Upchurch and E. Criado (eds.) *Aortic Aneurysms, Contemporary Cardiology*
DOI: 10.1007/978-1-60327-204-9_27, © Humana Press, a part of
Springer Science+Business Media, LLC 2009

Management

The natural history of isolated hypogastric artery aneurysms is not well known. Rate of growth has been estimated at 4 mm/year, similar to abdominal abdominal aortic aneurysms.[8] The rate of rupture for hypogastric aneurysms was 67% in a series of 14 patients reported in 1982 with an overall mortality of 71%.[9] Other authors have reported rupture rates of 38% at initial presentation.[10] One series of 50 patients with 71 isolated iliac aneurysms observed no ruptures in aneurysms smaller than 3.0 cm in diameter, and serial ultrasound every 6 months was recommended if the decision was made to observe the aneurysm.[8,10,11]

Various forms of treatment for hypogastric aneurysms have been described in the literature. These include simple proximal ligation of the hypogastric artery, complete resection with interposition grafting, proximal ligation with obliterative endoaneurysmorrhaphy, and endovascular repair.

Complete surgical excision of hypogastric aneurysm is unnecessary and rarely performed as it fraught with danger of deep pelvic vascular injury and uncontrollable pelvic hemorrhage. Simple proximal ligation may not be curative since patent distal branches continue to pressurize the aneurysm, and various reports have described continued expansion of the aneurysm following proximal ligation.[12]

Proximal ligation with obliterative endoaneurysmorrhaphy has also been described and several authors have recommended it as a repair of choice in low-risk patients.[13]

The least invasive method is a percutaneous transarterial approach with embolization of the distal branches and the aneurysmal sac, followed by coverage of the origin of the hypogastric artery by a stent graft from the common to the external iliac, or placement of a plug in the proximal hypogastric artery if the anatomy allows. Complications to this approach include distal embolization to the lower limb.[14] In addition, endoluminal therapy does not remove the mass effect of giant hypogastric aneurysms. Incomplete thrombosis may also result in continued expansion and eventual rupture. In a recent report of isolated iliac aneurysms (including ten hypogastric aneurysms), surgical repair showed better intraoperative and early postoperative outcomes as well as more durable midterm results compared with endoluminal repair.[15]

References

1. Brunkwall J, Hauksson H, Bengtsson H, Bergvist D, Takolander R,Bergentz S-E. Solitary aneurysms of the iliac system: An estimate of their frequency of occurrence. J Vasc Surg 1989; 10:381–384.
2. Frank IN, Thompson HT, Robb C, Schwartz SI. Aneurysm of the internal iliac artery. Arch Surg 1961; 83:178–180.
3. Wirthlin L, Warshaw AL. Ruptured aneurysms of the hypogastric artery. Surgery 1973; 73:629–633.
4. Markowitz AM, Norman JC. Aneurysms of the iliac artery. Ann Surg 1961; 154:777–87.
5. Rennick JM, Link DP, Palmer JM. Spontaneous rupture of an iliac artery aneurysm into a ureter: A case report and review of the literature. J Urol 1976; 116(1): 111–113.
6. Kirldand K, Start KW. Aneurysm of the right internal iliac artery: Five years' cure. Med J Aust 1953; 2:299–300.

7. Richardson JW, Greenfield LJ. Natural history and management of iliac aneurysms. J Vasc Surg 1988; 8:165–171.

8. McCready RA, Pairolero PC, Gilmore JC et-al. Isolated iliac artery aneurysms. Surgery 1983; 5:688–693.

9. Brin BJ, Busuttil RW . Isolated hypogastric artery aneurysms.Arch Surg 1982; 117:1329–1333.

10. Parry DJ, Kessel D, Scott DJ. Simplifying the internal iliac artery aneurysm.Ann R Coll Surg Engl 2001; 83:302–308.

11. Krupski WC, Selzman CH, Floridia R, Strecker PK, Nehler MR, Whitehill TA. Contemporary management of isolated iliac aneurysms. J Vasc Surg 1998; 28:1–13.

12. Nachbur BH, Inderbitzi RGC, Bar W. Isolated iliac aneurysms. Eur J Vasc Surg 1991; 5:375–381.

13. Zimmer PW, Raker EJ, Quigley TM. Isolated hypogastric artery aneurysms. Ann Vasc Surg. 1999; 13:545–549.

14. Hollis HW, Luethke JM, Yakes WF, et al. Percutaneous embolization of an internal iliac artery aneurysm: technical considerations and literature review. J Vasc Interv Radiol 1994; 5:449–451.

15. Pitoulias GA, Donas KP et al. Isolated iliac artery aneurysms: endovascular versus open elective repair.J Vasc Surg. 2007; 46:648–654.

Chapter 28

True Femoral and Popliteal Artery Aneurysms: Clinical Features and Treatment

K. Barry Deatrick and Peter K. Henke

Abstract Arterial aneurysms (AAs) of the periphery are uncommon, are likely under diagnosed, and primarily confer a risk for limb loss. This is in contrast to abdominal and thoracic AA that confers a significant risk to life, depending on size and growth rates. Peripheral aneurysms occurs often in patients with more proximal arterial tree AA, and thus evaluation of synchronous disease in these patients is important. A peripheral AA is traditionally defined as an increased size 150% of the proximal normal artery; for most patients, this is a dilation greater than 1.5 cm for the popliteal artery and ~2.5 for a common femoral artery. This chapter will focus on the modern evaluation and treatment of true peripheral AA, and will not discuss pseudoaneurysms.

Keywords Femoral/popliteal artery aneurysms, Peripheral AA, Risk factors for peripheral AA, Peripheral AA pathogenesis, Peripheral AA diagnosis, Open surgical treatment of PAA

True Peripheral Artery Aneurysms

Popliteal artery aneurysms (PAAs) are relatively rare, occurring in an estimated 0.1–1% of the population.[1] Nevertheless, they represent the most common form of peripheral AA, accounting for 70–80% of peripheral aneurysms.[2] True common femoral artery aneurysms (CFAAs) remain relatively uncommon as compared with PAA. Overall, few large series have been published in the last decade, in part because the evaluation and treatment is straightforward, safe, and durable. Further, the location is not as amendable for endovascular therapies. The benefit from an endovascular repair of an isolated CFAA is unlikely to be achieved, given the branching of the profunda and the fact that these can be repaired under local anesthesia (if need be) with excellent long-term results. The increased number of abdominal aortic aneurysms (AAAs) repaired via an endovascular approach, which mandates femoral artery exposure in many cases, allows the CFAA to be easily repaired in the same setting.

G. Upchurch and E. Criado (eds.) *Aortic Aneurysms, Contemporary Cardiology*
DOI: 10.1007/978-1-60327-204-9_28, © Humana Press, a part of
Springer Science+Business Media, LLC 2009

Demographics

Peripheral AAs predominantly occur in men, which make up nearly 96% of this population. Other risk factors for these aneurysms include: hypertension, smoking, the presence of coronary artery disease, hyperlipidemia, and chronic obstructive pulmonary disease. Other factors which are known to be associated with peripheral AA include abdominal aortic and iliac aneurysms.

More than 60% of PAA patients have concomitant AAAs, and almost 40% have femoral aneurysms.[3] Nearly 65% of patients with PAA disease have bilateral involvement.[4–6] Patients with CFAA have the highest concordance with proximal AA, up to 85% incidence, and associated PAAs are found in 40–50%.[7] Conversely, those with AAA have up to 14% peripheral AA incidence.[8]

Pathogenesis

Peripheral AAs have historically been linked to degenerative changes that accumulate as the result of atherosclerosis. Atherosclerotic changes are present in histological analysis of human peripheral AA tissue, similar to that observed with aortic atherosclerosis and AAA. Further studies, however, have suggested a more specific association with inflammatory changes in the vessel wall, primarily defined from PAA specimens.

Disruption of elastic lamellae and active proteolysis have been shown in excised aneurysmal tissue.[4] Additionally, the expression of molecules linked to apoptosis is increased. Bax, CPP-32, and Fas are significantly elevated in PAA specimens, particularly within vascular smooth muscle cells.[4] Another study found increased expression of CPP-32 in T cells located within the PAA wall itself.[5] The suggested mechanism is that T-cell-induced apoptosis leads to a degradation of the arterial wall matrix. It is unclear, however, whether the apoptotic pathway has a causative role in AA formation, or whether it is merely associated with the degenerative changes that occur.

Anatomical factors may also play a role. The popliteal artery arises from the superficial femoral artery as it passes through the adductor (Hunter's) canal, and continues into the popliteal fossa. Unique structural stresses on the popliteal artery that may contribute to PAA formation include turbulent blood flow associated with branching points and wall fatigue secondary to repeated knee flexion. This may also be a factor in the groin with flexion of the CFA and the branching of profunda feveris artery (PFA) and superficial fermoral artery (SFA).

Diagnosis

Diagnosis of a peripheral AA is fairly straightforward, even in the case of an asymptomatic lesion, but due to obesity or other patient features, may be missed on physical examination.[8] A prominent femoral or popliteal pulse or pulsatile mass in the inguinal or popliteal fossa in a patient should arouse suspicion, particularly if the patient is male, older than 50 years of age, has used tobacco, and/or has risk factors for coronary artery disease. Although the CFA is usually not difficult to palpate, it is a different situation with the popliteal artery. Because the popliteal pulse is rarely easily palpable, some practitioners recommend screening for all persons with an easily detectable popliteal pulse. If the aneurysm is thrombosed, a nonpulsatile mass may be present, which should also prompt further diagnostic evaluation.[9,10] In either scenario, the examination is performed with the knee in a relaxed, flexed position, and the aneurysm itself is defined in relation to the knee joint.

The differential diagnosis hinges mainly on whether the lesion detected on physical examination is pulsatile. Hypertrophic or malignant lymph nodes, incarcerated hernias (including femoral hernias), Baker's cysts, deep venous thrombosis, hematoma, lipoma, and sarcoma are all possible differential diagnoses for a mass in the inguinal or popliteal fossa, but are rarely pulsatile. Once the distinction is made, the lesion in question may be further evaluated with duplex ultrasound (DU). For screening, contrast-enhanced computed tomography (CT) and magnetic resonance imaging is rarely indicated. Because of the invasive nature of the procedure, angiography is not an appropriate initial diagnostic test, and the presence of intraluminal thrombus makes it inaccurate for assessing the presence or size of an aneurysm.

Diagnostic DU has several advantages as an initial mode of evaluation. First, it is relatively inexpensive and available in the clinic. Second, DU is accurate in determining the size of the aneurysm and for assessment of intraluminal thrombus.[1,5] Third, addition of DU measurements can be used postoperatively to detect flow within the aneurysm sac following exclusion.[11,12] It can also be applied as a screening technique for AAA and other peripheral aneurysms. Finally, DU can be used to map the availability of saphenous vein for arterial bypass, as well as to image the proximal and distal arterial tree, sometimes obviating the need for invasive arteriography (Fig. 1).

Although not appropriate for screening, angiography has an important role in selected preoperative evaluation of PAA, but perhaps less so in CFAA patients. Angiography allows evaluation of arterial inflow, popliteal artery patency, and distal runoff (Fig. 2). Although inflow disease does not appear to affect symptoms from the aneurysm, the presence of a proximal stenosis does alter the operative approach, and can increase the complexity of a repair. Knowledge of the lower extremity arterial runoff is important, as the bypass requires a distal

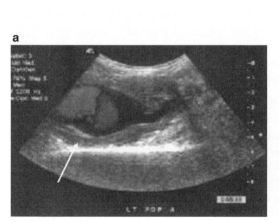
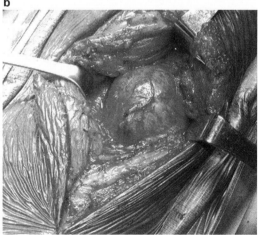

Fig. 1 (**a**) Gray scale ultrasound image of a large left popliteal aneurysm (*white arrow*). (**b**) A large popliteal aneurysm after surgical exposure. Note this is a posterior approach, and proximal and distal arteries appear of reasonable size (*See Color Plates*)

a   b   c

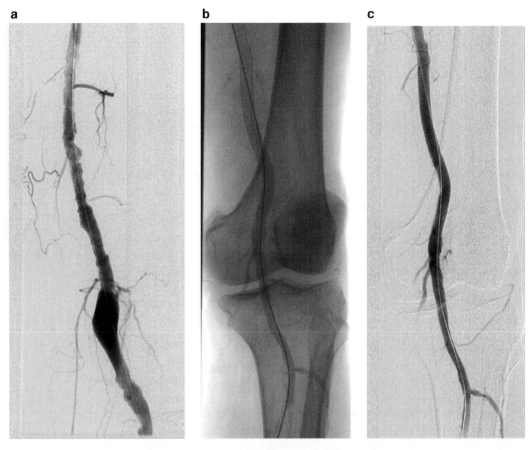

Fig. 2 (**a**) Preoperative angiogram showing a focal proximal popliteal aneurysm with intact distal arterial runoff. (**b**) Intraoperative angiogram showing placement of an ePTFE covered stent graft to exclude the aneurysm. (**c**) Postplacement balloon angioplasty of the graft. Note small collaterals that still fill the sac on this DSA image

target which may be at the level of a tibial artery. Alternatively, CT angiography is sufficiently reliable to base operative decisions in many cases, depending on the surgeon's comfort level and is particularly useful for planning CFAA repair (Fig. 3).

Presentation and Indications for Repair

Between 30% and 50% of patients with peripheral AA are asymptomatic, whereas 50% will present initially with some form of limb ischemia, embolic process, or local pain.[4,6,13,14] Arterial ischemic symptoms include claudication, rest pain, and tissue loss, and these are reported in 20–40% of patients, more commonly associated with PAAs.[6,9] Apart from complete vascular occlusion, peripheral AA may present with a "blue toe syndrome" resulting from repeated embolization of thrombotic debris to the distal extremity, and may occur in up to 12% of patients presenting with PAA.[10,15,16] Local compression from a sizable AA may result in a femoral or tibial nerve neuropathy, or venous obstruction resulting in edema, pain, and potentially deep venous thrombosis.

The complication rate for PAA ranges between 18% and 77%, depending on the definition used and the series reported. Amputation rates in some series are as high as 20%, but more recent studies have demonstrated improved limb salvage rates.[10–13] Even if the aneurysm is asymptomatic at the time of presentation, most patients will require intervention for a complication (such as acute ischemia or embolization) within several years after diagnosis. These patients will frequently require operative intervention to preserve the affected limb.[13,15,17]

Acute limb ischemia (ALI) is the most common limb-threatening presentation of a peripheral AA, and is distinctly more common with PAA, as compared with CFAA. Between 18% and 30% of PAA will present with some form of an ischemic limb.[3,13,14,17] Patients presenting with an ischemic limb in the setting of a PAA usually present with grade IIB ischemia (cool, painful, pulseless limb)[13] as the result of acute thrombosis of the popliteal artery, or a combination of acute thrombosis in the setting of outflow occlusion as the result of chronic embolization.[4–6,18] Less frequently, patients may present with a ruptured PAA. In either circumstance, immediate intervention is required for limb salvage.

In spite of the known risks of repeated thrombosis and embolization, consensus on repair of asymptomatic or incidentally discovered PAA is lacking, at least in part because the natural history of these aneurysms is poorly defined. It is therefore difficult to predict which PAA will become symptomatic, and thus no absolute standard for when to intervene in the case of the small aneurysm.[12,14,15,18] A diameter greater than 2 cm, presence of intraluminal thrombus, and poor distal runoff (absence of distal pulses or one vessel visualized on angiography) are all suggestive of complications.[15] Similarly, factors which may complicate repair of PAA include symptoms of ischemia, extension of the aneurysm into the tibial arteries, deterioration of distal runoff, lack of adequate vein for bypass, and associated coronary artery disease.[16] It is clear, however, that patients who undergo elective repair of an asymptomatic AA have better rates of limb salvage than those who undergo emergency revascularization for acute ischemia.[1,17–21] For this reason, there are many proponents of repair of PAA, even if less than 2 cm in diameter. Ascher et al. suggested that even small aneurysms tend to be lined with thrombus, and that there can be an ongoing embolization to distal arteries. This study found that 64% of small PAA were partially thrombosed, similar to a 70% thrombosis rate in larger PAA.[9] Further, they were not able to identify any connection between thrombosis and aneurysm size. This corresponds with other studies that have found significant rates of thrombosis in small PAA.[3,14] There is not yet a prospective investigation evaluating aneurysm diameter with symptoms and complications.

Although PAA are clearly associated with other aneurysms, it is not known whether the presence of other aneurysms affects long-term outcome for PAA repair. In one study, when PAA patients had a high rate of either bilateral PAA or extrapopliteal aneurysms, 10-year survival was worse in patients with multiple aneurysms (16% vs. 66%) compared with those who had isolated disease.[5] Mortality in this study, however, was the result of coronary artery disease rather than aneurysmal disease, suggesting a relationship between overall atherosclerotic burden and predisposition to aneurysm formation.

CFAAs are classified as either Type I or Type II. Type I is the most common and isolated to the common femoral artery whereas Type II involves the

PFA as well as the common femoral artery. A definitive size criteria for repair has not been defined, but generally those over 2.5–3 cm who are otherwise a good operative candidate should be repaired.[7,22] Again, CFAA are less often associated with ALI, but whether this is due to a more benign process or less reporting is not clear.

Treatment: Popliteal Artery Aneurysms

Endovascular Treatment

The advent of catheter-based interventions has spurred an increase in the number of centers and surgeons applying endovascular techniques to the management of PAA. This is especially popular in the management of patients, who based on comorbid conditions or lack of conduit would not otherwise be considered ideal operative candidates. Much of the enthusiasm for this technique is based on the success of AAA exclusion with endovascular graft placement. Although trials testing these techniques are still accumulating, evidence for the efficacy of these devices remains in flux as the devices continue to evolve (Table 1). The first such devices used were handmade devices, metallic stents covered with vein, or synthetic graft material.[17,23,24] There are now commercially available covered stent grafts, which both simplify placement and should standardize technique and outcomes (Fig. 2).

The most commonly used stent graft is made of a polytetrafluoroethylene-lined nitinol stent with thermal memory (Viabahn, Gore, Tempe, AZ).[18,25–27] Several variations of this exist. The location of the popliteal artery stent grafts requires several considerations not relevant to AAA, including flexibility and graft compliance, given the proximity to the knee joint. The mobility of the joint increases the risk of graft migration and graft kinking. Other potential complications include graft separation following deployment, and endoleaks from incompletely excluded vessels. Neointimal hyperplasia may result in narrowing of the lumen at the proximal and distal endpoints.

In general, the endovascular approach has been shown to be both safe and effective, and a prospective randomized study demonstrated similar patency rates with open repair. The largest series of endovascular repairs thus reported was that of Tielliu et al., with a series of 57 PAA treated with endovascular repair including 5 treated for acute ischemia.[25] A retrospective review of midterm outcomes from Curi et al. demonstrated no significant difference in primary patency, secondary patency, or survival between patients treated with

Table 1 Selected series of popliteal artery aneurysms treated by endovascular repair.

Authors	Year	Number of PAAs	Acute symptoms	Assisted patency (%)	Number with stent thrombosis	Limb salvage (%)	Mean follow-up (months)
Henry et al.[23]	2000	12	NA	58	5	NA	21
Howell et al.[35]	2002	13	NA	69	4	NA	12
Tielliu et al.[36]	2003	23	2	74	5	100	15
Gerasimidis et al.[18]	2003	9	3	75	4	NA	14
Antonello et al.[26]	2005	15	0	100	1	NA	46
Teilliu et al.[25]	2005	57	5	87	12	NA	24
Mohan et al.[24]	2006	35	NA	83	NA	100	36
Rajasinghe et al.[37]	2007	23	NA	100	1	NA	7
Curi et al.[27]	2007	15	0	100	6	NA	14

NA not available, *PAAs* popliteal artery aneurysms

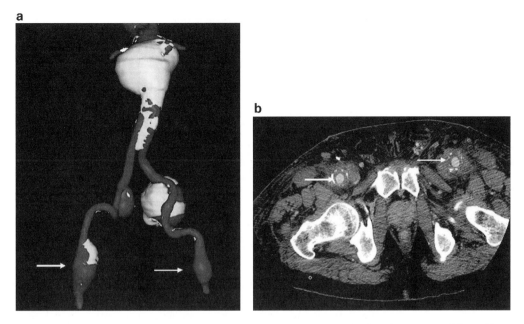

Fig. 3 (**a**) Preoperative 3D image in a patient with a Type IV thoracoabdominal aortic aneurysm, bilateral internal iliac artery aneurysms, and bilateral common femoral aneurysms (*white arrows*). (**b**) After an aortic debranching procedure, during stent graft placement, the bilateral common femoral artery aneurysms (*CFAA*) were repaired with 10-mm ePTFE grafts. A postprocedure computed tomography (*CT*) shows the grafts intact covered by the surrounding aneurysm sacs at closure (*white arrows*)

open repair or endovascular exclusion.[27] Confounding these studies, however, are the changes in graft design over the study periods described, and the changing role of antithrombotic medications, notably antiplatelet medications, such as clopidogrel.

Surgical Treatment

Open surgical intervention remains the gold standard treatment for PAA in good risk patients, and includes exclusion of the aneurysm by proximal and distal artery ligation, combined with revascularization (Table 2).

Three techniques of PAA exclusion have been described. One method involves proximal and distal ligation of the PAA with short segment revascularization. This technique is typically employed when there is a focal PAA and when the superficial femoral artery is relatively disease-free so that it can be used as an inflow source. Another technique also involves proximal and distal ligation of the aneurysm but with long segment exclusion (e.g., proximal ligation in upper superficial femoral artery with a common femoral to below-knee popliteal bypass). This procedure is usually performed when an extensive fusiform aneurysm is present, or when there is significant femoral-popliteal artery occlusive disease. A third method involves a single proximal ligature of the aneurysm and revascularization.[19,20] Most surgeons agree that full PAA exclusion by proximal and distal ligation is critical for long-term success and this later method has been discounted.[19]

Two anatomic approaches can be used for PAA repair. Most repairs are performed using the medial leg approach. Many surgeons prefer this approach due to its familiarity and the greater number of options available in the supine

Table 2 Selected surgically treated popliteal artery aneurysm series.

Authors	Year	Number of PAAs	Acute symptoms (%)	Autologous graft (%)	Assisted patency (%)	Limb salvage (%)	Mean follow-up (months)
Szilagyi et al.[38]	1981	50	82	58	68	96	48
Vermilion et al.[3]	1981	99	66	52	78	95	44
Whitehouse et al.[29]	1983	56	55	68	86	84	62
Anton et al.[14]	1986	123	52	36	56	83	120
Dawson et al.[5]	1991	57	86	60	64	95	60
Shortell et al.[10]	1991	51	71	96	67	94	60
Carpenter et al.[6]	1994	45	61	89	71	90	60
Varga et al.[33]	1994	126	63	76	91	94	22
Ascher et al.[9]	2003	29	69	83	72	94	13
Martelli et al.[39]	2004	42	71	81	78	96	48
Blanco et al.[40]	2004	70	53	76	80	NA	120

PAAs popliteal artery aneurysms

patient. The greater saphenous vein is easily accessible as are the tibial vessels, in the case a more distal arterial bypass is required. Additionally, the superficial or common femoral artery can be used for inflow, which may be necessary if the above-knee popliteal artery is found to be more diseased than expected from the preoperative studies. The posterior approach to PAA repair is typically used when the aneurysm is confined to the popliteal fossa. It is associated with an increased incidence of popliteal vein and tibial nerve injury, as these structures may be adherent to the aneurysm, but the bypass graft is shorter and the incision is smaller.

When selecting the conduit for bypass, autologous vein, specifically the greater saphenous vein, is preferred. Any adequately sized autologous vein, however (including cephalic or lesser saphenous), is associated with good long-term graft patency and limb salvage. Prosthetic grafts may also be employed, but only as a last resort for symptomatic PAA as patency rates are inferior.[10,13] However, some have reported good success with the posterior approach using a short ePTFE interposition graft.[28]

Outcomes for patients undergoing elective repair of their PAA are favorable, especially when in asymptomatic patients with preserved distal vessel runoff. In multiple studies, the range of 5- and 10-year graft patency rates is reported as 90–95% and 64–75%, respectively.[4,5,10,13] Five- and 10-year limb salvage rates are higher. In contrast to these results for asymptomatic aneurysm repair, amputation rates are high for patients presenting with ALI from a PAA. Despite attempts at urgent revascularization and emergent bypass grafting, long-term amputation rates are as high as 25%.[3,6] Operative mortality for PAA repair is low, with estimates from 0% to 2% overall.[1,29]

Treatment: Common Femoral Artery Aneurysms

Surgical

This aneurysm is approached through a standard groin exposure. Perioperative antibiotics are administered prior to incision and discontinued within 24 h. Isolation and control of the distal external iliac, SFA, and PFA is obtained. Only in rare circumstance is it necessary to obtain separate proximal external iliac artery control through a separate incision. Intravenous heparin is administered to achieve an ACT of more than 250. The AA sac is opened, and an appropriately sized graft is chosen (generally 8–10 mm Dacron or ePTFE). It is essential to preserve the PFA and most of the time the graft is sewn distally at the SFA–PFA junction. Occasionally, a side graft to the PFA is needed, or a transposed PFA patch can be sewn onto the side of the graft. These repairs provide a durable, short segment, modest sized graft with excellent patency.[22]

Profunda femoral aneurysms may actually be more dangerous to the patient as they often grow to a significant size[30] and may present with rupture or ALI in the setting of an occluded SFA.[31] These aneurysms are also more challenging to repair, particularly in a setting of a chronic SFA occlusion. It is important to maintain as many outflow branches with the repair as possible, but occasionally ligation and a femoral to distal bypass may be needed for limb salvage. In brief, a prosthetic graft (6–8 mm) is sewn between the inflow PFA neck and the first- or second-order PFA outflow nonaneurysmal branches. Several series are published on these AA, although the overall number of patients with isolated profunda aneurysms is very rare.[30,31] Graft patency and limb salvage for CFAA repair is more than 80% at 5 years follow-up.[22]

Thrombolysis for Acute Ischemia Related to AA

Peripheral AA may present with ALI resulting from either a thrombosed AA or a chronic embolization, and requires urgent intervention to reestablish flow. This may take the form of open thrombectomy and embolectomy or catheter-directed intra-arterial thrombolysis. As with other forms of ALI, all patients presenting with acute occlusion of a peripheral AA must be given systemic IV Heparin. Unfortunately, for patients who present with critical limb ischemia, the risk of eventual amputation is high, between 9% and 36%.[21]

Catheter-directed intra-arterial thrombolysis has replaced open thrombectomy as the primary treatment for PAA, and is less commonly used for acute CFAA occlusions. In addition to avoiding the morbidity of open operation and preserving the options (and conduit) for future bypass, thrombolysis may help improve the patency of the runoff vessels (tibial and peroneal), improving the success of eventual open repair. Thrombolysis also allows the repair to be performed on an elective rather than emergent basis. At least one study has suggested that preoperative thrombolysis is superior to primary open repair, with a 100% limb salvage rate, compared with a 57% salvage rate in the case of unassisted open repair.[6] This seems to be particularly true in the case of patients with poor arterial outflow at the time of presentation. One series demonstrated that thrombolysis was successful in establishing runoff in 10 of 13 patients where none had been present at the time of initial evaluation.[32]

Selection criteria for thrombolytic therapy are specific. Patients who undergo preoperative thrombolytic therapy have ischemic limbs that need to be able to withstand an additional period of ischemia due to slower return of perfusion than occurs with operative revascularization (thrombectomy, bypass). Therefore, advanced limb ischemia (grade IIb or grade III) is a contraindication to thrombolytic therapy. Patients presenting with such advanced ischemia should undergo immediate operation, including bypass, intraoperative thromboembolectomy, and fasciotomy.

The risks of thrombolysis are local (access site) and systemic bleeding complications (hematoma, intracerebral hemorrhage), as well as embolic complications of dislodged thrombotic debris. The overall risk of intracerebral hemorrhage with lysis is estimated as 0.1%. The risk of thrombolytic embolic complications is greater than 10%, presenting with pain, loss of signals, or even progression to compartment syndrome. Further, catheter-directed intra-arterial thrombolysis requires intensive monitoring and often several trips to the endovascular suite.

Thrombolytic therapy, while helpful in reestablishing outflow, does have limitations and may fail in 23% of patients.[33,34] It is most likely to be successful in clearing acute thrombi, and less likely to succeed in clearing those which are >14 days old.[34] If thrombolytic therapy is unsuccessful, this is associated with a high rate of limb loss, often due to embolization of thrombotic debris into an already compromised distal circulation bed. In spite of this, however, embolectomy and bypass are also rarely successful in these patients and emergency procedures are associated with amputation rates of 27%.[21]

Nonoperative Treatment

Not all patients diagnosed with peripheral AA are candidates for any surgical or endovascular intervention. Either open or endograft failure may create a worse situation for the patient than the natural history of their untreated peripheral AA. Several criteria may be used to select patients for nonoperative management, and the patients' general health and suitability for intervention must be considered. Patients with small (≤2 cm) asymptomatic aneurysms without thrombus and thrombosed PAA with stable claudication are reasonable nonoperative candidates. However, a thrombosed CFAA is usually symptomatic. Although no data exist to support the benefit of anticoagulation therapy with Coumadin, it is the author's current practice to use anticoagulation selectively, carefully considering the bleeding risk. Regardless, patients should be followed closely and educated about possible signs/symptoms of emboli or arterial occlusion.

Conclusion

A diagnosis of a peripheral arterial aneurysm mandates evaluation of a more proximal AAA. Imaging is primarily with duplex ultrasonography, and CT angiography is supplanting angiography for operative planning. Peripheral arterial aneurysms are more often limb threatening than life threatening, and repair is recommended for PAA > 2.0 cm and for > 2.5 cm CFAA in good risk patients. Open surgical repair for PAA and CFAA is time tested, safe, and durable in properly selected patients. PAA endovascular repair is promising, but long-term patency data is needed.

References

1. Graham LM. Femoral and Popliteal Aneurysms. Philadelphia: Lippincott Williams & Wilkins Publishers; 2001.
2. Dent TL, Lindenauer SM, Ernst CB, Fry WJ. Multiple arteriosclerotic arterial aneurysms. Arch Surg 1972;105(2):338–44.
3. Vermilion BD, Kimmins SA, Pace WG, Evans WE. A review of one hundred forty-seven popliteal aneurysms with long-term follow-up. Surgery 1981;90(6):1009–14.

4. Jacob T, Ascher E, Hingorani A, Gunduz Y, Kallakuri S. Initial steps in the unifying theory of the pathogenesis of artery aneurysms. J Surg Res 2001;101(1):37–43.

5. Dawson I, van Bockel JH, Brand R, Terpstra JL. Popliteal artery aneurysms. Long-term follow-up of aneurysmal disease and results of surgical treatment. J Vasc Surg 1991;13(3):398–407.

6. Carpenter JP, Barker CF, Roberts B, Berkowitz HD, Lusk EJ, Perloff LJ. Popliteal artery aneurysms: current management and outcome. J Vasc Surg 1994;19(1):65–72; discussion 72–3.

7. Graham LM, Zelenock GB, Whitehouse WM, Jr., et al. Clinical significance of arteriosclerotic femoral artery aneurysms. Arch Surg 1980;115(4):502–7.

8. Diwan A, Sarkar R, Stanley JC, Zelenock GB, Wakefield TW. Incidence of femoral and popliteal artery aneurysms in patients with abdominal aortic aneurysms. J Vasc Surg 2000;31(5):863–9.

9. Ascher E, Markevich N, Schutzer RW, Kallakuri S, Jacob T, Hingorani AP. Small popliteal artery aneurysms: are they clinically significant? J Vasc Surg 2003;37(4):755–60.

10. Shortell CK, DeWeese JA, Ouriel K, Green RM. Popliteal artery aneurysms: a 25-year surgical experience. J Vasc Surg 1991;14(6):771–6; discussion 6–9.

11. Ebaugh JL, Morasch MD, Matsumura JS, Eskandari MK, Meadows WS, Pearce WH. Fate of excluded popliteal artery aneurysms. J Vasc Surg 2003;37(5):954–9.

12. Kirkpatrick UJ, McWilliams RG, Martin J, Brennan JA, Gilling-Smith GL, Harris PL. Late complications after ligation and bypass for popliteal aneurysm. Br J Surg 2004;91(2):174–7.

13. Rutherford RB, Baker JD, Ernst C, et al. Recommended standards for reports dealing with lower extremity ischemia: revised version. J Vasc Surg 1997;26(3):517–38.

14. Anton GE, Hertzer NR, Beven EG, O'Hara PJ, Krajewski LP. Surgical management of popliteal aneurysms. Trends in presentation, treatment, and results from 1952 to 1984. J Vasc Surg 1986;3(1):125–34.

15. Lowell RC, Gloviczki P, Hallett JW, Jr., et al. Popliteal artery aneurysms: the risk of nonoperative management. Ann Vasc Surg 1994;8(1):14–23.

16. Batt M, Scotti L, Gagliardi JM, et al. Popliteal aneurysms. Our experience apropos of 119 cases. J Chir (Paris) 1985;122(5):319–25.

17. Puech-Leao P, Kauffman P, Wolosker N, Anacleto AM. Endovascular grafting of a popliteal aneurysm using the saphenous vein. J Endovasc Surg 1998;5(1):64–70.

18. Gerasimidis T, Sfyroeras G, Papazoglou K, Trellopoulos G, Ntinas A, Karamanos D. Endovascular treatment of popliteal artery aneurysms. Eur J Vasc Endovasc Surg 2003;26(5):506–11.

19. Mehta M, Champagne B, Darling RC, 3rd, et al. Outcome of popliteal artery aneurysms after exclusion and bypass: significance of residual patent branches mimicking type II endoleaks. J Vasc Surg 2004;40(5):886–90.

20. Jones WT, 3rd, Hagino RT, Chiou AC, Decaprio JD, Franklin KS, Kashyap VS. Graft patency is not the only clinical predictor of success after exclusion and bypass of popliteal artery aneurysms. J Vasc Surg 2003;37(2):392–8.

21. Ravn H, Bjorck M. Popliteal artery aneurysm with acute ischemia in 229 patients. Outcome after thrombolytic and surgical therapy. Eur J Vasc Endovasc Surg 2007;33(6):690–5.

22. Sapienza P, Mingoli A, Feldhaus RJ, di Marzo L, Cavallari N, Cavallaro A. Femoral artery aneurysms: long-term follow-up and results of surgical treatment. Cardiovasc Surg 1996;4(2):181–84.

23. Henry M, Amor M, Henry I, et al. Percutaneous endovascular treatment of peripheral aneurysms. J Cardiovasc Surg (Torino) 2000;41(6):871–83.

24. Mohan IIV, Bray PPJ, Harris JJP, et al. Endovascular popliteal aneurysm repair: are the results comparable to open surgery?European journal of vascular and endovascular surgery 2006;32(2):149–54.

25. Tielliu IF, Verhoeven EL, Zeebregts CJ, Prins TR, Span MM, van den Dungen JJ. Endovascular treatment of popliteal artery aneurysms: results of a prospective cohort study. J Vasc Surg 2005;41(4):561–7.

26. Antonello MM, Frigatti PP, Battocchio PP, et al. Open repair versus endovascular treatment for asymptomatic popliteal artery aneurysm: results of a prospective randomized study. Journal of vascular surgery 2005;42(2):185–93.

27. Curi MAMA, Geraghty PJPJ, Merino OAOA, et al. Mid-term outcomes of endovascular popliteal artery aneurysm repair. Journal of vascular surgery 2007;45(3):505–10.

28. Beseth BD, Moore WS. The posterior approach for repair of popliteal artery aneurysms. J Vasc Surg 2006;43(5):940–4; discussion 4–5.

29. Whitehouse WM, Jr., Wakefield TW, Graham LM, et al. Limb-threatening potential of arteriosclerotic popliteal artery aneurysms. Surgery 1983;93(5):694–9.

30. Posner SR, Wilensky J, Dimick J, Henke PK. A true aneurysm of the profunda femoris artery: a case report and review of the English language literature. Ann Vasc Surg 2004;18(6):740–6.

31. Harbuzariu C, Duncan AA, Bower TC, Kalra M, Gloviczki P. Profunda femoris artery aneurysms: association with aneurysmal disease and limb ischemia. J Vasc Surg 2008;47(1):31–4; discussion 4–5.

32. Marty B, Wicky S, Ris HB, et al. Success of thrombolysis as a predictor of outcome in acute thrombosis of popliteal aneurysms. J Vasc Surg 2002;35(3):487–93.

33. Varga ZA, Locke-Edmunds JC, Baird RN. A multicenter study of popliteal aneurysms. Joint Vascular Research Group. J Vasc Surg 1994;20(2):171–7.

34. Ramesh S, Michaels JA, Galland RB. Popliteal aneurysm: morphology and management. Br J Surg 1993;80(12):1531–3.

35. Howell M, Krajcer Z, Diethrich EB, et al. Waligraft endoprosthesis for the percutaneous treatment of femoral and popliteal artery aneurysms. J Endovasc Ther 2002;9(1):76–81.

36. Tielliu IFIFJ, Verhoeven ELELG, Prins TRTR, Post WJWJ, Hulsebos RGRG, van den Dungen JJJJAM. Treatment of popliteal artery aneurysms with the Hemobahn stent-graft. Journal of endovascular therapy 2003;10(1):111–6.

37. Rajasinghe HAHA, Tzilinis AA, Keller TT, Schafer JJ, Urrea SS. Endovascular exclusion of popliteal artery aneurysms with expanded polytetrafluoroethylene stent-grafts: early results. Vascular and endovascular surgery 2006;40(6):460–6.

38. Szilagyi DE, Schwartz RL, Reddy, DJ. Popliteal arterial aneurysms. Their natural history and management. Arch Surg 1981;116(5):724–8.

39. Martelli E, Ippoliti A, Ventoruzzo G, De Vivo G, Ascoli Marchetti A, Pistolese GR. Popliteal artery aneurysms. Factors associated with thromboembolism and graft failure. Int Angiol 2004;23(1):54–65.

40. Blanco E, Serrano-Hernando FJ, Monux G, et al. Operative repair of popliteal aneurysms: effect of factors related to the bypass procedure on outcome. Ann Vasc Surg 2004;18(1):86–92.

Index

Printed in the United States of America